Myeloid Leukemia

METHODS IN MOLECULAR MEDICINE™

John M. Walker, SERIES EDITOR

METHODS IN MOLECULAR MEDICINE™

Myeloid Leukemia

Methods and Protocols

Edited by

Harry Iland

Institute of Haematology
Royal Prince Alfred Hospital
Camperdown, NSW, Australia

Mark Hertzberg

Haematology Department
Westmead Hospital
Westmead, NSW, Australia

Paula Marlton

Haematology Department
Princess Alexandra Hospital
Brisbane, QLD, Australia

HUMANA PRESS ✴ TOTOWA, NEW JERSEY

© 2006 Humana Press Inc.
999 Riverview Drive, Suite 208
Totowa, New Jersey 07512

www.humanapress.com

This publication is printed on acid-free paper. ∞
ANSI Z39.48-1984 (American Standards Institute)

Permanence of Paper for Printed Library Materials.

Production Editor: Tracy Catanese

Cover design by Patricia F. Cleary

For additional copies, pricing for bulk purchases, and/or information about other Humana titles, contact Humana at the above address or at any of the following numbers: Tel.: 973-256-1699; Fax: 973-256-8341; E-mail: orders@humanapr.com; or visit our Website: www.humanapress.com

Photocopy Authorization Policy:

Printed in the United States of America. 10 9 8 7 6 5 4 3 2 1

eISBN 1-59745-017-0

ISSN 1543-1894

Library of Congress Cataloging in Publication Data

Myeloid leukemia : methods and protocols / edited by Harry Iland, Mark Hertzberg, Paula Marlton.
    p. ; cm. -- (Methods in molecular medicine ; 125)
    Includes bibliographical references and index.
    ISBN 1-58829-485-4 (alk. paper)
    1. Acute myeloid leukemia. 2. Chronic myeloid leukemia.   I. Iland, Harry. II. Hertzberg, Mark. III. Marlton, Paula. IV. Series.
    [DNLM: 1. Leukemia, Myeloid--genetics. 2. Acute Disease.
    3. Leukemia, Myeloid--diagnosis. 4. Molecular Diagnostic Techniques.
    W1 ME9616JM v.125 2006 / WH 250 M9965 2006]
    RC643.M94 2006
    616.99'419--dc22

                        2005016686

Preface

Recurring, nonrandom cytogenetic abnormalities are common in hematological malignancies, and their recognition has paved the way for the identification and therapeutic exploitation of the clonal molecular lesions that are uniquely associated with specific subtypes of myeloid leukemia. Appreciation of the prognostic importance of these cytogenetic and molecular genetic abnormalities has provided the major thrust for the emergence of new genetically based leukemia classifications.

Myeloid Leukemia: Methods and Protocols is devoted to a review of those laboratory techniques that are most likely to assist laboratory scientists and hematologists in the investigation and management of patients with myeloid malignancies. Scientists will benefit from the provision of a wide range of protocols that are documented in sufficient detail to enable their rapid implementation in a routine molecular hematology laboratory. Clinicians will also be rewarded by a concise description of the relevance of the assays, combined with recommendations for how each assay should be integrated into the overall management plan.

The early chapters deal with generally applicable techniques for molecular biology, cytogenetics, and fluorescence *in situ* hybridization. A comprehensive overview of the expanding field of real-time quantitative polymerase chain reaction is also included, so as to provide a background for the large proportion of chapters that utilize variations of this technique. The remainder of *Myeloid Leukemia: Methods and Protocols* is primarily directed toward acute myeloid leukemia (AML), with particular attention to the molecular lesions that enable prognostic stratification and facilitate monitoring for minimal residual disease. In particular, qualitative and quantitative methodologies for assessment of core binding factor leukemias and acute promyelocytic leukemia are presented. In addition to gene rearrangements, other prognostically relevant molecular lesions, such as FLT3 mutations and WT-1 overexpression, are covered. The rapidly developing field of oligonucleotide microarrays is addressed with a detailed methodological description and a review of the complex range of applicable statistical tools. This is then supplemented by another chapter that deals with a novel monoclonal antibody microarray approach for the diagnosis and classification of AML.

In addition, chapters addressing important molecular aspects of chronic myeloid leukemia, polycythemia rubra vera, essential thrombocythemia, hypereosinophilia, and myelodysplasia have also been included. Finally, a comprehensive review of methods for the assessment of hemopoietic chimerism in the setting of nonmyeloablative stem cell transplantation has been provided, because transplantation is an important component of the overall management of patients with acute and chronic myeloid malignancies.

Although the topics covered do not include all of the molecular abnormalities associated with myeloid malignancies, they broadly encompass those assays of immediate clinical relevance, and provide helpful strategies that are adaptable now and in the future for other molecular lesions that might be considered equally relevant.

The contributions of the many authors writing in *Myeloid Leukemia: Methods and Protocols* are gratefully acknowledged; they have generously shared the techniques that have proved so successful in their own laboratories. As with other volumes in the Methods in Molecular Medicine series, a collection of invaluable Notes accompanies each chapter to highlight specific technical issues, with the aim of facilitating the rapid establishment of the assays in the reader's own facility. Finally, we would also like to acknowledge the helpful assistance of Amy Nixon in coordinating the assembly of this volume.

Harry Iland
Mark Hertzberg
Paula Marlton

Contents

Contributors

TANYA L. APPLEGATE • *Johnson & Johnson Research Pty. Limited, NSW, Australia*

NICOLE BARBER • *School of Molecular and Microbial Biosciences, University of Sydney, NSW, Australia*

E. JOANNA BAXTER • *Department of Haematology, University of Cambridge, Cambridge, UK*

LARISSA BELOV • *School of Molecular and Microbial Biosciences, University of Sydney, NSW, Australia*

ANTHONY J. BENCH • *Department of Haematology, Addenbrooke's Hospital, Cambridge University Hospitals NHS Foundation Trust, Cambridge, UK*

LINDA BENDALL • *Westmead Institute for Cancer Research, Westmead Millennium Institute, Westmead, NSW, Australia*

ANDREA BIONDI • *Centro Ricerca M. Tettamanti, Clinica Pediatrica Università di Milano Bicocca and Dipartimento di Medicina Clinica, Prevenzione e Biotecnologie Sanitarie, Ospedale San Gerardo, Monza, Italy*

SUSAN BRANFORD • *Division of Molecular Pathology, Institute of Medical and Veterinary Science, South Australia, Australia*

LYNDA J. CAMPBELL • *Cytogenetics Department, St. Vincent's Hospital, Victoria, Australia*

PETER J. CAMPBELL • *Department of Haematology, University of Cambridge, Cambridge, UK*

RICHARD I. CHRISTOPHERSON • *School of Molecular and Microbial Biosciences, University of Sydney, NSW, Australia*

DANIELA CILLONI • *Department of Clinical and Biological Sciences, University of Turin, Turin, Italy*

JAN COOLS • *Department of Human Genetics, Flanders Interuniversity Institute for Biotechnology (VIB), University of Leuven, Leuven, Belgium*

WENDY N. ERBER • *Department of Haematology, Addenbrooke's Hospital, Cambridge University Hospitals NHS Foundation Trust, Cambridge, UK*

CAROLINE J. FUERY • *Johnson & Johnson Research Pty. Limited, NSW, Australia*

JEAN GABERT • *Department of Biochemistry & Molecular Biology, Hôpital Universitaire Nord (AP-HM), ERT-MEIDIA-IFR Jean Roche-Université de la Méditerranée, Marseille, France*

D. GARY GILLILAND • *Brigham and Women's Hospital, Harvard Medical School, and Howard Hughes Medical Institute, Harvard University, Boston, Massachusetts*

ENRICO GOTTARDI • *Department of Clinical and Biological Sciences, University of Turin, Turin, Italy*

ANTHONY R. GREEN • *Department of Haematology, University of Cambridge, and Department of Haematology, Addenbrooke's Hospital, Cambridge University Hospitals NHS Foundation Trust, Cambridge, UK*

TORSTEN HAFERLACH • *Laboratory for Leukemia Diagnostics, Department of Internal Medicine III, Ludwig-Maximilians-University, Munich, Germany*

WOLFGANG HIDDEMANN • *Laboratory for Leukemia Diagnostics, Department of Internal Medicine III, Ludwig-Maximilians-University, Munich, Germany*

TIMOTHY HUGHES • *Division of Hematology, Institute of Medical and Veterinary Science, South Australia, Australia*

JOOP H. JANSEN • *Central Hematology Laboratory, University Medical Center St. Raboud, The Netherlands*

WOLFGANG KERN • *Laboratory for Leukemia Diagnostics, Department of Internal Medicine III, Ludwig-Maximilians-University, Munich, Germany*

HITOSHI KIYOI • *Department of Infectious Diseases, Nagoya University School of Medicine, Nagoya, Japan*

ALEXANDER KOHLMANN • *Laboratory for Leukemia Diagnostics, Department of Internal Medicine III, Ludwig-Maximilians-University, Munich, Germany*

LUIGI M. LAROCCA • *Instituto di Anatomia Patologica and Ematologia, Università Cattolica del Sacro Cuore, Roma, Italy*

LAURA LEVATI • *Centro Ricerca M. Tettamanti, Clinica Pediatrica Università di Milano Bicocca and Dipartimento di Medicina Clinica, Prevenzione e Biotecnologie Sanitarie, Ospedale San Gerardo, Monza, Italy*

THOMAS LION • *Children's Cancer Research Institute (CCRI), Vienna, Austria*

MAURIZIO MARTINI • *Instituto di Anatomia Patologica and Ematologia, Università Cattolica del Sacro Cuore, Roma, Italy*

ELISA MOKANY • *Johnson & Johnson Research Pty. Limited, NSW, Australia*

STEPHEN P. MULLIGAN • *School of Molecular and Microbial Biosciences, University of Sydney, NSW, Australia*

TOMOKI NAOE • *Department of Hematology, Nagoya University Graduate School of Medicine, Nagoya, Japan*

CHRISTOPHE PICARD • *Department of Biochemistry & Molecular Biology, Hôpital Universitaire Nord (AP-HM), ERT-MEIDIA-IFR Jean Roche-Université de la Méditerranée, Marseille, France*
VINCENZO ROSSI • *Centro Ricerca M. Tettamanti, Clinica Pediatrica Università di Milano Bicocca and Dipartimento di Medicina Clinica, Prevenzione e Biotecnologie Sanitarie, Ospedale San Gerardo, Monza, Italy*
GIUSEPPE SAGLIO • *Department of Clinical and Biological Sciences, University of Turin, Turin, Italy*
LINDA M. SCOTT • *Department of Haematology, University of Cambridge, Cambridge, UK*
MIKE SCOTT • *Department of Haematology, Addenbrookes NHS Trust, Cambridge, UK*
MONIQUE SILVY • *Department of Biochemistry & Molecular Biology, Hôpital Universitaire Nord (AP-HM), ERT-MEIDIA-IFR Jean Roche-Université de la Méditerranée, Marseille, France*
KERRYN STONER • *Department of Haematology, Addenbrookes NHS Trust, Cambridge, UK*
ELIZABETH H. STOVER • *Brigham and Women's Hospital, Harvard Medical School, Boston, MA*
LUCIANA TEOFILI • *Instituti di Anatomia Patologica and Ematologia, Università Cattolica del Sacro Cuore, Roma, Italy*
KHALID TOBAL • *The Rayne Institute, King's College Hospital, London, United Kingdom*
ALISON V. TODD • *Johnson & Johnson Research Pty. Limited, NSW, Australia*
BERT A. VAN DER REIJDEN • *Central Hematology Laboratory, University Medical Center St. Raboud, Nijmegen, The Netherlands*
FRANZ WATZINGER • *Children's Cancer Research Institute (CCRI), Vienna, Austria*
ADRIAN WOOLFSON • *University of Cambridge School of Clinical Medicine, Addenbrooke's Hospital, Cambridge, United Kingdom*
JOHN A. LIU YIN • *Hematology Department, University of Manchester, Manchester, UK*

1

Isolation of RNA and DNA From Leukocytes and cDNA Synthesis

Joop H. Jansen and Bert A. van der Reijden

Summary

In this chapter, methods to isolate RNA and DNA from human leukocytes for the subsequent use in molecular diagnostic tests are described. In addition, protocols for cDNA synthesis are given, both for the use in conventional reverse transcription (RT)-polymerase chain reaction (PCR), and for the use in quantitative RT-PCR reactions. Because sensitive PCR methods are commonly used in molecular diagnostics, measures to avoid contamination are described. Finally, a simple procedure to control the quality of isolated RNA is described.

Key Words: RNA; DNA; cDNA synthesis; isolation; electrophoresis; spectrophotometry; integrity.

1. Introduction

Molecular diagnostics in hematological malignancies is often based on RNA or DNA that is isolated from the nucleated cells of the bone marrow or peripheral blood of the patient. The preparation of high-quality RNA and DNA using standardized methods is a crucial first step in the procedure. Several aspects require special attention.

Many assays are based on the detection of leukemia-specific genetic aberrations using amplification by polymerase chain reaction (PCR). This method is very sensitive, generally allowing the detection of one malignant cell among 100,000 normal cells. This extreme sensitivity allows the detection of minimal residual disease after treatment, but also carries the risk of false-positive results due to contamination of the sample during processing. If 40 cycles of PCR are performed, potentially 2^{40} molecules are generated from each single molecule that is present in the starting material. Obviously, the post-PCR product that is generated from positive patients forms the major contamination haz-

From: *Methods in Molecular Medicine, Vol. 125: Myeloid Leukemia: Methods and Protocols*
Edited by: H. Iland, M. Hertzberg, and P. Marlton © Humana Press Inc., Totowa, NJ

ard in laboratories that carry out these analyses on a regular basis. Because even minute quantities of post-PCR product contain more than enough molecules to yield a positive result in PCR, contamination may be spread through many routes, including laboratory equipment (like pipets), the hands of laboratory personnel, and aerosols that are generated from fluids that are spun at high speed in centrifuges. Monitoring of potential contamination (using several negative controls in each assay), and a regulated one-way traffic of materials from pre- to post-PCR laboratory space, are both necessary to minimize the risk of contamination. For negative controls, it may not be sufficient to simply include a template-negative sample (like water) in the PCR procedure. Where possible, negative blood or bone marrow samples should be processed alongside the patient samples during the complete procedure, from RNA or DNA isolation, reverse transcription (when RNA is analyzed), and the actual PCR reaction. For instance, if *BCR-ABL* is to be quantified in a patient with chronic myeloid leukemia, an appropriate negative control would be the simultaneous analysis of a sample from a known *BCR-ABL* negative patient (e.g., with acute myeloid leukemia) that is processed in the laboratory at the same time. Once a laboratory is contaminated, decontamination may prove very difficult. Small equipment (like pipets) may be decontaminated by ultraviolet (UV) irradiation. To avoid contamination, standard procedures should include a strict physical separation of pre- and post-PCR equipment, reagent stocks, and laboratory space. Ideally, the air control system of the laboratory should be set up and air pressure differences established in such a manner that the pre-PCR space is at higher pressure than the post-PCR space. Because it may be very laborious to track the source of a contamination, it is recommended that all reagents that are imported from different manufacturers (like primers, probes, enzymes, and so on) be received in a separate, dedicated laboratory space to which all traffic of equipment (including small laboratory items like pipets and tube racks), patient material, and, of course, post-PCR products is strictly prohibited at all times. In this contamination-free room, reagents can be aliquotted in small sample volumes and stored. When reagents are to be used, they can be taken from this room and opened at a different location, where the patient samples are handled and the reverse-transcription (RT)-PCR or PCR reactions are assembled. In the event of contamination, the small working stocks that are present in the lab can be completely disposed of, obviating the need to perform multiple test PCRs trying to track the source of contamination, without depleting costly bulk stock.

A second issue is the percentage of tumor cells present in the sample. Because patient samples may contain a mixture of normal and malignant cells, false-negative results may be produced if methods with limited sensitivity are used on samples with low numbers of malignant cells. If the goal is to determine the presence or absence of a specific mutation, the percentage of leukemic cells should be assessed to make sure that the method that is used is sensitive enough for the sample that is analyzed. At diagnosis, this information is usually readily available, as morphology and immunophenotyping are performed on these samples routinely. For very sensitive methods such as PCR, it may not be very problematic if only 1% of the cells belong to the leukemic clone. In contrast, if for instance Southern blotting is to be used to diagnose a specific genomic rearrangement, the number of malignant cells in the sample becomes a major issue. In that context, the type of material from which the RNA or DNA is isolated may be important. For instance, in chronic myeloid leukemia (CML), the level of BCR-ABL-positive cells in the bone marrow and blood is very much comparable, but in acute lymphoblastic leukemia (ALL), a 100-fold difference between bone marrow and blood is often observed. Furthermore, it is also important to realize that the method of red cell removal may have an impact on the percentage of malignant cells that is present in the cell sample used for RNA and/or DNA extraction. If cells are isolated using Ficoll 1.077 density gradient centrifugation, granulocytes are removed from the interphase cell fraction, enriching the sample for leukemic cells, whereas if NH_4Cl lysis of red cells is used, mature granulocytes will remain in the isolated cell fraction.

Molecular diagnostic procedures are often complex, consisting of multiple steps before a result is obtained. Because every step carries the risk of failure, a result is not always obtained in the first run even when standardized procedures are used. Because the patient material may be difficult to obtain, and may involve invasive procedures like bone marrow aspiration, it is highly recommended that samples be divided into aliquots at the start of the procedure, enabling the use of backup material if the procedure fails. Once the nucleated cells have been isolated, it is advisable to split the sample into several aliquots, which are stored until use in separate tubes. If samples are disqualified—for instance, as a result of either a contamination in a specific run or degradation—there will always be stored backup samples, greatly minimizing the number of failures. For PCR assays, we recommend four aliquots be prepared directly after isolation of the cells, two of which are worked up and analyzed to produce duplicate values, and two of which are stored as lysates that can be processed when necessary.

Finally, the cDNA reaction is an important step before PCR can be performed on RNA samples. Many different protocols exist using different brands of reverse transcription enzymes. In this chapter, we describe two general protocols, but as the optimal cDNA reaction may be different depending on the subsequent PCR reaction that is to be performed, the cDNA step must be optimized for individual assays.

2. Materials

1. Diethylpyrocarbonate (DEPC).
2. Guadinine thiocyanate (GTC) solution: 4 M guanidinium thiocyanate, 0.5% N-laurolylsarcosine, 25 mM sodium citrate (pH 7.0), 0.1 M 2-mercaptoethanol (added shortly before use).
3. CsCl solution for RNA ultracentrifugation: 5.7 M CsCl in 0.1 M sodium-ethylenediamine tetraacetic acid (EDTA) (pH 8.0). Treat with DEPC and autoclave.
4. DEPC-treated H_2O.
5. Ethanol.
6. Agarose.
7. Reverse transcriptase.
8. 0.1 M Diothiothreitol (DTT).
9. dNTPs, 25 mM each.
10. Random hexamers, 5 mg/mL.
11. RNasin ribonuclease (RNase) inhibitor.
12. 10X TBE buffer: 108 g Tris-base, 55 g boric acid, 40 mL 0.5 M EDTA (pH 8.0); add H_2O to 1 L.
13. Sodium dodecyl sulphate (SDS).
14. 6X loading buffer containing SDS: 0.25 g bromphenol blue, 0.25 g xylene cyanol, and 15 g Ficoll in 100 mL H_2O; add 10% SDS w/v.
15. Ethidium bromide.
16. SE buffer: 12.5 mL 100 mM EDTA plus 3.75 mL 1 M NaCl in 50 mL autoclaved H_2O.
17. Proteinase K, 20 mg/mL.
18. Saturated NaCl: 87.7 g NaCl in 250 mL.
19. TE buffer: 10 mM Tris-HCl, 1 mM EDTA (pH 8.0).
20. Microcentrifuge.
21. Ultracentrifuge.
22. Spectrophotometer.
23. Superscript II reverse transcriptase RNase H⁻, and buffer (Invitrogen).
24. Moloney murine leukemia virus (M-MLV) reverse transcriptase and buffer (Invitrogen).

3. Methods

In this section, the isolation of RNA and DNA, and the synthesis of cDNA are described.

3.1. Isolation of RNA

For the detection of most fusion genes and several other mutations that are recurrently found in hematological malignancies, total RNA can be used. Both bone marrow and peripheral blood nucleated cells may be used, depending on the question asked and the stage of the disease (*see also* Introduction). EDTA or citrate are preferred as anticoagulant (*see* **Note 1**). Various protocols to isolate RNA from mammalian cells exist. A commonly used protocol, on which various commercially available reagents (like Trizol® or RNABee®) are based, involves the use of acid guanidinium thiocyanate–phenol–chloroform extraction *(1)*. A second procedure involves the lysis of cells in denaturing guadinidium thiocyanate solution and separation of RNA by ultracentrifugation on a 5.7 *M* CsCl cushion *(2,3)*. The first method is very well suited for the simultaneous processing of multiple samples, and may be preferable in a routine diagnostic setting. The latter method yields very high-quality RNA, and allows the isolation of RNA from large numbers of cells in one tube. The drawbacks of this method are the long centrifugation times and the limited number of samples that can be processed in one run (most ultracentrifuge rotors fit six tubes). In addition, if open ultracentrifuge tubes are used (rather than the more difficult to handle sealable tubes), there may be an increased risk of cross-contamination. When handling RNA, it is important to take precautions to avoid degradation by ribonuclease activity (*see* **Notes 2–8**).

3.1.1. Decontamination of Solutions From Ribonuclease (RNAse) Activity Using Diethylpyrocarbonate (DEPC)

RNase activity can be inactivated by treatment of solutions with DEPC. Note that DEPC is toxic, and that buffers containing Tris should not be treated with DEPC (*see* **Notes 6–8**).

1. Add 0.1% DEPC (w/v).
2. Mix thoroughly and leave overnight at 37°C.
3. Because DEPC may also inhibit subsequent enzyme activity necessary for cDNA and PCR, it should be removed by autoclaving for 30 min, which causes hydrolysis of the DEPC (*see* **Notes 6–8**).

3.1.2. RNA Isolation Using Commercially Available Complete Reagent

Under this subheading, the isolation of total RNA using RNABee reagent is described. Several other commercially available kits are on the market that may be used as well.

1. If working with freshly isolated nucleated cells, proceed to **step 2**. If cryopreserved cells are used, rapidly thaw the cells at 37°C. Transfer them to a 15-mL tube on ice. Add medium (e.g., phosphate-buffered saline [PBS], HBBS, Dulbecco's modified Eagle's medium [DMEM]) supplemented with 1% fetal calf serum (FCS; 4°C) up to a total volume of 15 mL.
2. Spin down the cells at 350*g* for 5 min at 4°C. Discard the supernatant and resuspend the pellet in the remaining solution.
3. Add 10 mL ice-cold medium (PBS, HBBS, DMEM) with 1% FCS, and count the cells.
4. Spin down cells at 350*g* for 5 min at 4°C. Discard the supernatant and resuspend the pellet in the remaining solution.

5. Add 1 mL RNABee per 10 million cells on ice. Vortex thoroughly, leaving no clumps. As outlined in the introduction, we recommend aliquotting the lysate into four Eppendorf tubes (two samples for RNA isolation, generating a duplicate value, and two for backup that can be used in case of failure or contamination). At this point, the lysates can be stored at $-20°C$ or $-80°C$ until further extraction.

6. To 1 mL lysate, add 200 µL chloroform. Mix by vortexing and put on ice for 5 min.

7. Centrifuge for 15 min in a microcentrifuge at maximun speed (14,000g) at 4°C.

8. Prepare 1.5-mL Eppendorf tubes containing 500 µL isopropanol.

9. Transfer 750 µL of the upper phase from **step 7** to the tubes containing isopropanol. Take care not to transfer any of the lower (blue) solution or the interface.

10. Precipitate the RNA at 4°C for at least 15 min.

11. Centrifuge for 30 min at 14,000g at 4°C.

12. Wash the pellet with 70% ethanol at 4°C.

13. Centrifuge for 10 min at 14,000g.

14. Repeat **steps 12** and **13** once.

15. Discard the supernatant. Spin down once more and remove the rest of the ethanol.

16. Dry the pellet in air.

17. Dissolve the RNA in 20 µL DEPC-treated, RNAse-free water overnight at 4°C, or for 10 min at 65°C.

18. Measure spectroscopically the amount (optimal density $[OD]_{260}/OD_{280}$ ratio) of RNA. The concentration of RNA (µg/mL) = OD_{260} × dilution factor × 40. Ideally, the OD_{260}/OD_{280} ratio should be 2.0.

19. Determine the quality of the RNA on a 1.5% agarose gel (*see* **Subheading 3.1.4.**).

20. Store RNA samples at $-20°C$ or $-80°C$ in water. If preferred, RNA can also be stored as an ethanol precipitate (add 0.1 vol of 3 M sodium acetate, pH 5.2, and add ethanol to a final concentration of 70%). Note that repeated freeze-thawing will negatively affect the quality of the RNA (*see* **Note 9**).

3.1.3. RNA Isolation Using Guanidinium Thiocyanate Lysis and CsCl Ultracentrifugation

1. Spin down 5 to 50 million cells (5 min at 350g).

2. Discard the supernatant and resuspend the pellet in a minimal volume of remaining buffer.

3. Add 3.5 mL (if less than 25×10^6 cells are used) or 7.5 mL (if more than 25×10^6 cells are used) GTC solution containing freshly added 2-mercaptoethanol.

4. Vortex vigorously until all cells are completely lysed. If the cells do not lyse completely, more GTC solution must be added.

5. At this point, the lysate can be stored at $-80°C$ until further use.

6. Put 2 or 4 mL 5.7M CsCl solution in a polyallomer ultracentrifuge tube, depending on the volume of lysate produced at **step 4**.

7. Carefully layer the lysate on the CsCl.

8. Centrifuge (20°C) for 12–18 h at 170,000g (SW40 rotor), or 160,000g (SW50 rotor). Use a slow acceleration and do not use the brake, in order not to disturb the gradient.

9. Using an RNase-free disposable pipet, remove most of the supernatant, including the interface.
10. Invert the tubes to remove the remaining fluid and cut off the round bottom of the tube containing the pelleted RNA using an RNase-free razor blade.
11. Resuspend the RNA (which should be visible as a clear gelatinous pellet) in 200 µL DEPC-treated H_2O, and transfer to an Eppendorf tube.
12. Rinse the bottom of the cut polyallomer tube twice with 100 µL H_2O, and transfer to the Eppendorf tube.
13. To the 400 µL RNA solution add 40 µL 3 *M* sodium acetate (pH 5.2) and precipitate the RNA by adding 1 mL ethanol. Store for at least 30 min at –80°C and centrifuge for 10 min at 14,000g; discard the supernatant and dissolve the pellet in 400 µL H_2O.
14. Repeat the precipitation (**step 13**) once and resuspend the pellet in 100 µL DEPC-treated H_2O.
15. Determine the amount of RNA by measuring the OD_{260} and OD_{280}. The concentration of RNA (µg/mL) = OD_{260} × dilution factor × 40. Ideally, the OD_{260}/OD_{280} ratio should be 2.0.
16. As the OD gives only a rough indication of the quality of the sample, determine the quality of the RNA on a 1.5% agarose gel (*see* **Subheading 3.1.4.**).
17. Store RNA samples at –20°C or –80°C in water. If preferred, RNA can also be stored as an ethanol precipitate (add 0.1 volume of 3 *M* sodium acetate, pH 5.2, and add ethanol to a final concentration of 70%). Note that repeated freeze-thawing will negatively affect the quality of the RNA (*see* **Note 9**).

3.1.4. Quality Control of RNA by Gel Electrophoresis

The quality of RNA can be judged by visualization of 18S and 28S ribosomal RNA bands after gel electrophoresis. Instead of using formaldehyde-containing gels that are normally used for Northern blotting, a simple and fast protocol is described below using regular 0.5X TBE-containing agarose gels and SDS-containing loading buffer.

1. Pour a fresh 1.5% agarose gel in 0.5X TBE buffer containing 3.5 µL ethidium bromide per 100 mL.
2. Dilute 0.5–1 µg RNA in 10 µL H_2O.
3. Add 2 µL 6X loading buffer (dissolve 0.25 g bromphenol blue, 0.25 g xylene cyanol, and 15 g Ficoll in 100 mL H_2O, and add 10% SDS w/v).
4. Load the RNA on the gel and electrophorese in 0.5X TBE buffer.
5. Visualize the RNA using UV illumination. If the RNA is intact, the 18S and 28S ribosomal RNA should appear as two discrete bands, with the 28S band being approximately twice as intense as the 18S (**Fig. 1**).

3.2. Isolation of DNA

DNA can be extracted using many different protocols. For Southern blotting, high-molecular-weight DNA should be isolated, which can be achieved

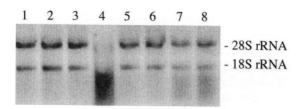

Fig. 1. Visualization of ribosomal RNA bands for assessment of RNA integrity. Visualization of 28S and 18S ribosomal RNA on a 0.5X TBE, 1.5% agarose gel using loading buffer to which 10% sodium dodecyl sulfate (w/v) is added. In lanes 1, 2, 3, 5, and 6, intact RNA is present. Lanes 7 and 8 show some RNA degradation, visualized as a low-molecular-weight smear. Lane 4 shows completely degraded RNA.

using protocols that are based on the salting-out procedure described by Miller et al. *(4)*. If PCR is to be performed, several commercially available columns can conveniently be used, which will rapidly yield DNA of somewhat smaller size (30–50 kb). Both methods can be applied on isolated nucleated cells from blood and bone marrow. High-molecular-weight DNA should be stored in TE buffer (10 mM Tris-HCl, 1 mM EDTA) at 4°C. Lower molecular weight DNA may also be stored as frozen solution.

3.2.1. Genomic DNA Isolation Using Commercially Available Spin Columns

Under this subheading, we describe the isolation of DNA using commercially available Qiagen® spin columns. Using different columns, DNA can be processed on different scales. Here we describe the small-scale isolation of DNA from a limited number of cells.

1. Pellet up to 10×10^6 isolated nucleated cells for 5 min at 300–350g.
2. Resuspend the pellet in 200 µL PBS/0.5% FCS at 4°C.
3. Add 20 µL protease supplied by the manufacturer, and mix.
4. Add 200 µL loading buffer (AL).
5. Vortex three times for at least 5 s to homogenize the sample.
6. Incubate for at least 10 min at 56°C.
7. Briefly spin down drops in a microcentrifuge.
8. Add 200 µL ethanol, vortex three times for 5 s.
9. Briefly spin down drops in a microcentrifuge.
10. Load the sample onto a Qiagen column.
11. Centrifuge in a microfuge for 1 min at 6000g.
12. Discard the eluate.
13. Add 500 µL washing buffer (AW1) onto the column.
14. Centrifuge for 1 min at 6000g, then discard the eluate.
15. Add 500 µL washing buffer (AW2) onto the column.

16. Centrifuge for 3 min at 14,000g, then discard the eluate.
17. Add 200 µL elution buffer (AE) or H$_2$O onto the column, depending on the number of cells that were used (200 µL elution buffer for 1×10^6 cells). If less than 5 $\times 10^6$ cells were used, load 50 µL elution buffer.
18. Incubate 1 min at room temperature.
19. Centrifuge for 1 min at 6000g.
20. Collect the eluate and measure the OD$_{260}$ and OD$_{280}$. Calculate the amount of DNA. The concentration of DNA (µg/mL) = OD$_{260}$ × dilution factor × 50. Ideally, the OD$_{260}$/OD$_{280}$ ratio should be 1.8.

3.2.2. Isolation of High-Molecular-Weight Genomic DNA Using High Salt Extraction

In this subheading, a commonly used method to isolate genomic DNA by high-salt/ethanol precipitation is described (based on **ref. 4**).

1. Isolate white blood cells from bone marrow or blood.
2. Resuspend $10–100 \times 10^6$ cells in a 15-mL tube in 3 mL SE buffer (12.5 mL 100 mM EDTA and 3.75 mL 1 M NaCl in 50 mL autoclaved H$_2$O).
3. Add 25 µL proteinase K (20 mg/mL) and mix gently.
4. Add 150 µL SDS (20%) and mix gently.
5. Incubate overnight at 37°C.
6. Add 1 mL saturated NaCl (87.7 g NaCl in 250 mL) and vortex for 15 s.
7. Spin for 15 min 1380g.
8. Transfer the supernatant to a new tube.
9. Repeat **steps 7** and **8** until the supernatant is clear.
10. Carefully add exactly two volumes ethanol (room temperature) to the supernatant.
11. Invert the tube several times.
12. Fish out the precipitated DNA with a disposable plastic pipet tip or spatula.
13. Transfer the DNA to a microcentrifuge tube and wash briefly in 70% ethanol by inversion of the tube several times followed by centrifugation at 14,000g for 1 min.
14. Discard the supernatant and air-dry the pellet.
15. Dissolve the DNA in 100–350 µL TE (10 mM Tris-HCl, 1 mM EDTA) overnight at room temperature.
16. Store at 4°C.

3.3. cDNA Synthesis

For the detection of mutations and leukemia-specific fusion genes by RT-PCR, RNA first needs to be reverse transcribed into cDNA. The cDNA synthesis efficiency depends upon the relative concentrations of random hexamers/oligo-dT primers, reverse transcriptase, and RNA. The following protocols are based on an input of 1 µg RNA. If less RNA is available, the cDNA synthesis ingredients can be downscaled proportionally. We recommend the use of random hexamers rather than oligo-dT primers (*see* **Note 10**).

3.3.1. General Protocol for cDNA Synthesis

Under this subheading, a commonly used method for cDNA synthesis is described. This method generates longer cDNA fragments and is therefore especially suitable for the detection of longer PCR fragments in conventional PCR (e.g., *PML-RARA* and *CBFB-MYH11* RT-PCR).

1. Denature 1 µg RNA in a volume of 20 µL H_2O for 5 min at 65°C.
2. Cool the denatured RNA on ice and spin down briefly.
3. Add the following components to the denatured RNA: 6.7 µL H_2O, 8.0 µL 5X SuperScript II RNase H⁻ reverse transcriptase buffer (Invitrogen), 0.4 µL DTT (0.1 *M*), 1.6 µL dNTPs (25 m*M* each), 0.8 µL random hexamers (5 mg/mL), 1.5 µL SuperScript II RNase H⁻ reverse transcriptase (Invitrogen), and 1.0 µL RNasin ribonuclease inhibitor (e.g., Promega, 33 U/µL).
4. Mix, spin down, and incubate for 1.5 h at 42°C.
5. The cDNA can be directly used in PCR or stored at –20°C (*see* **Note 9**).

3.3.2. Alternative cDNA Synthesis Method for Use With Real-Time PCR

Under this subheading, an alternative method for cDNA synthesis is described. This method results in more efficient real-time PCR amplifications and consistently lower threshold cycle (Ct) values (average 2 Cts) compared with the preceding version (**Subheading 3.3.1.**).

1. Denature 1 µg RNA in a volume of 20 µL H_2O for 5 min at 65°C.
2. Cool denatured RNA on ice and spin down briefly.
3. Add the following components to 5 µL of RNA (1 µg): 6.0 µL H_2O, 1.0 µL M-MLV reverse transcriptase (Invitrogen), 4.0 µL reverse transcriptase buffer (Invitrogen), 2.0 µL DTT (0.1 *M*), 0.5 µL dNTPs (25 m*M* each), 1.0 µL random hexamers (5 mg/mL), and 0.5 µL RNAsin ribonuclease inhibitor (e.g., Promega, 33 U/µL).
4. Mix, spin down, and incubate for 10 min at 20°C (priming).
5. Incubate for 45 min at 42°C.
6. Incubate for 10 min at 95°C (denaturation of the reverse transcriptase).
7. Add 5 µL H_2O.
8. Store cDNA at –20°C (*see* **Note 9**).
9. Use 5 µL for a PCR reaction.

4. Notes

1. Because heparin may inhibit subsequent PCR reactions, EDTA or citrate are preferred as anticoagulants.
2. As soon as RNA is taken up in nondenaturing solutions, it becomes very sensitive to RNase activity, resulting in degradation. Because human skin is an important source of RNase activity, always wear gloves when preparing and handling RNA.

3. Industrially produced plastics can be considered RNase-free, as long as they have been handled with gloves. In addition, several buffers and solutions can be purchased RNase-free.
4. Autoclaving does not inhibit, or only partially inhibits, RNase activity.
5. If glassware is used for the preparation and storage of buffers, inactivate RNases by baking at over 250°C for several hours.
6. Solutions can be made RNase free by treatment with DEPC (caution, this compound is toxic) (*see* **Subheading 3.1.1.**).
7. Because DEPC is highly unstable in the presence of Tris, buffers containing Tris cannot be treated with DEPC. Use RNase-free components and DEPC-treated water to prepare RNase-free buffers containing Tris.
8. After autoclaving, DEPC-treated buffers may smell sweet. This is caused by volatile esters that are produced by the decomposing DEPC and is not a sign that the DEPC has not been inactivated.
9. Repeated freezing and thawing of RNA or cDNA negatively affects its quality.
10. Because the target sequences that must be amplified may be located far away from the 3′ end of the gene, we recommend the use of random hexamers for the cDNA reaction rather than oligo-dT primers.

References

1. Chomczynski, P. and Sacchi, N. (1987) Single-step method of RNA isolation by acid guanidinium thiocyanate-phenol-chloroform extraction. *Anal. Biochem.* **162,** 156–159.
2. Glisin, V., Crkvenjakov, R., and Byus, C. (1974) Ribonucleic acid isolated by cesium chloride centrifugation. *Biochemistry* **13,** 2633–2637.
3. Chirgwin, J. M., Przybyla, A. E., MacDonald, R. J., and Rutter, W. J. (1979) Isolation of biologically active ribonucleic acid from sources enriched in ribonuclease. *Biochemistry* **18,** 5294–5299.
4. Miller, S. A., Dykes, D. D., and Polesky, H. F. (1988) A simple salting out procedure for extracting DNA from human nucleated cells. *Nucleic Acids Res.* **16,** 1215.

2

Cytogenetic and FISH Techniques in Myeloid Malignancies

Lynda J. Campbell

Summary

Chromosome analysis is an essential part of the diagnostic testing of myeloid malignancies. Good chromosome preparations are essential for a complete cytogenetic analysis. This means plentiful metaphase spreads with well-spread crisply banded chromosomes. To achieve such a result, several variables, including the growth rate of the leukemic cells, are critical. The method described in this chapter has been extensively tested and should produce reasonable results from most cases. Fluorescence *in situ* hybridization (FISH) is less influenced by sample variation and as a result may be obtained from either metaphase spreads or interphase cells. Moreover, FISH is capable of describing chromosome rearrangements at the gene level, rather than at the gross level shown by conventional cytogenetics. It does not, however, provide information on genetic rearrangements other than at the specific target site of the probe used, unlike conventional cytogenetics. Thus, these two techniques complement each other and are both now essential elements of chromosome analysis.

Key Words: Cytogenetic; karyotype; synchronization; harvest; metaphase; banding; fluorescence *in situ* hybridization.

1. Introduction

Over the past 40 yr, cytogenetic analysis has become an integral part of the diagnosis and management of patients with myeloid malignancies. Cytogenetic analysis is required to diagnose disorders such as chronic myeloid leukemia (CML) and to provide information regarding prognosis in acute myeloid leukemia (AML) and myelodysplastic syndromes (MDS) *(1–3)*. Although specific genetic targets can be detected using molecular techniques such as reverse-transcription polymerase chain reaction, cytogenetic analysis provides a global view of genetic rearrangements within the malignant cell. There are a number of different methods available for producing metaphase spreads suitable for cytogenetic analysis. The methods described below are in routine use in the Victorian Cancer Cytogenetics Service (VCCS). The number and type of cul-

From: *Methods in Molecular Medicine, Vol. 125: Myeloid Leukemia: Methods and Protocols*
Edited by: H. Iland, M. Hertzberg, and P. Marlton © Humana Press Inc., Totowa, NJ

tures established depends on the diagnosis, but good practice dictates the setting up, where possible, of at least two cultures for each sample. For most myeloid disorders, a culture using an agent to produce cell synchrony is preferred, and so if limited patient material enables the establishment of only one culture, a synchronized culture is recommended. With new acute leukemias, the subtype may not have been identified by the time the cultures are established, and so at the VCCS an overnight unsynchronized culture is established preferentially, and, if sample permits, a synchronized culture is set up as second choice. Synchronization requires a 48-h culture, and acute lymphoblastic leukemia cells are generally less capable than AML cells of surviving more than 24 h in culture.

Cell synchronization refers to a method of increasing the number of cells that have reached the metaphase part of the cell cycle, when harvesting of the culture is initiated. An agent is added to the culture to block DNA synthesis; the following method uses 5'-fluorodeoxyuridine (FdU) with added uridine. By blocking the cell cycle, a large number of cells are collected that have all arrived at the same point of division. Release of the blockage then allows them all to proceed through division together. FdU acts as an antagonist to thymidylate synthetase. BrdU (5-bromo-2'-deoxyuridine), an analog of thymidine, is then used to release the block. The harvest is timed for approx 7 h after release so that the maximum number of cells has arrived at metaphase *(4)*. Metaphase is the stage of mitosis at which chromosomes are most contracted, prior to the chromatids separating to travel to opposite poles of the cell; they are most distinguishable one from another at this point.

Cells are harvested by the addition of Colcemid®, a synthetic analog of colchicine, which prevents the formation of the cell spindle fibers and so prevents the onset of anaphase. The cells are treated with a hypotonic saline solution to increase the cell volume and so allow the chromosomes to disentangle from each other. Finally, the cells are fixed in a mixture of methanol and glacial acetic acid. The fixed suspension is dropped onto glass slides, which are then air-dried and ready for either G-banding or fluorescence *in situ* hybridization (FISH) studies. G-banding stands for Giemsa banding, named after the German chemist Gustav Giemsa, but the characteristic banding pattern of dark and light bands along each chromosome can be induced using a number of different stains. The method described here uses Leishman's stain. Prior to G-banding, the slides must be "aged." When banding methods were first introduced, it was discovered that G-bands could be induced in chromosome preparations only after the slides had been allowed to sit for several days or even weeks. The pressures on clinical cytogenetics laboratories today require rather speedier turn-around times than this leisurely practice would allow. It has therefore been necessary to simulate aging. The method below describes the heating of slides on a 100°C hotplate for a few minutes to "age" slides prior to immersing them in a weak trypsin solution and staining with Leishman's stain to produce G-banding. After air-drying, the slides are then cover-slipped and are ready for cytogenetic analysis *(5)*.

FISH is a method by which specific DNA sequences are labeled with a fluorescent tag and applied to metaphase chromosomes or interphase nuclei so that the DNA sequences or probes hybridize to their corresponding sequences within the target cell. The fluorescent tag indicates the presence and position of specific sequences within the cell. FISH may be performed on cytogenetic preparations, tissue imprints, bone marrow smears, or paraffin-embedded sections. FISH is a valuable complementary test to conventional cytogenetics. In cases of poor chromosome morphology, it is capable of accurately detecting subtle abnormalities that are of prognostic importance, such as the inversion 16 in acute myelomonocytic leukemia with abnormal eosinophils, and of detecting cryptic rearrangements and deletions such as the deletion that occurs at the *ABL/BCR* breakpoint in a proportion of CML cases *(6,7)*. The method described here refers to FISH performed on cytogenetic suspension dropped onto glass slides.

To allow hybridization, target and probe are both denatured to single-strand DNA. This is achieved by heat and in the presence of formamide and salt solution (both components of the hybridization buffer). The incubation time required for hybridization varies from a few hours to overnight. The specificity of hybridization to target DNA can be controlled by variations of temperature, pH, formamide, and salt concentration in the hybridization buffer. Despite a number of mismatched bases along the strands of DNA, stable duplexes can form under certain hybridization conditions, leading to cross-hybridization or "background." Under conditions of high stringency, only probes with high homology to the target sequence will form stable hybrids, resulting in low or no background hybridization. However, low-stringency conditions (reactions carried out at low temperature, high salt, or low formamide concentrations) may result in high background or nonspecific probe binding *(8)*.

Once the excess probe has been removed in a series of post-hybridization washes, the fluorescent signals are detected via a fluorescence microscope. Scoring of signals and interpretation of results varies according to the probes used and the initial indication for FISH studies.

The following methods outline (1) the establishment of both overnight and synchronized cultures of bone marrow cells from patients with myeloid disorders, and the harvesting of cells from each culture after varying periods of incubation; (2) slide making and the production of banded metaphase spreads for microscopic analysis; and (3) FISH performed on metaphase spreads and interphase cells.

2. Materials

The materials required for each step have been listed in separate sections according to the stage at which they are required.

2.1. Bone Marrow Culture and Harvest

1. Bone marrow aspirate, 0.5–1.0 mL, collected in a sterile syringe or tube containing approx 100 U of preservative-free heparin.
2. RPMI 1640 medium with L-glutamine and HEPES (*see* **Note 1**).
3. Fetal calf (bovine) serum (FCS): stored at –20°C in aliquots (i.e., 20-mL aliquots for addition to 200-mL bottles of medium to produce a 10% solution). This should be thawed and added to medium immediately before use.
4. L-Glutamine-penicillin-streptomycin (PSG): a mixture containing 200 mM L-glutamine, 10,000 U of penicillin, and 10 mg streptomycin per mL. PSG is stored at –20°C and 1 mL is added to a 200-mL bottle of medium immediately prior to use.
5. Sterile 50-mL tissue-culture flasks.
6. Sterile pipets.
7. FdU (5'-fluorodeoxyuridine, MW = 246.2) and uridine (MW = 244.2) working solution: 1 mL uridine solution (4×10^{-3} M) and 1 mL FdU solution (5×10^{-5} M) added to 8 mL sterile dH$_2$O to give working concentrations of 5×10^{-6} M FdU and 4×10^{-4} M uridine (stored at 4°C).
8. 5-Bromo-2'-deoxyuridine (BrdU): a 2×10^{-3} M working solution (stored at 4°C).
9. Colcemid: 10 μg/mL solution.
10. Hypotonic solution (potassium chloride 0.075 M): a 5.59 g/L solution of KCl (MW = 74.55).
11. Carnoy's solution: 3:1 (v/v) analar methanol/glacial acetic acid, made fresh just before use.
12. 15-mL plastic, nonsterile screw-top centrifuge tubes.
13. Microscope glass slides: 76 mm × 26 mm superfrost slides with ground edges.

2.2. Banding

1. Trypsin: desiccated tryptic enzyme rehydrated in 10 mL sterile distilled H$_2$O and aliquots stored at –20°C. The amount of desiccated trypsin provided by the manufacturer is based on its enzyme activity rather than weight, and so the solution is prepared according to the manufacturer's instructions to produce a 5% solution of trypsin (1:250). A working solution is made fresh daily by adding 0.25 mL trypsin solution to 35 mL trypsin diluent (discussed later) and 35 mL distilled H$_2$O in a Coplin jar.
2. Trypsin diluent: NaCl (8.0 g), KCl (0.4 g), Na$_2$HPO$_4$ (0.06 g), KH$_2$PO$_4$ (0.06 g), and NaHCO$_3$ (0.5 g) dissolved in 1 L distilled H$_2$O and stored at 4°C prior to use.
3. Ca^{2+}/Mg^{2+} free solution: NaCl (8.0 g), KCl (0.2 g), Na$_2$HPO$_4$ (1.15 g), and KH$_2$PO$_4$ (0.2 g) dissolved in 1 L distilled H$_2$O and stored at 4°C prior to use.
4. Leishman's solution (eosin methylene blue compound) (*see* **Note 2**) stored in powdered form at room temperature. Leishman's stain powder (2.8 g) is added to 1 L analytical-grade methanol and mixed with a magnetic stirrer for 3 h. The

resulting solution is incubated at 37°C for at least 1 wk. To prepare a working solution, 100 mL is filtered through Whatman No. 1 filter paper. The rest is stored in the dark at room temperature until required. The filtered Leishman's stain is then diluted 1 in 10 in stain buffer (discussed later) immediately prior to use.

5. Stain buffer: one Gurr® buffer tablet (pH 6.8) is dissolved in 1 L distilled H_2O and stored at 4°C prior to use.
6. DPX mounting solution, stored at room temperature.
7. Glass cover slips: 24 mm × 50 mm in size.

2.3. FISH

1. Microscope glass slides: 76 mm × 26 mm superfrost slides with ground edges; slides should be prepared as for conventional cytogenetic analysis.
2. Diamond pen for marking glass slides.
3. Dry block heater for co-denaturation of target and probe DNA. This heater should be capable of accurate temperature control at 72–74°C.
4. Hotplate heated to 37°C.
5. Hybridization box: a shallow plastic box with a sealable lid, microwavable and able to accommodate several slides laid inside horizontally.
6. Piece of absorbent foam to sit inside the hybridization box.
7. Cover slip of size determined by the amount of probe solution used (*see* **Note 3**). In general, the 24 mm square cover slip is recommended. The volumes described below refer to use of this size cover slip.
8. Glue/rubber cement (*see* **Note 4**).
9. Premixed probe/hybridization buffer solution: the product information recommends a mixture of 1 µL probe/2 µL purified H_2O/7 µL hybridization buffer (supplied with the probe and containing dextran sulphate, formamide, and SSC) (*see* **Note 5**).
10. 20X stock salt solution (SSC): 175.3 g NaCl and 88.2 g Na citrate dissolved in 1 L dH_2O and the pH adjusted to 7 using 1 N HCl and 1 N NaOH; all SSC solutions may be stored at room temperature (but discarded if turbidity develops).
11. 4X SSC: 200 mL 20X SSC diluted in 800 mL dH_2O and pH adjusted to 7.
12. 2X SSC: 100 mL 20X SSC diluted in 900 mL dH_2O and pH adjusted to 7.
13. 0.4X SSC/0.3% NP40: 100 mL 4X SSC, 900 mL dH_2O, and 3 mL NP40 combined in a glass bottle and stored at room temperature; inhalation of NP40 (polyethylene glycol octylphenyl ether) vapors should be avoided.
14. 2X SSC/0.1% NP40: 1 L 2X SSC and 1 mL NP40 combined in a 1-L sterile glass bottle and stored at room temperature.
15. DAPI counterstain: 20 µg/mL 4',6'-diamidino-2-phenylindole (DAPI) stock solution prepared.
16. DAPI/anti-fade working solution (*p*-phenylene diamine dihydrochloride): 100 mg *p*-phenylene diamine dihydrochloride (powder stored in a tightly sealed light-proof container at room temperature) added to 10 mL PBS and the pH adjusted to 8.0 with 0.5 M carbonate-bicarbonate buffer. The solution should have a slight pink tinge (if the color turns yellow/orange, the solution should be discarded).

The solution is filtered using a 0.22-μm filter to remove undissolved particles. 10 mL of filtered *p*-phenylene diamine dihydrochloride/PBS solution is added to 90 mL glycerol and mixed (inversion or vortex). A 3-μL aliquot of DAPI counterstain is added to 10 mL anti-fade to give a final concentration of 0.006 μg/mL (*see* **Note 6**).

3. Methods

3.1. Conventional Cytogenetics

3.1.1. Culture 1: Overnight Culture

1. Place 10 mL RPMI 1640 medium supplemented with PSG and 10% FCS into a sterile 50-mL tissue-culture flask.
2. Using a sterile pipet, inoculate medium with appropriate amount of bone marrow (*see* **Note 7**).
3. Lay flask flat and incubate at 37°C for approx 24 h.
4. Add 0.2 mL of 10 μg/mL Colcemid to culture and incubate at 37°C for a further 30 min.
5. Transfer culture to harvesting tube and centrifuge for 10 min at approx 200*g* in a sealed bucket centrifuge.
6. Discard supernatant.
7. Resuspend cell pellet in 8 mL of KCl and place in 37°C water bath for 20 min.
8. Centrifuge for 10 min at 200*g*.
9. Discard supernatant.
10. Resuspend in 5 mL of fresh fixative (3:1 analar methanol:glacial acetic acid) by adding the fix drop by drop initially with thorough mixing to avoid cell clumping (*see* **Note 8**).
11. Refrigerate cell suspension at 4°C for 15 min.
12. Repeat **steps 8–10** at least once. The fixative should be replaced until suspension appears clear without any trace of a brown tinge. Finally, the suspension is spun and diluted if necessary with fixative to produce a slightly cloudy appearance (*see* **Note 9**). The cell suspension should be stored at –20°C until slide making (*see* **Subheading 3.2.**).

3.1.2. Culture 2: 48-Hour Synchronized Culture

1. Place 10 mL RPMI 1640 medium supplemented with PSG and 10% FCS into a sterile 50-mL tissue-culture flask.
2. Using a sterile pipet, inoculate medium with appropriate amount of bone marrow (*see* **Note 7**).
3. Lay flask flat and incubate at 37°C for approx 24 h.
4. After incubation for 24 h, add 100 μL of combined FdU/uridine solution to the flask and incubate at 37°C overnight (*see* **Note 10**).
5. The following morning, add 100 μL of BrdU (*see* **Note 11**) and incubate for a further 7 h.
6. To harvest, follow the procedure outline for an overnight culture from **step 4**.

3.1.3. Direct Harvest of Peripheral Blood

When a peripheral blood sample is referred solely for interphase FISH analysis, a direct harvest of the buffy coat cells by the following method provides a fixed suspension of interphase cells suitable for interphase FISH.

1. Into a labeled, nonsterile centrifuge tube place 8 mL KCl and warm to 37°C for a minimum of 10 min.
2. Centrifuge peripheral blood tube in a sealed bucket for 10 min at 200*g*.
3. Take all the buffy coat from all tubes provided and add to warmed KCl.
4. Follow **steps 7** to **12** of the harvest procedure.
5. Store tube in –20°C freezer awaiting FISH analysis.

3.2. Slide Making and G-Banding

Slide preparation is important for optimal G-banding. Ideally, slides are made when the temperature is 22°C and the humidity is 40–45% (*see* **Note 12**).

1. Place cell suspension on the bench and allow it to warm to room temperature. This usually takes approx 15 min (*see* **Note 13**).
2. Clean slides by filling a Coplin jar with 100% ethanol, dipping slides into ethanol, wiping clean with a lint-free tissue, and allowing to air dry.
3. Using a clean Pasteur pipet, drop three to five drops of suspension evenly along the slide. Allow the slide to air dry.
4. Assess slide quality by phase-contrast microscopy. The chromosomes should appear medium gray in contrast and be well spread (*see* **Note 14**).
5. The slides should be aged prior to banding to reduce fuzziness and to produce clear, crisp G-bands. There are a number of methods available. The following steps are designed to produce successful G-banding on the day slides are made (*see* **Note 15**).
6. Allow the freshly made slide to air-dry at room temperature for 30 min (*see* **Note 16**).
7. Prior to commencing banding, set up one Coplin jar with a working solution of diluted trypsin and two Coplin jars with Ca^{2+}/Mg^{2+}-free solution and stand at room temperature.
8. Place slide on hotplate at 100°C for 8 to 10 min (*see* **Note 17**).
9. Without allowing the slide to cool, dip into the diluted trypsin and agitate for approx 8–10 s (*see* **Note 18**).
10. Rinse in two changes of Ca^{2+}/Mg^{2+}-free solution.
11. Shake off excess moisture and place slide on a staining rack. Pipet Leishman's solution onto the slide and let stand for 8 to 10 min or longer if necessary (*see* **Note 19**).
12. Rinse stain off under running tap water.
13. Allow slide to air-dry.
14. Cover slip slide by placing three small drops of DPX mounting medium at intervals along the cover slip. Gently place the air-dried slide face down onto the coverslip, invert and place the slide onto a 37°C hotplate for sufficient time to allow the DPX to set.

15. The G-banded slide is now ready for microscopic analysis. All abnormalities are described according to the International System for Human Cytogenetic Nomenclature (ISCN) (1995) (*see* **Note 20**). An analysis may require more than one slide to be examined per culture, depending on the number and quality of metaphases available. Malignant cells tend to produce metaphase spreads with shorter chromosomes and poorer morphology than their normal counterparts. Abnormal clones may be overlooked if only well-banded metaphases of good morphology are analyzed. The number of metaphases available for analysis on each slide varies greatly. Ideally, the 20 to 40 metaphases required for an adequate analysis will be found on one slide, but it may be necessary to band several slides to obtain sufficient metaphases (*see* **Note 21**).

3.3. Fluorescence In Situ Hybridization

The following method is optimized for Vysis® translocation probes. It includes a co-denaturation step of both probe and target DNA. This method works well for cytogenetic preparations, tissue imprints, and bone marrow smears.

1. Slides should ideally be prepared in advance and aged at least 24 h (*see* **Note 22**).
2. When making slides, there should be adequate numbers of metaphases or interphase cells for FISH analysis. Place one to three drops of suspension, depending on cellularity, on one area of the slide (*see* **Note 23**).
3. Locate an interphase/metaphase-rich area of the slide and mark the top of this area with a diamond pencil on the underneath surface of the slide (*see* **Note 24**).
4. Calculate the volume of probe/hybridization buffer mixture required for the size of cover slip to be used (*see* **Note 3**).
5. Turn on the dry block heater to 72°C and hotplate to 37°C.
6. Prepare the hybridization box by placing a sponge dampened with 2X SSC in the bottom of the box, heat for 10 s in a microwave, and then place the box into the 37°C incubator.
7. Apply 10 μL premixed probe mixture to each slide using the mark underneath the slide as a guide.
8. Cover with a 24-mm square cover slip and seal the edges with glue/rubber cement immediately after the probe mixture has been applied to avoid drying.
9. Place slides (no more than six at one time) on the 72°C hotplate and denature for 2 min (it is critical that it be no longer than 2 min).
10. Transfer slides to the 37°C hotplate until all slides have been denatured and are ready to place in the hybridization box.
11. Incubate at 37°C. The probe manufacturer recommends that hybridization occur over a 6- to 16-h period; we have obtained successful results using a 3.5-h incubation.
12. Prewarm a Coplin jar filled with 0.4X SCC/0.3% NP40 in the water bath, to the temperature appropriate for each probe (74°C for Vysis translocation probes).
13. Carefully peel off glue from the slide and remove the cover slip.
14. Immediately, immerse the slide in the posthybridization wash solution. Slides (no more than four at a time) should be placed in 0.4X SCC/0.3% NP40 for 2 min.

15. Wash slides in 2X SCC/0.1% NP40 at room temperature for no more than 1 min.
16. Air dry away from light and apply the DAPI/anti-fade counterstain. This should be applied sparingly—one drop is usually sufficient—using a Pasteur pipet.
17. Overlay with a 24 mm × 50 mm cover slip and press down gently with a tissue to spread the DAPI/anti-fade under the cover slip and remove any excess around the edges (*see* **Note 25**).
18. The slide is now ready for analysis.
19. All FISH studies should be scored by two scientists, preferably within 1 to 2 d of hybridization. For unique sequence probes on diagnostic samples, a minimum of 5–10 metaphases and/or 50 interphase nuclei should be scored. For follow-up cases or suspected mosaicism, a minimum of 200–300 interphase cells should be scored. If signals are too faint or a significant number of cells are unscorable and the control slides are also unscorable, the experiment should be repeated. There are a number of variables that will affect the final FISH result (*see* **Note 26**). Ultimately, however, a poor result may relate to specimen factors beyond the control of the laboratory.
20. Images should be captured and saved as a record. The VCCS protocol advocates the capture of at least one image for cases with a normal result and at least two images representing clonal abnormalities.
21. FISH reports should include the probe type, the number of cells scored, and a karyotype according to the ISCN (1995) *(9)* (*see* **Note 27**).
22. When interphase FISH results are reported, the results should be compared with normal control values. This is particularly important when loss of signals is identified.

4. Notes

1. RPMI 1640 medium, modified with HEPES buffer, is commercially available in liquid form. At the VCCS, medium is made up from powder: 16.4 g RPMI 1640 powder is dissolved in 1 L distilled H_2O with 2 g sodium bicarbonate, adjusting the pH to 7.2–7.3 using 1 N HCl or 1 N NaOH and sterilizing by filtration through a 0.20-µm filter. It is aseptically decanted into sterile bottles and stored at 4°C for 1 to 2 wk. It should not be used if it becomes opaque, changes color, or has floating particles. This is certainly the most cost-effective method. However, if only small numbers of samples are being cultured, it may be simpler to purchase liquid medium. Once a bottle of medium is opened and ready for use, it will last only a few days at 4°C in the dark. One way to avoid wasting expensive medium is to place 10-mL complete medium aliquots into tissue-culture flasks and freeze at –20°C until required.
2. The G-banding method given here uses Leishman's solution, as we have found this method to be the most reliable and least given to fading over time. However, other methods commonly used in cytogenetics laboratories involve the use of Giemsa stain or Wright's stain.
3. Cover slip size: to ensure adequate coverage of the hybridization area on the slide while avoiding wastage of expensive probe, the minimum possible volume of hybridization mixture plus probe applied to the slide is used with the appropriate-

Table 1
Probe/Buffer Volume Determins the Cover Slip Size
Required

Recommended cover slip size	Volume of probe/buffer mixture
12 mm round	3 µL
18 mm square	6 µL
24 mm square	10 µL
24 mm × 50 mm rectangular	20 µL

sized cover slip. Too little probe mixture applied under a large cover slip causes air pockets, drying out of the specimen, and areas of no hybridization. Too much probe with a small cover slip causes probe mixture to seep out around the cover slip (*see* **Table 1**).

4. The glue or rubber cement used must be able to seal the edges of the cover slip to ensure an adequate seal but also be readily removed. We have found bicycle tube glue to be the easiest to use.

5. Premixing of probe with hybridization mixture allows more accurate pipetting of the small volumes of probe required for each experiment and allows the probe to be aliquotted into small volumes to reduce the number of times the probe stock is thawed and re-frozen. It is possible to dilute most probes considerably more than recommended and still achieve good results. The high cost of probes dictates that most laboratories will attempt to use as little as possible. We have successfully used most probes at half the recommended concentration. Using only 3 µL probe mixture with a 12-mm round cover slip further reduces the amount of probe used per slide and hence the overall cost of the test. However, all FISH methods should first be established using the recommended concentration of probe.

6. If the DAPI counterstain appears to fluoresce too strongly, such that target signals are being overpowered, it can be diluted further with anti-fade. The final DAPI/anti-fade solution is aliquotted into Eppendorf tubes and stored in the dark at –20°C.

7. The amount of bone marrow aspirate inoculated into each culture is dependent on the cellularity of the aspirate and the degree of blood dilution. If a cell count is performed on the aspirate, approx 1×10^7 nucleated cells should be added to each 10-mL culture. Alternatively, an assessment of the viscosity of the marrow specimen may be made. If the marrow appears to be quite thick and viscous, add 5 to 7 drops to each culture using a sterile pipet; if only slightly viscous, add 8 to 11 drops; and if quite thin and blood diluted, add 12 to 14 drops of marrow. Bone marrow from a new case of CML may readily overgrow; if the marrow specimen is thick and sticky, use only one to three drops; if of medium viscosity, three to four drops; and if thin or very thin, five to eight drops of marrow. In general, care should be taken not to exceed approx 12 to 14 drops of marrow, as an excess of red cells added to the culture may affect cell growth. If bone marrow is not avail-

able, peripheral blood may be used, provided there are sufficient cells capable of spontaneous division in the peripheral blood. Peripheral blood samples should be inoculated as for thin marrow, taking into account the white blood cell count (WBC) (i.e., fewer drops when high WBC). Note, however, that greater than eight drops tends to result in excessive red cell contamination and a poor suspension after fixing. When the WBC is not given, the specimen should be spun at 200*g* for 10 min and the size of buffy coat observed. If there is a small buffy coat layer, indicating a low WBC, set up from the buffy coat interface. If the buffy coat layer is large, remix the sample and use whole blood. In the case of a newly diagnosed CML specimen, when only peripheral blood is available, whole blood should always be used rather than buffy coat. Occasionally, bone marrow trephine samples may be induced to yield analyzable metaphases, but the success rate with trephines is generally low. Trephine specimens should be scraped or chopped up under sterile conditions, to produce a single-cell suspension that can then be used for inoculation.

8. All harvesting to the point of first adding fixative, should be performed wearing disposable gloves and in a class II biohazard cabinet. All centrifuging to the first fix stage should be in a centrifuge with sealed, autoclavable buckets.

9. An overcrowded suspension indicates that the culture was over-inoculated. If a culture yields more than 8 mL of cloudy cytogenetic suspension, a repeat culture should be attempted using less marrow, if possible. Overcrowding may result in few metaphases of poor morphology.

10. The blocking period should not be less than 14 h or greater than 17 h (*10*).

11. The incorporation of BrdU into the DNA renders the chromosomes susceptible to degradation on exposure to ultraviolet light; therefore, the culture should be shielded from light. Because modern incubators are light-proof, no special precautions are required. However, with an incubator that allows light entry when the door is closed, the flasks should be placed in a light-proof box inside the incubator after the addition of BrdU.

12. High humidity causes slides to dry too slowly and thus chromosomes to overspread. If humidity is above 45–50%, the slide may be warmed briefly on a hotplate prior to dropping suspension onto the slide. Alternatively, low humidity causes slides to dry too fast, and so chromosomes become clumped and underspread. Below 40% humidity, slides may be rested on a freezer block for a few seconds prior to dropping suspension onto the slide. An alternate method of slide making when the humidity is low is to use cell suspension that has just been removed from the freezer, rather than allowing the suspension to warm to room temperature.

13. Small amounts of suspension should not be left uncapped on the bench at room temperature for long periods of time. As soon as slides have been made, recap and store suspension in the freezer.

14. The following steps may be tried to enhance spreading: (1) breathe warm, moist air onto a clean slide and drop sample onto the misted surface; (2) place clean slides in freezer until surface is misted, then drop as described previously; (3)

hold slide on an angle when dropping suspension; (4) dip slide in a 60% acetic acid solution and drop sample onto the wet slide. To reduce overspreading, the slide may be heated on a 60°C hotplate prior to dropping suspension onto slide. Traditionally, cytogeneticists claimed that the height from which the cell suspension was dropped onto the slide was critical for successful spreading. However, in truth, there is no advantage to dropping suspension from a great height and considerable disadvantage if the best metaphases end up on the floor.

15. Slides may be "aged" by a variety of methods, including placing slides in a 60°C oven or in a desiccator for 1–2 d or as long as required.

16. Slides can continue to be aged in this manner for a number of hours after being made (30 min is not a critical time period). However, it works well only if performed the same day on which slides are made.

17. While most slides require between 8 and 10 min on the 100°C hotplate to age sufficiently, up to 20 min may be required in some cases when banding is being attempted on the same day as slides are prepared.

18. The time needed for each slide to be immersed in trypsin may vary depending on the quality of the chromosome morphology; less time may be required for chromosome preparations of poor quality. One slide should be tested at a time to estimate the optimum time for producing satisfactory G-bands. If the banding is not distinct, the time in trypsin may be extended. If the chromosomes appear fuzzy, the slides may need to be aged longer, either by increasing the time on the 100°C hotplate or by leaving overnight in a 60°C oven.

19. Hotplate-aged slides tend to be paler staining than slides aged by alternative methods, and so may require a longer application of Leishman's solution.

20. Only clonal abnormalities can be included in the karyotype. Thus, structural abnormalities or gains of whole chromosomes must be observed in at least two metaphases, and loss of a whole chromosome must be observed in at least three metaphases to establish the clonality of an abnormality.

21. A failed culture may result from a number of factors. The cause may be sample related, with few cells capable of division due to relative aplasia or blood dilution of the sample, prior therapy with chemotherapy agents, too long in transit, inappropriate storage in transit (either too hot or too cold conditions), inappropriate anticoagulation (ethylenediamine tetraacetic acid [EDTA]), too much anticoagulant (hemolyzing the sample) or too little (allowing the marrow to clot). Of the laboratory factors that may contribute to culture failure, the medium is critical; it must be maintained at the correct pH, and a careful check of the color of the medium provides an indication of whether the pH has changed.

22. For an urgent FISH study using a freshly made slide, pre-treatment with 2X SSC will obviate the need for aging the slide. The slide is immersed in 2X SSC in a Coplin jar at 37°C for 30 min. The slide is then dehydrated through an ethanol series—placed for 1 min each in 70%, 80%, and finally 100% ethanol and then air dried.

23. To ensure that adequate numbers of metaphases and interphase cells are available for FISH analysis, there should be 20 or more interphase cells per low-power field and 30 or more metaphases in the area of a small cover slip (12 mm^2) if

metaphase FISH analysis is required. Optimally, at least 80 interphase cells and 2 or more metaphases per high-power field should be observed.

24. Slides should be marked on only one side of the hybridization area, as multiple marks with a diamond pencil render the slide more fragile and prone to breaking.

25. Any mixing of DAPI/anti-fade on the surface of the cover slip with oil used to visualize the slide through an oil-immersion lens creates an opaque smear, through which microscopic analysis is impossible.

26. FISH troubleshooting: if FISH results obtained are less than optimal, there are a number of areas that can be altered to improve results. Cross-hybridization may be improved by increasing the posthybridization wash temperature or decreasing co-denaturation time or temperature. High levels of background on the slide may be due to the slides not being cleaned sufficiently prior to dropping suspension, or inadequate posthybridization washes. Ensure that wash solutions are made up correctly and at the correct temperature, remove cover slip, and repeat wash. Weak or no signal may be caused by many factors. The slide and/or probe may be inadequately denatured; increase denaturation temperature or denaturation time by 2 to 4 min. The premixed probe may have been incorrectly diluted or not well mixed prior to use. The wash conditions may be too stringent, in which case, decrease hybridization temperature or increase salt concentration in posthybridization wash solutions to 0.2X SSC. Probe or specimen may have been stored improperly— probes must be stored at –20°C, protected from light; and if slides are made more than a few days in advance of FISH being performed, they should be stored at –20°C. Use of the incorrect filter set on the fluorescence microscope may lead to the inference that the experiment has been unsuccessful. The filter set on the fluorescence microscope must be appropriate for the probe fluorophore being used; multi-bandpass filter sets provide less light than single-bandpass filters, and so probes may appear fainter when viewed through a multi-bandpass filter.

27. FISH nomenclature was included in the 1995 version of the ISCN *(9)*. However, its use is problematic, with extraordinary variation observed in its application *(11)*.

References

1. Goldman, J. M. and Melo, J. V. (2003) Chronic myeloid leukemia—advances in biology and new approaches to treatment. *N. Engl. J. Med.* **349,** 1451–1464.

2. Byrd, J. C., Mrozek, K., Dodge, R. K., Carroll, A. J., Edwards, C. G., Arthur, D. C., et al; Cancer and Leukemia Group B (CALGB 8461). (2002) Pretreatment cytogenetic abnormalities are predictive of induction success, cumulative incidence of relapse, and overall survival in adult patients with de novo acute myeloid leukemia: results from Cancer and Leukemia Group B (CALGB 8461). *Blood* **100,** 4325–4336.

3. Greenberg, P., Cox, C., LeBeau, M. M., Fenaux, P., Morel, P., Sanz, G., et al. (1997) International scoring system for evaluating prognosis in myelodysplastic syndromes. *Blood* **89,** 2079–2088.

4. Webber, L. M. and Garson, O. M. (1983) Fluorodeoxyuridine synchronization of bone marrow cultures. *Cancer Genet. Cytogenet.* **8,** 123–132.

5. Barch, M. J., Knutsen, T., and Spurbeck, J. L. (1997) *The AGT Cytogenetics Laboratory Manual*, third ed. Philadelphia: Lippincott-Raven Publishers.
6. Frohling, S., Skelin, S., Liebisch, C., Scholl, C., Schlenk, R. F., Dohner, H., et al; Acute Myeloid Leukemia Study Group, Ulm. (2002) Comparison of cytogenetic and molecular cytogenetic detection of chromosome abnormalities in 240 consecutive adult patients with acute myeloid leukemia. *J. Clin. Oncol.* **20**, 2480–2485.
7. Sinclair, P. B., Nacheva, E. P., Leversha, M., Telford, N., Chang, J., Reid, A., et al. (2000) Large deletions at the t(9;22) breakpoint are common and may identify a poor-prognosis subgroup of patients with chronic myeloid leukemia. *Blood* **95**, 738–744.
8. Andreeff, M. and Pinkel, D. (1999) *Introduction to Fluorescence in situ Hybridization*. Wiley-Liss, New York.
9. Mitelman, F. (ed) (1995) *An International System for Human Cytogenetic Nomenclature*. S. Karger, Basel.
10. Rooney, D. E. (2001) *Human Cytogenetics: Malignancy and Acquired Abnormalities*, third ed. Oxford University Press, Oxford, UK.
11. Mascarello, J. T., Brothman, A. R., Davison, K., Dewald, G. W., Herrman, M., McCandless, D., et al; Cytogenetics Resource Committee of the College of American Pathologists and American College of Medical Genetics. (2002) Proficiency testing for laboratories performing fluorescence in situ hybridization with chromosome-specific DNA probes. *Arch. Pathol. Lab. Med.* **126**, 1458–1462.

3

Overview of Real-Time RT-PCR Strategies for Quantification of Gene Rearrangements in the Myeloid Malignancies

Christophe Picard, Monique Silvy, and Jean Gabert

Summary

In acute myeloid leukemia (AML), molecular diagnosis for the optimal management of patients and for minimal residual disease (MRD) monitoring is of extreme importance. Cumulative data suggest that quantitative monitoring or MRD in AML with fusion transcripts corresponding to 5(I;21), inv(16), and t(15;17) is useful in distinguishing patients at high risk of relapse from those in durable remission. Real-time quantitative polymerase chain reaction (RQ-PCR) is by far the most sensitive assay in the context of MRD detection. We present herein an overview of the principles of RQ-PCR encompassing both the chemistries (double-stranded DNA detection or specific fragment detection) and the instruments. The absolute and relative quantification and the most commonly used methods for calculation of MRD results in absolute quantification are also described.

Key Words: Real-time quantitative PCR; fusion transcript; acute myeloid leukemia; chemistry; results interpretation.

1. Introduction

Nucleic acid amplification and quantification methods play an increasing role in medical diagnostics and drug discovery. Since the early 1990s, quantitative reverse transcription (RT)-polymerase chain reaction (PCR) has been used for determining the amount of mRNA transcripts in biological samples. The method has evolved from a low-throughput gel-based format to the use of fluorescence techniques that do not require separation of the reaction products ("closed tube" format). These fluorescent techniques are faster (less than 3 h) and reduce contamination risk. The amount of cDNA amplified by PCR correlates with an increase in the fluorescent signal. Thus, this new technology provides higher performance than other PCR techniques, such as competitive PCR.

From: *Methods in Molecular Medicine, Vol. 125: Myeloid Leukemia: Methods and Protocols*
Edited by: H. Iland, M. Hertzberg, and P. Marlton © Humana Press Inc., Totowa, NJ

However, like all PCR, inaccurate results may occur because of either false-positives due to contamination, or false-negatives as a result of (1) poor RNA quality, (2) failure of the RT and PCR steps, or (3) inappropriate primers.

In acute myeloid leukemia (AML), molecular diagnosis for the optimal management of patients and for minimal residual disease (MRD) monitoring is of extreme importance. In the mid-1990s, competitive RT-PCR was successfully applied to quantify the level of fusion gene transcripts in CML and AML with either t(8;21) or inv(16). Based on the results of this method, the risk of relapse among patients with *AML1-ETO* and *CBFB-MYH11* transcripts detected in clinical remission is correlated with the relative level of residual disease, and the kinetic of achievement of molecular remission is an independent prognostic factor *(1,2)*. However, competitive RT-PCR is end-point PCR, requires many controls, lacks reproducibility, and necessitates labor-intensive and time-consuming practices, which prohibit both standardization and large-scale multicenter analysis.

Real-time quantitative PCR (RQ-PCR) is by far the most sensitive assay in the context of MRD detection. It can detect a single leukemia cell in a background of 10^5–10^6 normal cells. Therefore, it is quantitative to seven orders of magnitude and is up to five orders of magnitude more sensitive than other conventional methods. The inter-assay and intra-assay sensitivity of RQ-PCR is controlled by quantification of housekeeping genes. Some laboratories have demonstrated the reliability of this technology and its potential clinical value for MRD studies using fusion gene (FG) transcripts.

The detection of fusion transcripts (*PML-RARA, AML1–ETO*, and *CBFB-MYH11*) by RQ-PCR both at diagnosis and for MRD analysis plays an increasing role in the management of AML patients and is prospectively being incorporated into many clinical trials. However, the real predictive clinical value of MRD detection remains to be confirmed.

After an overview of the principles of RQ-PCR encompassing the chemistry, the instruments, and the primer and probe design, we will focus on more practical considerations "at the bench" and finish this overview with comments on RQ-PCR results (their expression and their interpretation).

Fig. 1. Example of amplification on ABI 7700 instrument of a plasmid standard curve (100,000 to 10 copies) using TaqMan chemistry and following the Europe Against Cancer protocol. (**A**) ΔRn vs cycle in a linear scale—the threshold (black line) was set in the exponential phase of polymerase chain reaction (PCR); (**B**) ΔRn vs cycle in a logarithmic scale—the threshold (black line) was set in the exponential phase of the PCR reaction; (**C**) standard curve obtained by plotting Ct of different dilutions vs log of initial concentration. The slope is −3.341 with a correlation coefficient of 0.996, and the y-intercept is 38.833, indicating that the experiment is valid and allowing further quantification and analysis of this experiment.

A

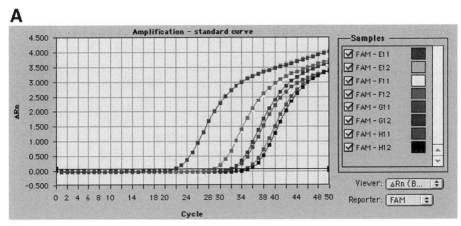

B

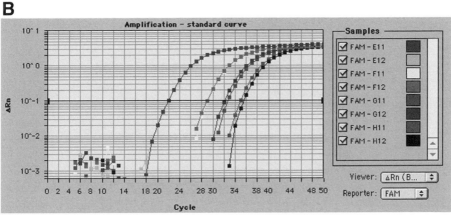

C

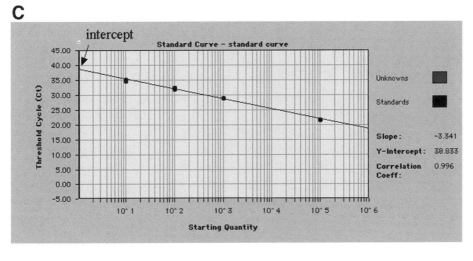

2. Principles of RQ-PCR

Typical PCR amplification curves have three segments: an early background, an exponential growth phase (or a log-linear phase) and a plateau phase. The exponential growth phase begins when sufficient product has accumulated to be detected above background and ends when the reaction efficiency falls. During this phase, the increase in signal corresponds directly to an increase in PCR product and is dependent on the amount of starting material (**Fig. 1A**).

The general principles for quantification by RQ-PCR are identical whatever the chemistry and instrument used. The amplification plot is visualized in a format of ΔRn vs cycle number, where ΔRn is the normalized reporter signal relative to the baseline signal established in the first few cycles of PCR. Rn represents the fluorescent signal of the reporter dye divided by the fluorescent signal of the reference dye (generally Rox). The presence of this dye is obligatory for RQ-PCR on Applied Biosystems (ABI) machines but may be omitted on other instruments. The background fluorescence is detected in all wells that contain the PCR reaction during the first few PCR cycles. A threshold level is then defined as a level of fluorescence above the background Rn, and is typically a multiple of the standard deviation of the background (e.g., 10-fold for ABI instruments). This threshold, which can be manually readjusted, defines the threshold cycle (Ct). The Ct is the cycle number in the exponential phase of PCR for which the fluorescence emitted by the reporter dye crosses the threshold. It is dependent on the starting template copy number, the efficiency of DNA amplification, the PCR system, and the type of chemistry used.

Either absolute or relative quantification methods can be employed. A standard curve is required for absolute quantification and for one of the two possible methods of relative quantification (*see* **Subheading 4.**). The standard curve is constructed using 1:10 serial dilutions of a positive control (e.g., a plasmid containing the target sequence, or DNA or cDNA from an appropriate cell line). The Ct of these 10-fold serial dilutions vs $\log_{10}$ of their initial concentrations produces a linear curve, which is defined by several characteristics: (1) the y-intercept, which provides the Ct value equivalent to one target copy in the case of a plasmid standard curve (**Fig. 1C**), and (2) the slope, which is indicative of the difference in Ct values equivalent to a 1-log difference in the initial quantity of target sequence (i.e., the efficiency of amplification). Theoretically, the slope of the standard curve should be −3.3, because for a PCR with 100% efficiency, the Ct value decreases by one cycle when the concentration of template is doubled. Thus the difference of one log or 10X in the initial template concentration is equivalent to a Ct difference of 3.3 (**Fig. 1B**).

2.1. Chemistry

There are various kinds of fluorescence techniques used in PCR-based detection. The most common methods use either a DNA-binding dye (nonspecific detection) or an oligonucleotide labeled with a fluorophore and a quencher moiety (specific detection). In 2004, the most frequently used chemistry for detection and quantification of fusion gene transcripts in AML utilizes dual labeled probes (TaqMan probes). Only a few articles have described other chemistries for these applications *(3)*. However, this situation may change with the advance of new chemistries. Indeed, all chemistries allow quantification, and some of them provide other advantages such as multiplexing or greater specificity (double-stranded DNA detection vs specific fragment detection). The aim of this chapter is to give an overview of the various possibilities either with double-stranded DNA detection or with specific fragment detection.

2.1.1. Double-Stranded DNA Detection

For systems employing double-stranded DNA detection, the detection is not specific for the amplified sequences. Rather, the specificity relies on the primers chosen and the PCR conditions. At least four different chemistries can be described.

2.1.1.1. SYBRGREEN I

SybrGreen I is an intercalating dye that binds only to the minor groove of double-stranded DNA (dsDNA) in a sequence-independent manner (**Fig. 2**). SybrGreen I fluorescence increases over 100-fold upon binding. This dye is excited at 497 nm and emits at 520 nm. Increasing fluorescence is observed during the polymerization step and decreases during DNA denaturation. Accordingly, in RQ-PCR, fluorescence measurements are performed at the end of the elongation step *(4,5)*.

This method is inexpensive and easy to set up. However, only one target can be amplified, therefore precluding multiplexing. Furthermore, longer amplicons create stronger amplification signals, occasionally causing charge-coupled device (CCD) camera saturation. The advantage and disadvantage of SybrGreen I is that it binds to any dsDNA. Therefore design and optimization of probes are not required. However, all amplifications, specific or not, are detected equally well. Primer dimers are the most frequent cause of nonspecific amplification and limit the sensitivity of assays. To reduce the formation of primer dimers, a Roche technical note (LC 1/1999) provides different optimization strategies. The use of two step reactions (reverse transcription and PCR) and DNAase treatment of RNA prior to cDNA synthesis decreases the formation of primer dimers *(6)*.

Generation of a melting curve at the end of the reaction is indispensable for identifying amplification products *(7)*. dsDNA amplification is melted into ssDNA by a stepwise increase in temperature from 40°C to 95°C while continuously monitoring the fluorescence. PCR products of different length and sequence will be melted at different temperatures and will be observed as dis-

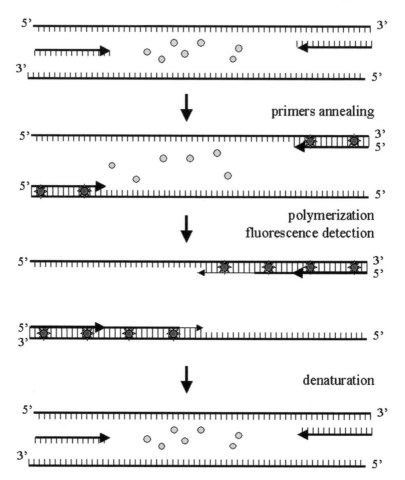

Fig. 2. Double-stranded DNA detection with SYBR Green I dye incorporation. During denaturation, unbound SYBR Green I dye exhibits little fluorescence. At the annealing temperature, a few dye molecules bind to the primer-target double strand, resulting in light emission upon excitation. During the polymerization step, more and more dye molecules bind to the newly synthesized DNA and the increasing fluorescence can be monitored. On denaturation, the dye molecules are released and the fluorescence signal returns to background.

tinct peaks when plotting the first negative derivative of fluorescence vs temperature. If only the specific PCR product has been formed, a single peak should be visible in the melting peak profile.

2.1.1.2. LIGHT-UP PROBE

Some reporters are intercalating asymmetric cyanine dyes that exhibit a large increase in fluorescence intensity upon binding to DNA: oxazole yellow (YO), thiazole orange, and 4-[(3-methyl-6-(benzothiazol-2-yl)-2,3-dihydro-(benzo-1,3-thiazole)-2-methylidene)]-1-methyl-pyridinium iodide (BEBO) *(8,9)*. The light-up probe is a peptide nucleic acid (PNA) that consists of a sequence-recognizing element linked to a single fluorescent dye that serves as a group reporter. The PNA is an uncharged nucleic acid analog to which an asymmetric cyanine dye (thiazole orange) is tethered *(10)*. The light-up probe is flexible, allowing the dye to interact with the target nucleic acid upon hybridization. PNA are uncharged analogs to minimize internal complex formation. Upon probe hybridization, PNA binds specifically to the target nucleic acid, bringing the dye to it, which results in a large enhancement in dye fluorescence *(10,11)*.

2.1.1.3. AMPLIFLUOR HAIRPIN PRIMERS

Amplifluor hairpin primers (Amplifluor Technology) are designed so that a fluorescent signal is generated only when the primer is unfolded during its incorporation into an amplification product *(12)*. The fluorescence signal produced directly correlates with the accumulation of PCR product at each cycle. Each Amplifluor primer consists of a 3′ 18-base oligonucleotide tail (Z sequence) and a 5′ intracomplementary sequence labeled with paired energy-transfer molecules (the fluophore and the quencher DABSYL). The Z sequence acts as a universal PCR primer and is specifically designed to reduce PCR background due to heterodimer formation. The Z sequence is added to the 5′ end of one of the target-specific primers. At the annealing temperature, the Z sequence anneals to the complementary sequence contained in an amplicon generated in the initial cycles of the reaction. The hairpin is unfolded, allowing an increase in fluorescence emission (**Fig. 3**).

Light upon extension (LUX) primers (Invitrogen) are a variation on hairpin primers. They are oligonucleotides of 20–30 bases labeled with a single fluorophore (FAM or JOE) close to the 5′ end in a hairpin structure *(13)*. This fluorogenic primer has a short sequence tail of 4–6 nucleotides on the 3′ end that is complementary to the 5′ end of the primer (**Fig. 4**). This configuration intrinsically renders fluorescence quenching capability, so that a separate quenching moiety is not needed. When the primer is incorporated into the double-stranded PCR product, the PCR LUX primer is dequenched, resulting in a significant increase in fluorescence signal. The fluorogenic primer may be the forward or the reverse primer. The characteristics of the primers, such as length and Tm, are included in the primer design by proprietary software, called LUX Designer (Invitrogen, http://www.invitrogen.com/lux). These design rules enable the software to output numerous primer pairs that are located throughout the target (input) sequence.

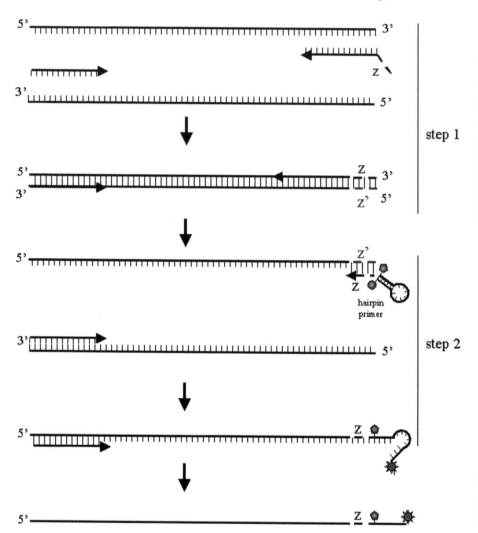

Fig. 3. Double-stranded DNA detection with Amplifluor hairpin primers. One of the target-specific primers possesses at its 5′ end the Z sequence, which acts as a universal polymerase chain reaction primer. During the initial cycle of the reaction, an amplicon is generated that contains the complement sequence to the Z sequence (Z′ sequence). The Z′ sequence specifically anneals to a hairpin primer. This hairpin amplifluor primer consists of a 3′ oligonucleotide tail (Z sequence) and a 5′ intracomplementary sequence labeled with a pair of energy-transfer molecules. As the hairpin amplifluor primer is incorporated, the hairpin is unfolded; quenching is no longer possible as a result of increased distance between the reporter (circle) and the quencher (pentagon).

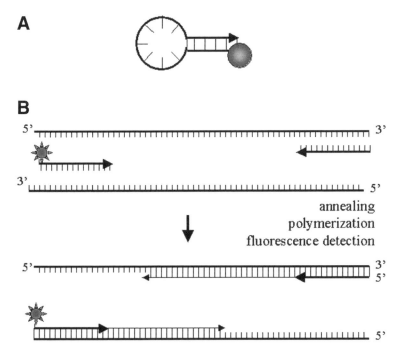

Fig. 4. Double-stranded DNA detection with light upon extension (LUX) primers. **(A)** Structure of a native LUX primer. **(B)** During the denaturation step, the LUX primer assumes a random coil configuration and emits low fluorescence upon excitation. During the polymerization step, double-stranded DNA is formed, leading to an increase in the fluorescence emitted by the reporter (circle), which can be monitored.

2.1.1.4. DzyNA OR BD QZyme (BD Biosciences)

The 10–23 DNAzyme is capable of cleaving nucleic acid substrates at specific RNA phosphodiester bonds under simulated physiological conditions. This DNAzyme has a catalytic domain of 15 deoxynucleotides flanked by two substrate-recognition domains (arms). The DNAzyme interacts with the substrate through Watson-Crick pairing and cleaves between an unpaired purine and a paired pyrimidine. DNAzymes can facilitate the detection of products of in vitro amplification by PCR. PCR is performed using a DzyNA PCR primer that contains a target-specific sequence and the complementary (antisense) sequence of a 10–23 DNAzyme. During PCR, amplicons are generated that contain both target sequence and active (sense) copies of DNAzymes. A DNA/ RNA chimeric reporter substrate, containing fluorescence resonance energy transfer fluorophores incorporated on either side of a DNAzyme cleavage site, is included in the reaction mixture. Cleavage of this reporter substrate pro-

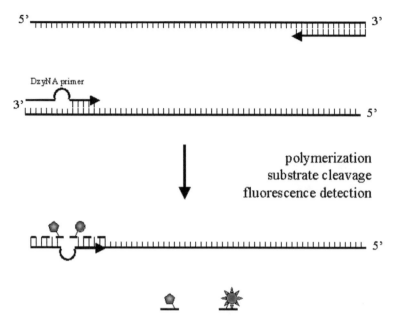

Fig. 5. Double-stranded DNA detection with DzyNA. Reverse transcription of the transcript from total RNA and amplification of cDNA occur sequentially in a single tube. cDNA amplification is achieved by using both the standard and a DzyNA primer containing both target sequence and 5′ tag sequences that are complementary to 10–23 deoxyribozymes (DNAzymes). During polymerase chain reaction (PCR), amplicons are synthesized that contain the target sequences linked to catalytic (sense) DNAzymes, which cleave reporter substrates included in the PCR mixture. The accumulation of amplicon is monitored during PCR by the change in fluorescence produced by separation of the reporter (circle) and the quencher (pentagon) moieties incorporated into opposite sides of DNAzyme cleavage sites within the generic substrates (dotted line) *(14)*.

duces an increase in fluorescence that is indicative of successful amplification of the target gene or transcript (**Fig. 5**).

The accumulation of amplicons during PCR is monitored by an increase in reporter fluorescence produced by separation of fluoro/quencher dye molecules incorporated into opposite sides of the DNAzyme cleavage site within the reporter substrate. The DNAzyme and reporter substrate sequences can be generic and hence can be adapted for use with primer sets targeting various genes or transcripts. This technology has been used at diagnosis and for molecular monitoring of acute promyelocytic leukemia to quantify *PML/RARA* fusion transcripts *(14)*.

2.1.2. Specific Fragment Detection

In order to add further specificity to quantitative PCR, specific fragment detection must be employed. Six variant chemistries are reported.

2.1.2.1. TAQMAN PROBES OR HYDROLYSIS PROBES

The TaqMan assay (Perkin-Elmer–Applied Biosystems) is characterized by using three oligonucleotides (two template-specific primers and one probe) and a DNA polymerase with 5' exo-nuclease activity *(15)*. Taq and Tht polymerase are the two polymerases used most commonly.

The probe is characterized by a fluorophore that is covalently attached to one end and by a quencher that is covalently attached to the other end (**Fig. 6**). Upon excitation, the reporter passes its energy, via fluorescent resonance energy transfer (FRET; or, Förster-type energy transfer), to the quencher while the probe is intact *(16)*. The principle is that when a high-energy dye is in close proximity to a low-energy dye, energy transfers from high to low. The quencher reduces the fluorescence of the fluorophore when the two moieties are separated by <100 Å *(17)*. Traditionally, for TaqMan assays, the FRET pair is FAM (6-carboxyfluorescein) as the reporter and TAMRA (6-carboxytetramethylrhodamine) as the quencher. TAMRA is excited by the energy from the FAM and fluoresces. As the fluorescence of TAMRA is detected at a different wavelength from that of FAM, the background level of FAM is low. After denaturation in each PCR cycle, the probe hybridizes to the amplicon between the forward and the reverse primers. The DNA polymerase extends the primers until it reaches the hybridized probe, when it displaces its 5' end to hold it in a forked structure. The polymerase continues to move from the now free end to the new bifurcation, and the 5'-3' exonuclease activity of DNA polymerase leads to cleavage of the probe *(18)*. The effect is a dislocation of the reporter dye and, as a result of the decrease in energy transfer to the quencher, a rise of the reporter's fluorescence. The resulting relative increase of the reporter dye's fluorescent emission is measured in the course of every PCR cycle. The TaqMan technology is more specific for the target amplicon and more sensitive than SybrGreen. However, this technology requires optimization for each target sequence.

2.1.2.2. MINOR GROOVE BINDER (MGB)

An MGB is a small crescent-shaped molecule (dihydrocyclopyrroloindole tripeptide, or DPI3) that fits snugly into the minor groove of a duplex DNA *(19)*. Increases in melting temperature (Tm) of as much as 49°C have been observed for A/T-rich octanucleotides in the presence of MGB. In TaqMan probes, the MGB group is attached at the 3' end along with the nonfluorescent quencher dye and allows a very short probe (typically 13–20mer). This tech-

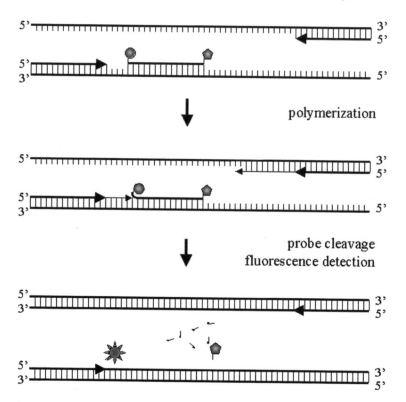

Fig. 6. Specific fragment detection with dual labeled probe (TaqMan assay). After denaturation, primers and probe anneal. The proximity of the two dyes quenches the signal from the reporter dye at the 5′ end of the probe. Polymerization proceeds at the same temperature as the annealing step. The polymerase hydrolyzes the labeled probe, leading to the release of the reporter dye (circle) from the proximity of the quencher (pentagon). The fluorescence of the reporter is detected.

nology is actually used by Applied Biosystems for Taqman Assays-on-demand gene expression products, which are predesigned primer and probe sets allowing quick and easy quantification expression studies in humans. Unfortunately, assays for the common leukemia FG are not yet available in the ABI catalog, and only certain control genes (CG) are included.

2.1.2.3. LOCKED NUCLEIC ACID (LNA)

LNA is a type of nucleic acid analog that contains nucleosides whose major distinguishing characteristic is the presence of a methylene bridge that connects the 2′ oxygen with the 4′ carbon. When this bridge is locked in a 3′-endo conformation, it restricts the flexibility of the ribofuranose ring and locks the structure into a rigid bicyclic formation, conferring an increased thermal stability and hybridization specificity *(20)*. These LNA can be included in the sequence of primers and/or probes such as hydrolysis probes, hybridization probes, or molecular beacon probes. The LNA hydrolysis probes seem to have sensitivity and specificity comparable to MGB probes *(21)*.

2.1.2.4. HYBRIDIZATION PROBES

RQ-PCR analysis with hybridization probes is based on the detection of two adjacent oligonucleotide probes, whose fluorescent labels "communicate" through FRET *(22,23)*. The detection of a given nucleic acid is achieved by the adjacent hybridization of two probes, or by an internal labeled PCR strand and a detection probe located on the opposite strand. In practice, probes are designed to hybridize to the amplified DNA fragment in a "head to tail" arrangement within 5 bp of each other. The probe that possesses a fluophore in the 3' end (donor) is excited by a light source. Its emission spectrum excites the fluophore that is covalently attached to the 5' end of the adjacent second probe (acceptor). The acceptor probe's fluorophore then emits a fluorescent signal, which is measured after the annealing step (**Fig. 7**). The second probe is also modified at the 3' end to prevent its extension during the annealing step. Generally, the 3' label is FAM and the 5' label is LC red 640 or 705 (ROX or Cy5).

2.1.2.5. MOLECULAR BEACON (MB)

Molecular Beacons (Stratagene) are synthetic short oligonucleotides that possess a loop and a stem structure *(24)*. The loop portion of a MB is a probe sequence complementary to a target nucleic acid. The arms flanking either side of the probe are complementary to one another. A fluorophore and a quencher (non-fluorescent chromophore) are attached to the termini (**Fig. 8A**). When the MB is free in solution, it assumes a hairpin structure, bringing the end-bound fluorophore and quencher into close proximity, thereby allowing quenching of the fluorescence signal. At the annealing temperature, the probe hybridizes with the target disrupting the hairpin structure, resulting in the separation of the fluophore and the quencher, leading to the restoration of fluorescence emission (**Fig. 8B**).

A real time detection system can also be generated by using a fluorescein-conjugated molecular beacon in combination with the nucleic acid sequence based amplification (NASBA) system. NASBA is a single-step isothermal RNA-specific amplification that amplifies single-stranded nucleic acids (mRNA) in a dsDNA background. A NASBA reaction is based on the simultaneous activity of avian myeloblastosis virus (AMV) reverse transcriptase, RNase H, and T7 RNA polymerase with two oligonucleotide primers to produce amplification of the targeted fragment in 90 to 120 min *(25)*.

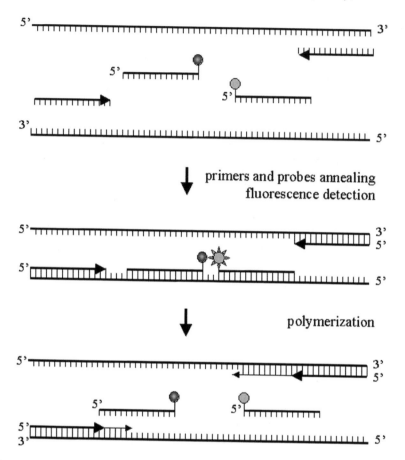

Fig. 7. Specific fragment detection with hybridization probes. During the denaturation step, both probes remain separate in solution. During the annealing step, the probes hybridize and the two dyes come into close proximity. The energy emitted by the excited probe is transferred to the second probe, which emits red fluorescent light at a longer wavelength. At the polymerization step, both probes return into solution and the fluorescence signal returns to background.

2.1.2.6. SCORPION PROBE

Scorpion probe/primer systems combine sequence-specific primers and hybridization probes into a single structure, theoretically improving the kinetics of fluorescent signal generation (26,27). **Fig. 9A** shows the basic elements of a Scorpion probe. It consists of (1) a target-specific probe sequence held in a hairpin loop configuration by complementary 5′ and 3′ arms, (2) a

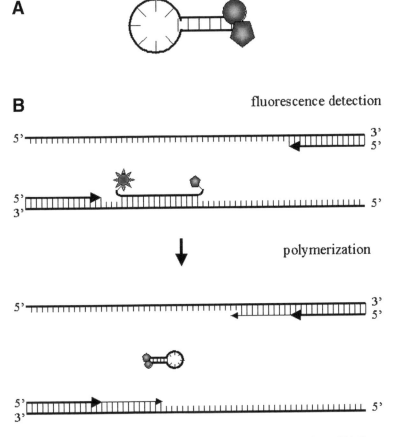

Fig. 8. Specific fragment detection with molecular beacon probes. **(A)** Structure of a molecular beacon probe, which consists of a hairpin loop structure where the loop is a single-stranded probe that is complementary to the amplicon. The arm sequences flanking either side of the probe are complementary to one another. A fluorophore (circle) and a quencher (pentagon) nonfluorescent chromophore are attached to the termini. **(B)** During the denaturation step, the hairpin is opened out and the fluorophore and quencher are separated. During annealing step, the probe binds to target sequence and fluorescence can be monitored. During primer extension, the molecular beacons dissociate from their targets, and fluorescence is again quenched.

fluorophore at the 5' end, (3) a quencher at the 3' end, and (4) a target-specific PCR primer linked to the 3' end of the hairpin loop structure via (5) a PCR stopper *(26,27)*. The PCR stopper prevents read-through of the probe element.

After PCR extension of the scorpion primer, the resultant amplicon contains a sequence that is complementary to the probe, which is rendered single stranded

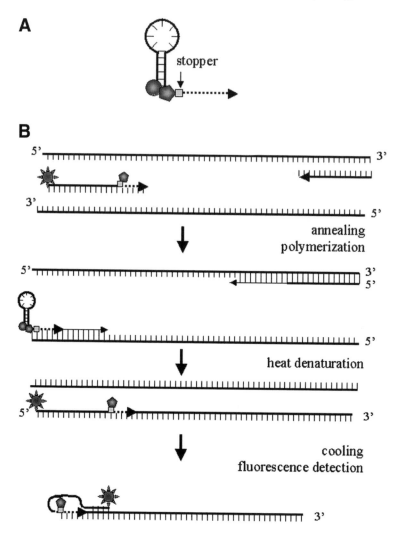

Fig. 9. Specific fragment detection with scorpion primers. (A) Structure of a scorpion primer: in the hairpin loop structure, the reporter (circle) and the quencher (pentagon) are in close proximity, and the signal from the reporter dye at the 5′ end of the probe is quenched. The hairpin loop is linked to the 5′ end of a specific primer (dotted line). (B) During polymerase chain reaction (PCR), the scorpion primers are extended to become part of the amplicon. After extension of the primer during PCR amplification, the specific probe is able to bind to its complement within the same strand of DNA. This hybridization event opens the hairpin loop so that fluorescence is no longer quenched, and increases in signal are observed.

during the denaturation stage of each PCR cycle. On cooling, the probe is free to bind to this complementary sequence, producing an increase in fluorescence, as the quencher is no longer in the vicinity of the fluorophore (**Fig. 9**).

Further improvement of the Scorpion system is also possible. In the duplex Scorpion, the hairpin structure is replaced by two oligonucleotides *(28)*. The target-specific probe element has a fluorophore attached at its 5' end, and at its 3' end is again linked via a PCR stopper to a target-specific primer. In addition, a separate oligonucleotide with a quencher at its 3' end is included in the reaction; this oligonucleotide is complementary to the Scorpion probe. Like simplex scorpion probes, following PCR primer extension and cooling, the probe element is separated from the quencher oligonucleotide and binds to its complement on the same strand, and fluorescence is then observed. Duplex Scorpions produce a more intense fluorescent signal because of the vastly increased separation between fluorophore and quencher in the active form. Furthermore, duplex Scorpions are easier to synthesize and to purify by high-performance liquid chromatography (HPLC) than simplex Scorpion primers.

2.2. Instruments

The quantitative PCR machines currently on the market can be classified into two categories based on the needs of the user: flexible or low-throughput instruments and high-throughput instruments. The flexible or low-throughput instruments are systems primarily dedicated for smaller batches of samples, but they are faster and present more opportunity for flexibility, allowing the user to use different parameters. The high-throughput instruments (96-well plate format) are dedicated for laboratories running large series of samples and few different parameters. The principal characteristics of several RQ-PCR machines are listed in **Table 1**.

Among the flexible instruments, the Smart Cycler (Cepheid) is based on a modular model of 16 independent reaction sites (each containing one sample), allowing the performance of 16 independent PCRs simultaneously. To increase the number of samples analyzed to 96, it is possible to combine up to six modules. This machine, which is fast, is ideal for PCR optimization. The Rotor-Gene (Corbett Research) uses a system of centrifugation to ensure the homogeneity of the temperature. It is possible to analyze 36 or 72 samples simultaneously, depending on the rotor used. Moreover, the use of 0.1 mL tubes allows reduction of the reaction volume to 10 µL, leading to a reduction in sample consumption and cost of each experiment. This machine, which is also very fast, can detect many fluorophores, because it contains four excitation sources (light-emitting diodes [LEDs] that emit at 470 nm, 530 nm, 585 nm, and 625 nm) and six detection channels (from 510 to 660 nm) without spectral overlap, thus allowing the use of the instrument in multiplexing. The third flexible RQ-PCR

Table 1
Characteristics of Different Instruments for Real-Time Polymerase Chain Reaction

Company	Name	Excitation	Detection	Wells	Cycling system
Cepheid	Smart Cycler	Light-emitting diodes (LEDs)—4 channel (450–495, 500–550, 565–590, 630–650 nm)	4 channels (510–527, 565–590, 606–650, 670–750 nm)	16	I-CORE® modules
Idaho Technology Inc.	R.A.P.I.D.™ System	450–490 nm	3 channels (520–540, 630–650, 690–730 nm)	32	Fan & heating coil
Roche Applied Science	LightCycler®	Blue LED light (470 nm)	3 channels (530 nm, 640 nm, 710 nm)	32	Heated air
	LightCycler® 2.0	Blue LED light (470 nm)	6 channels (53, 560, 610, 640, 710 nm)	32	Heated air
Corbett Research	Rotor-Gene 3000	LED four excitation filters (470, 530, 585, 625 nm)	PMT 510, 555, 610, 580 hp, 610 hp, 660 hp nm	36 & 72	
Applied Biosystems	ABI prism 7000	Tungsten-halogen	Four-position filter wheel and CCD camera	96	Peltier
	ABI prism 7300	Single excitation	Four emission filters CCD camera	96	Peltier
	ABI prism 7500	Five excitation	Five emission filters CCD camera	96	Peltier
	ABI prism 7900	488 nm argon-ion laser	CCD	96/384	Peltier
Bio-Rad	iCycler	Tungsten-halogen lamp (400–700 nm)	CCD	96	Peltier

Company	Instrument	Light source	Detection	Wells	Thermal system
Biogene	MyiQ single color	400 nm	585 nm	96	Peltier & Joule
	InSyte	Solid-stable Blue laser (473 nm)	Multichannel PMT (520–720 nm)	96	Electrically Conducting Polymer (ECP)
MJ Research	Chromo 4™	4 channels (450–490, 500–535, 555–585, 620–650 nm)	4 channels (515–530, 560–580, 610–650, 675–730 nm)	96	Peltier
	Opticon®	470–505 nm	2 channels (523–543, 540–700 nm)	96	Peltier
Stratagene	Mx3000P	Quartz tungsten Halogen lamp (350 nm–750 nm)	1 scanning PMT— Four-position filter wheel	96	
	Mx4000™	Tungsten Halogen lamp (350 nm–750 nm)	4 PMT (350–830 nm)	96	
Techne	Quantica*	Halogen white lamp (470–650 nm)	PMT (500–710 nm)	96	
CLP (Continental Laboratory Products)	ATC901*	400–650 nm	450–700 nm	96	

In the upper panel are presented the more flexible instruments (i.e., low-throughput machines), in the middle panel are reported the high-throughput machines, and in the lower panel are noted the instruments actually in development (* coming soon). PMT, photomultiplier tube.

machine is the LightCycler® instrument (Roche Diagnostics). The use of tubes
or plastic plates is replaced by 32 glass capillaries. This constraint requires the
use of specific buffers but makes this system very fast (20°C per s). Dye excitation
is from a single LED at 470 nm, and it detects only at 530 nm (FAM or
SybrGreen I), 640 nm, and 710 nm. There are very few dyes that are excited at
470 nm and emit at 640 nm or particularly 710 nm. The instrument was originally set up for hybridization probes, which use FRET, but is also suitable for
fast cycling using a FAM double-dye oligonucleotide probe or SybrGreen I.
Recently, the LightCycler 2.0 instrument was released. Although it retains the
advantages of the LightCycler, it offers greater possibilities for fluorophore
use, because six detection channels are available.

With regard to the high-throughput instruments, by utilizing a 96-well plate
format, they allow the simultaneous analysis of up to 384 wells for ABI 7900
systems. Their method of fluorescence detection can be by CCD detector on
the ABI 7000 or 7900 (Applied Biosystems) and the iCycler (Bio-Rad), or by
an optical fiber system for the ABI 7700 (Applied Biosystems) and the
MX4000 (Stratagene). Because of its broad spectra of excitation (350 to 750
nm) and of reading (350 to 830 nm), the MX4000 allows the use of a greater
number of fluorophores and thus remains very open to the development of new
fluorophores. Others factors are important. For example, the ABI instruments
allow the collection of data from a passive reference signal to normalize each
reaction for variances in the optics of the system.

The performances of seven of these machines were compared using the Europe Against Cancer (EAC) program protocol (ABI 7000, ABI 7700, iCycler,
Smart Cycler, Rotor-Gene, LightCycler, and MX4000). No differences were
observed in results obtained from cell line dilutions *(28a)*. However, an increasing number of RQ-PCR machines are now available (**Table 1**), more or
less adapted to different chemistries and fluorophores, and the choice of an
instrument is primarily dependent upon the requirements of the user. The cost
should not be the only factor in making a decision.

In AML studies (diagnostic or MRD), the majority of authors have used the
ABI 7700. This instrument is particularly adapted for quantification. However,
it seems less powerful than others to detect multiple PCR products within a
single reaction (i.e., multiplex PCR). Newer versions of all these instruments
are appearing on a regular basis, and the available features are steadily being
upgraded.

2.3. Primer and Probe Design

A successful run of real-time PCR relies heavily on the primers and probes,
and the conditions of the PCR reaction. Specificity is always of primary concern when designing the primers and probes; however, there are several con-

siderations to be kept in mind. If the assay is to be used to study gene expression levels, it is advised to design the primers and probe across an exon/exon boundary. For mutation detection, the probe must obviously be designed around the mutation site. Considering that G-T mismatches are very stable, ideally the probe will need to be fairly short to make the mismatch significant enough to prevent the probe binding. The sequence surrounding the mutation will also affect the stability of a mismatch. However, as primer and probe design and experimental evaluation are time-consuming, a public database application for storage and retrieval of validated real-time PCR primer and probe sequences has been developed *(29)*. This includes a range of detection chemistries such as intercalating dyes, hydrolysis probes (TaqMan), hybridization probes, and molecular beacons.

In any real-time application, it is desirable to obtain 100% efficiency of the amplification reaction. Thus, attention should be paid to secondary structures (hairpins), because these could affect the efficiency of the reaction. Indeed, if the secondary structure is thermodynamically more stable than the oligo-target hybridization, hybridization to the target will be discouraged. A program to test for secondary structures is called "mfold" (http://www.bioinfo.rpi.edu/applications/mfold/old/dna/form1.cgi).

Some generally accepted guidelines for dual labeled probe and primer selection are as follows:

- Select the probe first and design the primers as close as possible to the probe without overlapping it.
- Amplicon size 50–150 bp range, because small amplicons promote high-efficiency assays (not longer than 300 bp).
- G-C content between 20 and 80%.
- Avoid G being on the 59 end of the probe, because the quenching effect of a G base in this position will be present even after probe cleavage.
- To maximize normalized fluorescence values (ΔRn), probes should contain more C than G.
- Melting temperature (Tm) should be 68–70°C for probes and 58–60°C for primers.
- To reduce the possibility of nonspecific product formation, the five nucleotides at the 39 end of each primer should have no more than two G or C bases.
- Test primers and probes against each other to avoid formation of dimers and stem loop structures.

Selecting primers and probes with recommended Tm is one of the factors that allow the use of universal cycling parameters. Moreover, the Tm of primers (between 58 and 60°C) is important, because dual labeled probe assays are usually run at an annealing temperature of 60°C. This is where the required 5′ exonuclease has its highest activity. Having the probe Tm 8–10°C higher than that of the primers ensures that the probe is fully hybridized during primer extension.

Some companies produce probes (Applied Biosystems, Genset Corp, Eurogentec, Operon Technologies, Sigma-Genosys) and some offer design and synthesis (MWG, Proligo). Some software applications are available for the design of primers and probes. Among these, Primer Express (Applied Biosystems) allows the design of dual labeled probes, and the LightCycler Probe Design software allows the design of hybridization probes. Additional primer programs for real-time PCR primer and probe design are available online (http://www.molecular-beacons.org; http://www.genome.wi.mit.edu/ cgi-bin/primer/primer3_www.cgi; http://alces.med.umn.edu/webprimer.html).

Many sequences of primers and probes for fusion gene transcripts or control genes are relatively comparable between the various AML studies. This is explained principally by the use of the same software for their design. It should be noted that certain published sequences (**Table 2**) are false or comprise various errors, whereas the probe and primer sequences we have reported within the EAC program can be used immediately *(30,31)*.

3. At the Bench

3.1. Preparation of a Run

Depending on the RQ-PCR instrument used, real-time PCR is carried out in 96-well reaction plates, in 32 glass capillaries, or in single tubes. However, general considerations are identical in all cases. The PCR mix can be prepared at room temperature, because the DNA polymerase is inactivated either by chemical modification or by an antibody. For clinical evaluation, the use of a master mix (containing buffer, $MgCl_2$, dNTPs, SybrGreen (if used), and enzyme) is preferred to minimize handling and subsequent inter-assay variations. The optimal probe concentration is 50–200 nM (ideally 100 nM), and the primer concentration is 100–900 nM (ideally 300 nM for reverse and forward primers). These variations in concentration are generally dependent on the company that synthesizes the primers and probes. PCR amplifications are performed in a total volume that varies depending on the instrument used (for example, 50 µL or 25 µL for 7700/7000 ABI, 20µL for LightCycler). Patient samples are ideally analyzed in duplicate for control genes and in triplicate for fusion gene transcripts. However, when using low-throughput instruments, a single control gene analysis and a duplicate for fusion genes can be performed. PCR conditions are 10 min at 94°C followed by a total of 40–50 two-temperature cycles (15 s at 94°C and 1min at 60°C).

For absolute quantification using plasmid standards, a calibration curve for each transcript is generated. For control gene amplification, three plasmid dilutions between 100,000 and 1000 copies are sufficient, because for lower copy number, the quantity/quality of sample is low, leading to either a loss of

Table 2
Real-Time Quantitative Polymerase Chain Reaction Studies for Detection of Fusion Transcripts in Acute Myeloid Leukemia

Instruments	Primers	Results	Standard Curve	Control gene	Fusion gene	Ref.
ABI 7700	home made	NCN	plasmids	β-actin	AML1-ETO	50
ABI 7700	home made (Primer Express)	NCN	plasmids	PBGD	PML-RARA	51
ABI 7700	home made (Primer Express)	NCN	plasmids	GAPDH	AML1-ETO	52
ABI 7700	home made (Primer Express)	NCN	cell lines	GAPDH	AML1-MTG8	53
LightCycler	Published (66)	NCN	plasmids	AML	AML1-ETO	3
ABI 7700	home made (Primer Express)	NCN	plasmids	GAPDH	CBFB-MYH11	54
ABI 7700	home made (Primer Express)	NCN	patient diagnostic	GAPDH	PML-RARA	55
ABI 7700	home made (Primer Express)	NCN	plasmids	18S	CBFB-MYH11	56
ABI 7700	home made (Primer Express)	NCN	plasmids	GAPDH	PML-RARA	57
ABI 7700	home made (Primer Express)	NCN	cell lines	ABL	PML-RARA	58
ABI 7700	home made (Primer Express)	NCN	plasmids	ABL	CBFB-MYH11	59
ABI 7700	EAC	NCN	plasmids	ABL	CBFB-MYH11; AML1-ETO	60
ABI 7700	EAC	NCN	plasmids	ABL	CBFB-MYH11	61
ABI 7700	EAC	NCN	plasmids	ABL; GUS	PML-RARA;CBFB-MYH11; AML1-ETO	30
ABI 7700	Published (57)	NCN	plasmids	GAPDH	PML-RARA	62
ABI 7700	EAC	NCN	plasmids	ABL	CBFB-MYH11	63
ABI 7700	home made (Primer Express)	NCN	plasmids	PBGD	MLL/AF9	64
ABI 7700	home made (Primer Express)	NCN	plasmids	ABL	AML1-ETO	65

NCN, normalized copy number; EAC, Europe Against Cancer.

quantification or a poor sensitivity of analysis (discussed later). For fusion gene transcripts, at least four dilutions are recommended (100,000 to 10 copies), because the FG assay must be sensitive. To avoid contamination, careful attention is required, notably when using plasmids. Thus, we recommend separate locations for handling cDNA samples and plasmids. For cell line dilutions, all dilutions are required.

As for any PCR analysis, negative and positive controls are required for RQ-PCR assays. Negative controls (like water or Tris-EDTA) allow identification of contamination of reaction mix. A no-amplification control that contains sample and no enzyme could be necessary to rule out the presence of fluorescent contaminants in the sample or in the block of the thermal cycler. To monitor sample contamination, we recommend performing a negative control for each sample—i.e., an RT sample in which reverse transcriptase has been omitted. Positive PCR controls, such as a cell line dilution, can also be used as a calibrator. Moreover, to control the extraction step, which is probably the most variable part of a PCR assay, an aliquot of a frozen pool of PBMCs spiked with a cell line positive for the fusion transcript can be added to each extraction batch and can be run in each RQ-PCR analysis.

Ideally, all samples, standard curve and negative as well as positive controls, should be amplified at minimum in duplicate in order to limit experimental pitfalls in a well. It is noted that one well is generally used in LightCycler for CG detection.

3.2. Fusion Gene Transcripts and AML

Thirty percent of AML cases express one of three fusion gene (FG) transcripts: *PML-RARA*, *AML1-ETO*, or *CBFB-MYH11*. In the literature, different sequences for FG transcript primers and probes are described (**Table 2**). However, only one study has led to the development of standardized RQ-PCR achieving sensitivities of at least 10^{-5}, suitable for detection of MRD as well as diagnostic screening *(30)*. Therefore, in 2004, standardization of RQ-PCR is possible by two means: the EAC protocol or diagnostic kits.

3.2.1. The EAC Protocol

In 1999, 26 laboratories from 10 European countries designed a joint project of the health and consumer protection of the European Commission (SANCO) via the EAC program in order to develop standardization and quality control for RQ-PCR analysis, based on the ABI 7700 platform (Applied Biosystems). The major aim was to establish a standardized protocol allowing comparison of MRD data within multicenter therapeutic trials in order to assess the relative efficiency of each therapeutic strategy for leukemias bearing an appropriate marker *(30,31)*. The EAC primers and probes for amplification of *PML-RARA*,

AML-ETO, and *CBFB-MYH11*, which were based on Taqman chemistry, were designed during the first meeting in Rotterdam, and were then optimized during phase II, for a definitive selection during phase III, and overall testing in phase IV *(30)*. For *PML-RARA* transcripts, the three breakpoint regions bcr1, bcr2, and bcr3 can be detected by the different sets designed by the EAC program. Similarly, three different sets were developed for the most frequently occurring *CBFB-MYH11* fusion gene transcripts—types A, D, and E.

This EAC protocol can be transferred directly with no adaptation onto different instruments, like the ABI 7000/7700, Light Cycler, Smart Cycler, Rotor-Gene, iCycler, and MX4000 *(28a)*.

3.2.2. Several Kits Are Commercially Available

AME Biosciences and Roboscreen have developed a quantification kit: Amplitect *PML-RARA* cDNA quantification module, which detects breakpoint region bcr1. Its use requires the housekeeping gene quantification module: *GAPDH*, 18S rRNA, or *ABL* cDNA. Each lot of amplitect consists of FG control DNA at different concentrations per eight-well control strip, and FG real time reagent mix (primers and probe). The TaqMan chemistry is used with ABI 7000/7700, GeneAmp 5700, iCycler, Smart Cycler, and Rotor-Gene.

Roche Diagnostics promotes a number of quantification kits for the Light-Cycler:

- LightCycler Inv(16) quantification kit.
- LightCycler t(8;21) quantification kit.
- LightCycler t(15;17) quantification kit.

These kits are specifically adapted for PCR in glass capillaries using the LightCycler instrument. Each lot provides all reagents required for the quantification of the FG RNA in a two-step procedure (RT and PCR). The amplicon is detected by using a specific pair of hybridization probes. Results are expressed as the ratio of FG/*G6PDH* in the sample, relative to the ratio of FG/*G6PDH* in the calibrator. For analysis, a calibrator provided with the parameter-specific LightCycler quantification kits is included in each LightCycler run. For inv(16) quantification, the LightCycler Inv(16) quantification kit and the EAC protocol have identical detection sensitivities (unpublished data).

3.3. Quality Controls

RQ-PCR has become an important tool in research as well as in clinical diagnostics. However, the RT-PCR reaction is fraught with hazards *(32)* and is characterized by significant variation and nonreproducibility between different laboratories, even with identical samples *(33,34)*. Clearly, there is an urgent requirement for stringent quality control and standardization of sample acquisition and processing, especially as multicenter protocols are currently being developed.

Nucleic acid amplification techniques are prone to variation in results, because the sensitivity of these assays makes them very susceptible to small changes in assay conditions, leading to false-positive or false-negative results. Standardization and validation of biological assays are necessary before routine use in order to control inter- and intra-laboratory variations in results, to reduce errors, and to detect critical loss of assay sensitivity.

The reference material should resemble, as closely as possible, the test material, which in this case is cellular material from patients undergoing therapy or not. Thus, the use of cellular material as a reference material would be preferable to cDNA or plasmid, as this would allow control of the extraction step, which is probably the most variable part of a PCR assay.

For example, reference reagents and World Health Organization (WHO) international standards have been established for nucleic acid amplification assays for the detection of several viruses in human plasma. These reagents consist of virus diluted in pooled plasma, and closely resemble the samples routinely tested by blood banks and blood product manufacturers. These reagents are lyophilized for greater long-term stability and ease of transport *(35–37)*.

Collaborative work between the National Institute for Biological Controls and Standards (NIBSC; http//:www.nibsc.ac.uk) and a study group of Professor Gabert has been performed to develop international standards for real-time *BCR-ABL* transcript PCR dosage using lyophilized cells. This procedure permits the control of the extraction phase, the reverse transcription, and the RQ-PCR. In 2004, a reference value was established for *BCR-ABL* expression in a lyophilized K562 cell line. Experiments in accelerated aging of lyophilized cells have shown that the material, transported at room temperature, is stable for 3 yr for RQ-PCR application. A French patent was obtained by the University of the Méditerranée and the NIBSC in March 2003, and a European Patent Cooperation Treaty (PCT) extension was applied for a year later.

Fusion gene-positive cell line RNA, or negative cell line RNA spiked with in vitro synthesized fusion gene, RNA, or plasmid DNA (EAC plasmid, Ipsogen, France) can be used as controls for cDNA synthesis and most importantly for amplification using the TaqMan primer sets. In the same way, Roboscreen has created a standard, the "intelligent reaction tube." In this system, common glass capillaries or plastic tubes required for either standardized nucleic acid purification or quantification are precoated with defined amounts of distinct control DNA or RNA, respectively *(38)*. However, these controls suffer from the limitation that they do not reliably evaluate sample handling and RNA extraction steps, which may also have an important bearing on assay sensitivity. Another method of RNA conservation is the use of the Fast Technology for Analysis (FTA) card system (Whatman), which is a chemically treated filter paper designed for storing blood samples for subsequent DNA and RNA testing *(39,40)*. The FTA cards are impregnated with a chemical formula that lyses cell membranes and denatures proteins upon contact. Nucleic acids are physically entrapped, immobilized, and stabilized for storage at room temperature. Furthermore, cards protect nucleic acids from nucleases, oxidation, ultraviolet damage, and infectious pathogens. The stability of genomic DNA on FTA cards for at least 14 yr has been demonstrated. RNA stability depends on the storage temperature and the type of biological specimen. RNA of mammalian cells stored on FTA cards is stable for over 1 yr at temperatures below $-20°C$ and for 2–3 mo in samples stored at room temperature.

3.4. Normalization and Quantification

3.4.1. Normalization

For normalization, one challenge is to choose one or more endogenous control gene(s) which take into account factors influencing the different steps of RQ-PCR. Crucial parameters such as RNA quality and quantity should be evaluated. This is generally accomplished by amplification, in parallel with the target gene, of one or more CGs, also called housekeeping or endogenous reference genes. In the literature, numerous CGs for MRD detection by RQ-PCR are in use: *ABL, BCR, β-actin, GAPDH, PBGD, TBP*, and 18S rRNA (**Table 2**).

A suitable CG in any application of RQ-PCR analysis can be defined as a gene (1) that is stably expressed in all the nucleated cells among different analyzed samples and is unaffected by any experimental treatment; (2) that is not associated with any pseudogenes, in order to avoid genomic DNA amplification; (3) whose amplification would reflect variations in RNA quality, quantity, and/or cDNA synthesis efficiency; (4) whose stability should be equivalent to that of the target gene transcript(s), or whose impaired amplification should be accompanied by a corresponding reduction in the quantity of target gene transcript(s); and (5) whose expression should not be very low ($Ct > 30$) or very high ($Ct < 15$).

Generally, one CG is not sufficient for all situations. In order to address the stability of a given control gene in a series of tissue samples, a robust gene-expression stability measure was developed by creating an algorithm to determine the most stable—and hence, reliable—housekeeping genes in a given tissue panel *(41)*. The algorithm is based on repeated gene stability measurements and subsequent elimination of the least stable control gene. To handle the large number of calculations, a visual basic application for Microsoft Excel, termed Genorm, was developed. Three to five control genes are required for each tissue (e.g., bone marrow) *(41)*.

Few studies have focused on the definition of control genes. A collaborative action was undertaken within the EAC program involving 6 laboratories among 26 from 10 member countries. This program defined and standardized RQ-PCR protocols suitable for measuring the levels of FG in leukemia with special reference to the selection and optimization of CGs *(31)*. This multicenter retrospective study on over 250 acute and chronic leukemia samples obtained at diagnosis and with an identified FG confirmed that three CGs (*ABL*, β-glucuronidase [*GUS*], and β-2-microglobulin [*B2M*]) had stable expression within the different samples. However, only *ABL* transcript expression did not differ significantly between normal and leukemic samples at diagnosis, and therefore the EAC proposes to use *ABL* as the CG for RQ-PCR-based diagnosis and MRD detection in leukemic patients.

It should be noted that Roche Diagnostics and Applied Biosystems market different kits that evaluate the expression of a variety of housekeeping genes.

3.4.2. Quantification

RQ-PCR can be subdivided into two basic categories: absolute and relative quantification.

3.4.2.1. ABSOLUTE QUANTIFICATION

Absolute quantification utilizes a standard curve derived from known amounts of a calibrator. If quantitation is normalized to an endogenous control, a second standard curve for the endogenous reference must also be prepared. Then, the target amount is divided by the endogenous reference amount to obtain a normalized target value. The calibration curves used in absolute quantification can be based on known concentrations of DNA standard molecules (recombinant plasmid DNA), genomic DNA, RT-PCR products, or commercially synthesized large oligonucleotides. Recombinant plasmid DNA dilutions in *Escherichia coli* 16S and 23S rRNA (20 ng/μL) are most widely used. This allows the determination of absolute gene-expression levels in unknown samples. Plasmids are robust and helpful for standardization and reproducibility of results within multicenter studies. Because the use of plasmids leads to highly reproducible results, the threshold can be fixed, allowing a direct comparison of Ct values or copy numbers (CN) for the same sample in different laboratories. Furthermore, their storage is very easy (they are stable for several years at −20°C). However, there are limitations to the use of plasmids. First, they allow validation of the PCR step but not of the reverse transcriptase step. Second, contamination risk is relatively important and requires a separate laboratory for handling plasmids, or the use of degradable dU-based DNA templates. Furthermore, plasmid design and construction is a relatively long process (involving standard synthesis, purification, cloning, transformation, plasmid preparation, linearization with restriction enzyme, verification, precise determination of standard concentration, and accurate preparation of dilutions).

3.4.2.2. RELATIVE QUANTIFICATION

Relative quantification can also be performed using a standard curve, with the results expressed relative to a calibrator. The standard curve may be prepared from dilutions of cell lines, or diagnostic patient bone marrow RNA may be serially diluted in water or in RNA from peripheral blood leucocytes (PBL), peripheral blood mononuclear cells (PBMC), FG-negative cell lines, or in *E. coli* rRNA. Dilutions of cell line RNA in PBL or PBMC RNA are preferred. The units of the standard are irrelevant, because quantification of the target sequence is expressed relative to the calibrator (which is also quantified from the same standard curve). In contrast with plasmid DNA, RNA is relatively unstable, and gene expression can vary according to culture conditions and between different laboratories. Moreover, fusion gene and control gene expression may differ among subclones of the same line in each laboratory and also from diagnostic patient samples. Accordingly, data comparison is difficult over time and between laboratories. The data obtained are expressed relative to an arbitrary calibrator and consequently do not directly reflect the proportion of malignant cells in a given test sample. However, all RT-PCR steps are precisely evaluated, their use is relatively easy, and the contamination risk is relatively low. As with absolute quantification, the expression level of the gene in question may be normalized to an endogenous control gene. Each of the normalized target values is then divided by the normalized calibrator target value to generate the relative expression levels.

Relative quantification can also be performed without a standard curve by using a comparative Ct method (also known as $\Delta\Delta$Ct). This method assesses the expression of a target gene relative to a control gene in both the test sample and in a comparator (calibrator) sample, and the expression in the test sample is given relative to the expression in the calibrator sample. The following formulae summarize the process of relative quantification without a standard curve:

$$\Delta Ct = Ct(\text{target gene}) - Ct(\text{control gene}) \qquad (1)$$

$$\Delta\Delta Ct = \Delta Ct(\text{test sample}) - \Delta Ct(\text{calibrator}) \qquad (2)$$

The relative expression level of the test sample is given by the formula $2^{-\Delta\Delta Ct}$ (3)

When the $\Delta\Delta$Ct method is employed, the PCR efficiency has a major impact on the fluorescence profile and the accuracy of the calculated expression result, and is critically influenced by PCR reaction components. Constant amplification efficiency in all samples being compared is one important criterion for reliable comparison between samples. Small efficiency differences between target and reference generate false expression ratios, and the true initial level of mRNA may be over- or underestimated. Several mathematical methods that determine real-time PCR efficiency have been described *(42–45)* and are compared online (http://www.gene-quantification.info/). The equivalence of PCR efficiency between test samples and calibrators should be validated in an independent experiment.

Efficiency-corrected quantifications should be included in the setup and calculations that are performed in relative quantification procedures. LightCycler Relative Expression, Q-gene, Rest, and Rest-XL software applications allow the evaluation of amplification efficiency plots. Q-gene, Rest, and Rest-XL software are available directly on the Web and are applicable on different instruments, whereas LightCycler Relative Expression is an application of LightCycler that permits the use of one to two calibration wells for each series. For example, the LightCycler kits are function tested using calibrator RNA derived from an immortalized cell line for each FG expression and do not require a standard curve. Instead, the amount of mRNA encoding the FG is expressed as a ratio relative to a reference gene (*G6PDH*) in that particular sample, and then compared to the FG:*G6PDH* ratio in the calibrator.

4. RQ-PCR Results

4.1. Expression of the Results

Based on the quantification of (1) CG expression in a patient's follow-up samples and (2) FG and CG expression in the patient's diagnostic sample, two methods are most commonly used for calculation of MRD results and experimental sensitivity: the $\Delta\Delta$Ct method and the normalized copy number (NCN) method.

With the $\Delta\Delta$Ct method, the results can be calculated using slopes and intercepts derived from previously generated plasmid standard curves. Based on the EAC results, average intercept and slope values of 40 and –3.4, respectively, can be used for such calculations.

Alternatively, the NCN method requires inclusion of plasmid standards in each quantitative PCR experiment. The NCN method has been most frequently used for reporting MRD data in the literature. The levels of expression of fusion transcripts in both patient and control samples are expressed as normalized copy numbers by calculating the ratio of fusion gene transcript copy number divided by the control gene transcript copy number, and adjusted as required for ease of interpretation (e.g., multiplication by 100 or 1000). The NCN method is robust and is the preferred method for standardization of results between various laboratories. This is crucial if RQ-PCR is to be used as a clinical tool for AML patients. Indeed, as shown by nucleic acid quantification technology in virology, the final goal is to define international units allowing data comparisons of different therapeutic strategies.

Few authors in the research field use the $\Delta\Delta$Ct relative quantification (relative expression) approach (described previously, and in more detail in the Applied Biosystems User's Bulletin #2). The Ct values are normalized for an endogenous reference control gene (ΔCt = Ct$_{FG}$ – Ct$_{CG}$) and compared with a calibrator ($\Delta\Delta$Ct = ΔCt$_{samples}$ – ΔCt$_{calibrator}$). The calibrator can be a dilution of a cell line, or the average Ct value of several bone marrow or blood samples from healthy volunteers. The comparative $\Delta\Delta$Ct method requires similar PCR efficiency (more than 90%) for both target and control genes. Different efficiencies may be observed between patients and standards; thus, a validation experiment is required. cDNA from randomly selected patients and healthy donor samples as well as from cell lines are serially diluted over a concentration of 1:1 to 1:1000. All samples are analyzed in triplicate and the resulting median used for further calculation. The resulting Ct values are plotted against the $\log_{10}$ concentration of total RNA. The slope of the fitted line is then determined. A slope of less than 0.1 indicates that the efficiency of amplification of the target or control genes between the various samples is equivalent.

In this area, it is worth noting that the LightCycler Relative Quantification software provides a tool for fully automated calculation of calibrator-normalized and PCR efficiency-corrected relative quantification of mRNA expression levels or gene dosage values. The great advantage of this system is that standards are not required in each LightCycler analysis run, because stored files containing fitted coefficients can be used instead. To generate analysis parameters for storage and use in subsequent assays, plasmid or cell line dilutions for both target and control genes are performed several times. The resultant Ct values are plotted against the log of the concentration, and two different regression fits are performed. A linear fit is calculated using LightCycler Data Analysis (LCDA) software, and a nonlinear fit is performed by exporting LCDA data into the coefficients module of the Relative Quantification software. The automatically calculated fit coefficient is stored in a file for subsequent analysis. This software provides a method to compensate for the observed "low concentration shift" of the Ct values. Relative concentrations of target and reference genes of each sample and calibrator are calculated automatically from this curve.

The calibrator can be a cell line or plasmid dilutions at known concentration. For example, for *AML1-ETO* detection, Kasumi cell RNA diluted to 10^{-3} or plasmid concentration of 1000 copies can be used. NB4 cells and ME-1 cells can be similarly used for *PML-RARA* bcr1 and *CBFB-MYH11* type A, respectively. The data of LCDA show both the concentration ratio and the normalized ratio. The final result is expressed as a normalized ratio (FG/CG in the sample, relative to the ratio of FG/CG in the calibrator). If the relevant standard curve is performed using plasmid dilutions, the concentration ratio corresponds to the NCN.

The LightCycler Relative Quantification software provides highly accurate and convenient calculations for an individual laboratory. However, it is not adapted for comparison of data between laboratories unless a universal calibrator is employed.

4.2. Interpretation of the Results in Absolute Quantification

To interpret RQ-PCR results with absolute quantification, different parameters for validation have to be checked: slope, CG expression level, and sensitivity.

The standard curve obtained from cell line or plasmid dilutions should have an acceptable slope and correlation coefficient. The slope should be between −3 and −3.6, corresponding to PCR efficiencies between 90% and 115%, provided the correlation coefficient is >0.95. In this case, as defined by the EAC group, the intercept should be lower than 40. Slope values <−3.6 with a good correlation coefficient may indicate problems in dilution of the standards. When the correlation coefficient is poor, the standards may be degraded. Slope values >−3.0 are sometimes due to pipetting errors.

The accuracy of RQ-PCR is very important, and therefore for any one sample, the duplicates should not differ by more than 0.5 Ct. Indeed, the coefficient of variation (CV) for Ct data has been shown to be less than 2% for ABI7700, and 0.4% for LightCycler *(46,22)*.

The RQ-PCR is quantitative in the exponential growth phase of the PCR reaction, requiring that the amplification is expressed in $\log_{10}$. For low copy number (CN < 10), the values are not reliable and are not accurate. Accordingly, positivity at 10^{-4} for cell line dilutions or 100 copies for plasmid dilutions is recommended. Furthermore, the specific amplification should be sufficiently distant from the nonspecific amplification (i.e., have a much lower Ct) so that if contamination occurs it can be readily identified, especially for low levels of molecular MRD. We recommend that to interpret these amplifications, a sample in which RNA was not reverse-transcribed into cDNA (in which reverse transcriptase was omitted from the reaction, "RT-") should always be analyzed in MRD assays.

For MRD quantification, CG expression offers the possibility of quantifying the sensitivity of experiments, which is a crucial point for FG-negative results. If *ABL* is used as the CG, the *ABL* CN for a sample should not be lower by more than 1 log (i.e., *ABL* CN <1000 according to EAC criteria *(31)*) of the average value of the laboratory. Others use the formula: $10^{\Delta Ct/3.3}$, where $\Delta Ct =$

$Ct_{CG,sample} - Ct_{CG,median}$; $Ct_{CG,sample}$ is the Ct of the CG in the sample, and $Ct_{CG,median}$ is the median Ct of the CG in the laboratory. A low *ABL* expression level could be due to RNA degradation or to faulty amplification due to the presence of PCR inhibitors. RNA degradation is not highlighted by the Agilent 2100 Bioanalyzer in the majority of such samples *(47)*. Therefore, the most likely explanation for low *ABL* expression is the presence of inhibitors and not RNA degradation *per se*. These inhibitors can be removed by dilution of cDNA, purification of cDNA on columns, or by the addition of an amplification facilitator such as bovine serum albumin (BSA) in the PCR buffer. It seems that the addition of 0.04% BSA to TaqMan-based RQ-PCR analysis is better than the other techniques for achieving satisfactory amplification of transcripts in poor quality samples *(47)*.

The FG levels in diagnostic samples are also important for calculating the sensitivity. Indeed, the expression level of an FG in a patient's diagnostic sample can vary considerably (up to 100-fold). Furthermore, FG transcripts have also been detected in the peripheral blood of healthy subjects *(30,48)*. A simple formula allows calculation of the sensitivity:

$$\text{dynamic range (log value)} = [Ct(FG_{LIMIT}) - Ct(FG_{DIA})]/\text{slope}$$

where $Ct(FG_{LIMIT})$ is the Ct limit for detection (the *y*-intercept if a plasmid standard curve is used), and $Ct(FG_{DIA})$ is the Ct of the FG at diagnosis. If the slope is −3.3 and $Ct(FG_{DIA})$ is 21, quantitative data are reliable to a dilution of 1 in 10,000. So, to determine the level of MRD in patient samples, the FG value at diagnosis is set to one, and the fraction of leukemic cells is calculated from the following equation:

$$10^x = (\Delta Ct_{MRD} - \Delta Ct_{DIA})/\text{slope}$$

where x is the fraction of leukemic cells, ΔCt_{MRD} is the normalized threshold cycle $[Ct(FG_{MRD}) - Ct(CG_{MRD})]$ at MRD, and ΔCt_{DIA} is the normalized threshold cycle at diagnosis.

The EAC protocol proposes an assessment of the sensitivity of RQ-PCR experiments. The sensitivity is calculated according to the normalized copy number (NCN = FG copy number/CG copy number) of the FG at diagnosis $(FG/CG)_{DIA}$, and from the level of CG expression (CG_{MRD}) in the follow-up sample being tested. Accordingly, the sensitivity of RQ-PCR experiments is $(CG_{CN,DIA}/FG_{CN,DIA} \times CG_{CN,MRD})$. Ideally, the calculation should be based on the patient's NCN at diagnosis, after correction for blast percentage. If these data are not available, EAC values can be used.

In routine practice, the interpretation of patient sample results is dependent on the control gene expression level to monitor the quality of the sample. Based on EAC data, samples with *ABL* CN > 1000 (i.e., $10^{\Delta Ct/3.3} < 10$) are "good quality samples" and samples with *ABL* CN < 1000 (i.e., $10^{\Delta Ct/3.3} > 10$) are "poor quality samples." However, at diagnosis, detection of the FG is almost independent of CG quantification, because EAC results have shown that FG expression can be more than 100 times the CG expression *(30)*. As an example, provided *ABL* CN > 100 (i.e., $10^{\Delta CT/3.3} < 100$), the expression of the FG can be monitored, but the result is not quantifiable and the sensitivity is low. For all positive results, a repeat RT and RQ-PCR are performed. For negative samples, a new patient sample must be obtained for the analysis.

MRD results are harder to interpret than diagnostic results. When the FG is amplified, results are interpreted based on the CN values of both the sample and the controls (RT- and water). In the case of good quality samples (*ABL* CN > 1000), quantification is accurate and the FG expression is interpretable. Thus, for FG amplification with a high CN value, the sample is "positive" (discussed later). For FG amplification with CN value <1 (i.e., Ct value > the *y*-intercept), the result is reported as a negative sample. In the case of low CN (i.e., high Ct value), the interpretation of a result is dependent on the sensitivity of the RQ-PCR analysis. Thus, for FG expression lower than 10 copies in EAC, the sample is considered "positive not quantifiable." A difference in CN between the sample and the negative controls (RT- and water) of more than 1 log (which corresponds to a difference of 3 Ct) is necessary in order to eliminate false-positives; if the difference in CN between the sample and the negative controls is <1 log, a new assay should be performed using a fresh patient sample.

When amplification is detected in only one well of the replicate, regardless of the Ct value, true amplification must be verified. The ABI 7000/7700 "Multicomponent view" allows true amplification to be distinguished from nonspecific baseline creeping. When baseline creeping is detected, the result is a negative sample. In all other cases, the PCR assay should be repeated using a new patient sample. Indeed, this amplification could be due to contamination with either cDNA or plasmid DNA introduced during or after nucleic acid extraction.

In the case of poor quality samples (*ABL* CN < 1000), the accuracy of RQ-PCR is not guaranteed. In such cases the lack of amplification of an FG is not interpretable and a positive amplification of FG is considered not quantifiable positive (**Fig. 10**).

MRD and sensitivity values can be plotted on a graph for presentation of MRD follow-up data. Results are depicted graphically with a time scale on the *x*-axis, whereas day to day sensitivity calculated from CG values and MRD results are plotted on the *y*-axis (**Fig. 11**). Results of diagnostic and follow-up samples are expressed relative to the median EAC values. The EAC value is set at 1 or 100% independent of the value in the diagnostic sample.

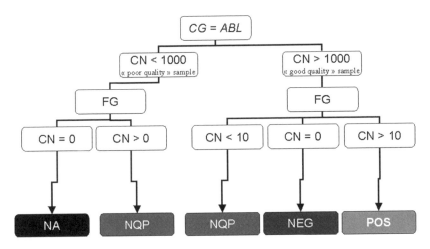

Fig. 10. Decision algorithm for the interpretation of real-time quantitative polymerase chain reaction results according to Europe Against Cancer criteria. For minimal residual disease follow-up monitoring, the interpretation of the results depends on the level of control gene expression for assessment of the quality of the sample. CG, control gene; FG, fusion gene; CN, copy number; NA, not amplifiable; NQP, not quantifiable positive; NEG, negative; POS, positive.

Thus, the interpretation of results varies depending on whether the sample was obtained at diagnosis or during serial assessments for MRD. In all cases, to ensure appropriate interpretation, it is essential that the RQ-PCR data that have been obtained be assessed within the clinical context of the AML patients. As an example, at diagnosis a low positivity result should always be suspected of being false data.

5. Conclusion and Future Steps

RQ-PCR is the method of choice for quantifying mRNA levels of FG and CG. This technology is fast, accurate, and sensitive compared to the other methods of nucleic acid detection. However, RQ-PCR necessitates optimization and control of the parameters relevant to the pre-analytic and analytical phases. Until now, all RQ-PCR results to detect FG and CG in AML were obtained by using dual labeled probe technology with relatively identical probes and primers and with an identical instrument (ABI 7700). This quantitative method is robust and accurate. However, the new chemistries and new instruments facilitate multiplexing that combines the quantification of control gene and fusion gene in a single PCR. Furthermore, they may give the same results with a lower cost.

In 2005, real-time PCR has become a technology that is essential in MRD studies in patients treated for AML. Cumulative data suggest that quantitative

FG : *AML1-ETO* (AML) // CG *ABL*

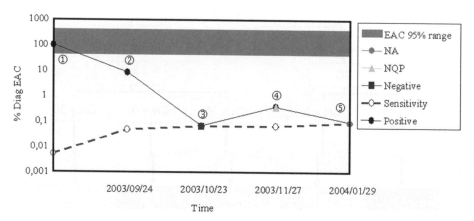

Fig. 11. Longitudinal minimal residual disease (MRD) monitoring of an *AML1-ETO*-positive patient using EAC *AML1-ETO* and *ABL* real-time quantitative polymerase chain reaction sets. For each sample, the MRD value is a normalized copy number (*AML1-ETO* copy number/*ABL* copy number) expressed as a percentage of the Europe Against Cancer (EAC) median for the fusion gene transcript. The gray area defines the EAC 95% range values for *AML1-ETO* normalized copy number (NCN). The sensitivity is calculated according to the relative expression of the fusion gene (FG) at diagnosis and control gene (CG) expression during follow-up. (1), EAC median value for *AML1-ETO* NCN is set to 100%; (2), patient diagnostic sample; (3), example of negative sample (i.e., "good quality sample" and absence of FG detection); (4), example of "not quantifiable positive" sample—the sensitivity is correct, indicating that *ABL* CN is >1000; therefore, the FG CN is <10; (5), example of "not amplifiable" sample with *ABL* CN < 1000 and FG not detected.

monitoring of MRD in AML with t(8;21), inv(16), and t(15;17) is useful in distinguishing patients at high risk of relapse from those in durable remission. This information is essential for defining risk stratification. Thus, the role of MRD monitoring by RQ-PCR is being prospectively evaluated in current clinical trials, and molecular response is being used to determine subsequent treatment approaches in some protocols such as the MRC AML 15 protocol (risk stratification of acute promyelocytic leukemia).

However, the major problem of RQ-PCR is that the interpretation of results and the quality control varies between the different studies. Quality control programs are required particularly for clinical use (routine diagnostic assays) to monitor the performance of the different laboratories. The advent of automation could be helpful. These tools will allow a standard to be provided in order to compare results from various laboratories and to facilitate studies to assess the value of MRD monitoring in a large number of patients enrolled in clinical trials. Common guidelines and quality controls should be developed within various international networks. This work is particularly essential for communication between clinicians and molecular biologists. This standardization should be obligatory for the assessment of prognostic value and for serial assessment of MRD by RQ-PCR for rare FG, such as *MLL-AF9*, *MLL-AF6*, or *DEK-CAN*. In these cases, centralization of results is recommended. This effort should be started immediately for new markers such as *WT1* or *ras* mutations.

In conclusion, it is evident that the technology is available for quantifying gene transcripts within the clinical setting for the benefit of large series of patients. In this way, it is possible to objectively document therapeutic efficacy (MRD studies). This technology will definitively evolve, and here we have described some variant approaches. However this technology is still in its infancy, and is not yet implemented routinely in large multicenter trials for myeloid malignancies. Two main limitations for its lack of penetration are likely: first, improvements in standardization and better quality controls are mandatory (such as the EAC program and the use of freeze-dried cells); second, it must be available for the majority of the patients. Currently, fusion gene transcripts are identifiable in only 35–45% of patients with AML. New markers have to be found (new fusion transcripts, *WT1*, gene-expression profiles, and so on). Very recently, Lossos et al. *(49)* showed that measurement of the expression of six genes using RQ-PCR and based on gene-profiling data is sufficient to predict overall survival in patients with large B-cell lymphoma. All together, these efforts should pave the way towards the definition of new biological markers—quantified gene transcript(s) for myeloid malignancies.

References

1. Laczika, K., Novak, M., Hilgarth, B., et al. (1998) Competitive CBFbeta/MYH11 reverse-transcriptase polymerase chain reaction for quantitative assessment of minimal residual disease during postremission therapy in acute myeloid leukemia with inversion(16): a pilot study. *J. Clin. Oncol.* **16,** 1519–1525.
2. Tobal, K. and Liu Yin, J. A. (1998) Molecular monitoring of minimal residual disease in acute myeloblastic leukemia with t(8;21) by RT-PCR. *Leuk. Lymphoma* **31,** 115–120.
3. Barragan, E., Bolufer, P., Moreno, I., et al. (2001) Quantitative detection of AML1-ETO rearrangement by real-time RT-PCR using fluorescently labeled probes. *Leuk. Lymphoma* **42,** 747–756.
4. Higuchi, R., Fockler, C., Dollinger, G., and Watson, R. (1993) Kinetic PCR analysis: real-time monitoring of DNA amplification reactions. *Biotechnology* **11,** 1026–1030.
5. Wittwer, C. T., Herrmann, M. G., Moss, A. A., and Rasmussen, R. P. (1997a) Continuous fluorescence monitoring of rapid cycle DNA amplification. *Biotechniques* **22,** 130–131, 134–138.

6. Vandesompele, J., De Paepe, A., and Speleman, F. (2002) Elimination of primer-dimer artifacts and genomic coamplification using a two-step SYBR green I real-time RT-PCR. *Anal. Biochem.* **303,** 95–98.

7. Ririe, K. M., Rasmussen, R. P., and Wittwer, C. T. (1997) Product differentiation by analysis of DNA melting curves during the polymerase chain reaction. *Anal. Biochem.* **245,** 154–160.

8. Nygren, J., Svanvik, N., and Kubista, M. (1998) The interactions between the fluorescent dye thiazole orange and DNA. *Biopolymers* **46,** 39–51.

9. Bengtsson, M., Karlsson, H. J., Westman, G., and Kubista, M. (2003) A new minor groove binding asymmetric cyanine reporter dye for real-time PCR. *Nucleic Acids Res.* **31,** e45.

10. Svanvik, N., Westman, G., Wang, D., and Kubista, M. (2000) Light-up probes: thiazole orange-conjugated peptide nucleic acid for detection of target nucleic acid in homogeneous solution. *Anal. Biochem.* **281,** 26–35.

11. Stahlberg, A., Aman, P., Ridell, B., Mostad, P., and Kubista, M. (2003) Quantitative real-time PCR method for detection of B-lymphocyte monoclonality by comparison of kappa and lambda immunoglobulin light chain expression. *Clin. Chem.* **49,** 51–59.

12. Nazarenko, I. A., Bhatnagar, S. K., and Hohman, R. J. (1997) A closed tube format for amplification and detection of DNA based on energy transfer. *Nucleic Acids Res.* **25,** 2516–2521.

13. Nazarenko, I., Pires, R., Lowe, B., Obaidy, M., and Rashtchian, A. (2002) Effect of primary and secondary structure of oligodeoxyribonucleotides on the fluorescent properties of conjugated dyes. *Nucleic Acids Res.* **30,** 2089–2195.

14. Applegate, T. L., Iland, H. J., Mokany, E., and Todd, A. V. (2002) Diagnosis and molecular monitoring of acute promyelocytic leukemia using DzyNA reverse transcription-PCR to quantify PML/RARalpha fusion transcripts. *Clin. Chem.* **48,** 1338–1343.

15. Holland, P. M., Abramson, R. D., Watson, R., and Gelfand, D. H. (1991) Detection of specific polymerase chain reaction product by utilizing the 5,Ä≤-3,Ä≤ exonuclease activity of *Thermus aquaticus* DNA polymerase. *Proc. Natl. Acad. Sci. USA* **88,** 7276–80.

16. Förster, V. (1948) Zwischenmolekular Energiewanderung und Fluoreszenz. *Ann. Phy.* **2,** 55–57.

17. Clegg, R. M., Murchie, A. I., Zechel, A., Carlberg, C., Diekmann, S., and Lilley, D. M. (1992) Fluorescence resonance energy transfer analysis of the structure of the four-way DNA junction. *Biochemistry* **31,** 4846–4856.

18. Lyamichev, V., Brow, M. A., and Dahlberg, J. E. (1993) Structure-specific endonucleolytic cleavage of nucleic acids by eubacterial DNA polymerases. *Science* **260,** 778–783.

19. de Kok, J. B., Wiegerinck, E. T., Giesendorf, B. A., and Swinkels, D. W. (2002) Rapid genotyping of single nucleotide polymorphisms using novel minor groove binding DNA oligonucleotides (MGB probes). *Hum. Mutat.* **19,** 554–559.

20. Latorra, D., Arar, K., and Hurley, J. M. (2003) Design considerations and effects of LNA in PCR primers. *Mol. Cell. Probes* **17,** 253–259.

21. Letertre, C., Perelle, S., Dilasser, F., Arar, K., and Fach, P.. (2003) Evaluation of the performance of LNA and MGB probes in 5'-nuclease PCR assays. *Mol. Cell. Probes* **17**, 307–311.

22. Wittwer, C. T., Ririe, K. M., Andrew, R. V., David, D. A., Gundry, R. A., and Balis, U. J. (1997b) The LightCycler: a microvolume multisample fluorimeter with rapid temperature control. *Biotechniques* **22**, 176–181.

23. Meuer, S. Wittwer, C., and Nakagawara, K. (eds) (2001) *Rapid Cycle Real-Time PCR: Methods and Applications.* Springer, Heidelberg.

24. Tyagi, S. and Kramer, F. R. (1996) Molecular beacons: probes that fluoresce upon hybridization. *Nat. Biotechnol.* **14**, 303–308.

25. Leone, G., van Schijndel, H., van Gemen, B., Kramer, F. R., and Schoen, C. D. (1998) Molecular beacon probes combined with amplification by NASBA enable homogeneous, real-time detection of RNA. *Nucleic Acids Res.* **26**, 2150–2155.

26. Whitcombe, D., Theaker, J., Guy, S. P., Brown, T., and Little, S. (1999) Detection of PCR products using self-probing amplicons and fluorescence. *Nat. Biotechnol.* **17**, 804–807.

27. Thelwell, N., Millington, S., Solinas, A., Booth, J., and Brown, T. (2000) Mode of action and application of Scorpion primers to mutation detection. *Nucleic Acids Res.* **28**, 3752–3761.

28. Solinas, A., Brown, L. J., McKeen, C., et al. (2001) Duplex Scorpion primers in SNP analysis and FRET applications. *Nucleic Acids Res.* **29**, E96.

28a. Silvy, M., Mancini, J., Thirion, X., Sigaux, F., and Gabert, J. (2005) Evaluation of real-time quantitative PCR machines for the monitoring of fusion gene transcripts using the Europe Against Cancer protocol. *Leukemia* **19**, 305–307.

29. Pattyn, F., Speleman, F., De Paepe, A., and Vandesompele, J. (2003) RTPrimerDB: the real-time PCR primer and probe database. *Nucleic Acids Res.* **31**, 122–123.

30. Gabert, J., Beillard, E., van der Velden, V. H., et al. (2003) Standardization and quality control studies of "real-time" quantitative reverse transcriptase polymerase chain reaction of fusion gene transcripts for residual disease detection in leukemia—a Europe Against Cancer program. *Leukemia* **17**, 2318–2357.

31. Beillard, E., Pallisgaard, N. van der Velden, V. H., et al. (2003) Evaluation of candidate control genes for diagnosis and residual disease detection in leukemic patients using "real-time" quantitative reverse-transcriptase polymerase chain reaction (RQ-PCR)—a Europe against cancer program. *Leukemia* **17**, 2474–2486.

32. Freeman, W. M., Walker, S. J., and Vrana, K. E. (1999) Quantitative RT-PCR: pitfalls and potential. *Biotechniques* **26**, 112–122, 124–125.

33. Keilholz, U., Willhauck, M., Rimoldi, D., et al. (1998) Reliability of reverse transcription-polymerase chain reaction (RT-PCR)-based assays for the detection of circulating tumour cells: a quality-assurance initiative of the EORTC Melanoma Cooperative Group. *Eur. J. Cancer* **34**, 750–753.

34. Bolufer, P., Lo Coco, F., Grimwade, D., et al. (2001) Variability in the levels of PML-RAR alpha fusion transcripts detected by the laboratories participating in an external quality control program using several reverse transcription polymerase chain reaction protocols. *Haematologica* **86**, 570–576.

35. Saldanha, J. (2001) Validation and standardisation of nucleic acid amplification technology (NAT) assays for the detection of viral contamination of blood and blood products. *J. Clin. Virol.* **20,** 7–13.
36. Saldanha, J., Lelie, N., Yu, M. W., and Heath, A. (2002) Establishment of the first World Health Organization International Standard for human parvovirus B19 DNA nucleic acid amplification techniques. *Vox Sang.* **82,** 24–31.
37. Saldanha, J. and Heath, A. (2003) Collaborative study to calibrate hepatitis C virus genotypes 2–6 against the HCV International Standard, 96/790 (genotype 1). *Vox Sang.* **84,** 20–27.
38. Köhler, T., Schill, C., Deininger, M. W., et al. (2002) High Bad and Bax mRNA expression correlate with negative outcome in acute myeloid leukemia (AML). *Leukemia* **16,** 22–29.
39. Dobbs, L. J., Madigan, M. N., Carter, A. B., and Earls, L. (2002) Use of FTA gene guard filter paper for the storage and transportation of tumor cells for molecular testing. *Arch. Pathol. Lab. Med.* **126,** 56–63.
40. Kline, M. C., Duewer, D. L., Redman, J. W., Butler, J. M., and Boyer, D. A. (2002) Polymerase chain reaction amplification of DNA from aged blood stains: quantitative evaluation of the "suitability for purpose" of four filter papers as archival media. *Anal. Chem.* **74,** 1863–1869.
41. Vandesompele, J., De Preter, K., Pattyn, F., et al. (2003) Accurate normalization of real-time quantitative RT-PCR data by geometric averaging of multiple internal control genes. *Genome Biol.* **3,** RESEARCH0034.
42. Pfaffl, M. W. (2001) A new mathematical model for relative quantification in real-time RT-PCR. *Nucleic Acids Res.* **29,** e45.
43. Liu, W. and Saint, D. A. (2002) A new quantitative method of real time reverse transcription polymerase chain reaction assay based on simulation of polymerase chain reaction kinetics. *Anal. Biochem.* **302,** 52–59.
44. Ramakers, C., Ruijter, J. M., Deprez, R. H., and Moorman, A. F. (2003) Assumption-free analysis of quantitative real-time polymerase chain reaction (PCR) data. *Neurosci. Lett.* **339,** 62–66.
45. Tichopad, A., Dilger, M., Schwarz, G., and Pfaffl, M. W. (2003) Standardized determination of real-time PCR efficiency from a single reaction set-up. *Nucleic Acids Res.* **31,** e122.
46. Gerard, C. J., Olsson, K., Ramanathan, R., Reading, C., and Hanania, E. G. (1998) Improved quantitation of minimal residual disease in multiple myeloma using real-time polymerase chain reaction and plasmid-DNA complementarity determining region III standards. *Cancer Res.* **58,** 3957–3964.
47. Silvy, M., Pic, G, Gabert, J., and Picard, C. (2004) Improvement of gene expression analysis by RQ-PCR technology: addition of BSA. *Leukemia* **18,** 1022–1025.
48. Quina, A. S., Gameiro, P., Sa da Costa, M., Telhada, M., and Parreira, L. (2000) PML-RARA fusion transcripts in irradiated and normal hematopoietic cells. *Genes Chromosomes Cancer* **29,** 266–275.
49. Lossos, I. S, Czerwinski, D. K., Alizadeh, A. A., et al. (2004) Prediction of survival in diffuse large-B-cell lymphoma based on the expression of six genes. *N. Engl. J. Med.* **350,** 1828–1837.

50. Marcucci, G., Livak, K. J., Bi, W., Strout, M. P., Bloomfield, C. D., and Caligiuri, M. A. (1998) Detection of minimal residual disease in patients with AML1/ETO-associated acute myeloid leukemia using a novel quantitative reverse transcription polymerase chain reaction assay. *Leukemia* **12**, 1482–1489.

51. Cassinat, B., Zassadowski, F., Balitrand, N., et al. (2000) Quantitation of minimal residual disease in acute promyelocytic leukemia patients with t(15;17) translocation using real-time RT-PCR. *Leukemia* **14**, 324–328.

52. Fujimaki, S., Funato, T., Harigae, H., et al. (2000) A quantitative reverse transcriptase polymerase chain reaction method for the detection of leukaemic cells with t(8;21) in peripheral blood. *Eur. J. Haematol.* **64**, 252–258.

53. Sugimoto, T., Das, H., Imoto, S., et al. (2000) Quantitation of minimal residual disease in t(8;21)-positive acute myelogenous leukemia patients using real-time quantitative RT-PCR. *Am. J. Hematol.* **64**, 101–106.

54. Krauter, J., Hoellge, W., Wattjes, M. P., et al. (2001) Detection and quantification of CBFB/MYH11 fusion transcripts in patients with inv(16)-positive acute myeloblastic leukemia by real-time RT-PCR. *Genes Chromosomes Cancer* **30**, 342–348.

55. Kwong, Y. L., Au, W. Y., Chim, C. S., Pang, A., Suen, C., and Liang, R. (2001) Arsenic trioxide- and idarubicin-induced remissions in relapsed acute promyelocytic leukaemia: clinicopathological and molecular features of a pilot study. *Am. J. Hematol.* **66**, 274–279.

56. Marcucci, G., Caligiuri, M. A., Dohner, H., et al. (2001) Quantification of CBFbeta/MYH11 fusion transcript by real time RT-PCR in patients with INV(16) acute myeloid leukemia. *Leukemia* **15**, 1072–1080.

57. Slack, J. L., Bi, W., Livak, K. J., et al. (2001) Pre-clinical validation of a novel, highly sensitive assay to detect PML-RARalpha mRNA using real-time reverse-transcription polymerase chain reaction. *J. Mol. Diagn.* **3**, 141–149.

58. Visani, G., Buonamici, S., Malagola, M., et al. (2001) Pulsed ATRA as single therapy restores long-term remission in PML-RARalpha-positive acute promyelocytic leukemia patients: real time quantification of minimal residual disease. A pilot study. *Leukemia* **15**, 1696–1700.

59. Buonamici, S., Ottaviani, E., Testoni, N., et al. (2002) Real-time quantitation of minimal residual disease in inv(16)-positive acute myeloid leukemia may indicate risk for clinical relapse and may identify patients in a curable state. *Blood* **99**, 443–449.

60. Cilloni, D., Gottardi, E., De Micheli, D., et al. (2002) Quantitative assessment of WT1 expression by real time quantitative PCR may be a useful tool for monitoring minimal residual disease in acute leukemia patients. *Leukemia* **16**, 2115–2121.

61. Guerrasio, A., Pilatrino, C., De Micheli, D., et al. (2002) Assessment of minimal residual disease (MRD) in CBFbeta/MYH11-positive acute myeloid leukemias by qualitative and quantitative RT-PCR amplification of fusion transcripts. *Leukemia* **16**, 1176–1181.

62. Gallagher, R. E., Yeap, B. Y., Bi, W., et al. (2003) Quantitative real-time RT-PCR analysis of PML-RAR alpha mRNA in acute promyelocytic leukemia: assessment of prognostic significance in adult patients from intergroup protocol 0129. *Blood* **101**, 2521–2528.

63. Martinelli, G., Buonamici, S., Visani, G., et al. (2003) Molecular monitoring of acute myeloid leukemia associated with inv(16): threshold of CBFbeta/MYH11 transcript copy number above which relapse occurs and below which continuous complete remission is likely. *Leukemia* **17,** 650–651.
64. Scholl, C., Breitinger, H., Schlenk, R. F., Dohner, H., Frohling, S., and Dohner, K. (2003) AML Study Group Ulm. Development of a real-time RT-PCR assay for the quantification of the most frequent MLL/AF9 fusion types resulting from translocation t(9;11)(p22;q23) in acute myeloid leukemia. *Genes Chromosomes Cancer* **38,** 274–280.
65. Viehmann, S., Teigler-Schlegel, A., Bruch, J., Langebrake, C., Reinhardt, D., and Harbott, J. (2003) Monitoring of minimal residual disease (MRD) by real-time quantitative reverse transcription PCR (RQ-RT-PCR) in childhood acute myeloid leukemia with AML1/ETO rearrangement. *Leukemia* **17,** 1130–1136.
66. Satake, N., Maseki, N., Kozu, T., et al. (1995) Disappearance of AML1-MTG8(ETO) fusion transcript in acute myeloid leukaemia patients with t(8;21) in long-term remission. *Br. J. Haematol.* **91,** 892–898.

4

Diagnosis and Monitoring of Chronic Myeloid Leukemia by Qualitative and Quantitative RT-PCR

Susan Branford and Timothy Hughes

Summary

Real-time quantitative reverse-transcription polymerase chain reaction (RQ-PCR) methods for the quantitation of *BCR-ABL* mRNA in the blood of patients with chronic myeloid leukemia (CML) has become the predominant molecular monitoring technique. The *BCR-ABL* fusion gene is expressed in over 95% of patients with CML, and RQ-PCR provides a reliable, high-throughput method to accurately assess the level of treatment response and provides an early indication of emerging drug resistance. The ABI Prism 7700 Sequence Detection System uses TaqMan® fluorogenic probes to quantitate specific nucleic acid sequences using RQ-PCR. The analyzer monitors an increase in fluorescence during the PCR cycle, which is proportional to the amount of accumulated product. The starting copy number is calculated relative to a series of standards. The copy number is normalized to a control gene that compensates for variations in the efficiency of the RT step and for the degree of RNA degradation. In our experience, reliable and consistent RQ-PCR requires thorough validation of all aspects of the procedure, including the selection of an appropriate control gene, careful assay design to avoid polymorphisms in primer or probe binding sites and to exclude the amplification of contaminating DNA, and monitoring the performance of the RQ-PCR by the use of quality control samples.

Key Words: Chronic myeloid leukemia; *BCR-ABL*; real-time quantitative PCR; TaqMan; imatinib mesylate; quality control; atypical; fluorescent probes.

1. Introduction

Chronic myeloid leukemia (CML) is a clonal myeloproliferative disorder of the hemopoietic stem cell, which is characterized by the Philadelphia chromosome translocation (t(9;22)) in approx 95% of patients. The translocation produces the *BCR-ABL* gene by juxtaposing part of the *ABL* proto-oncogene to the 5′ portion of the *BCR* gene. The Bcr-Abl protein is an activated tyrosine kinase that is causally associated with CML *(1,2)*. The level of *BCR-ABL* transcript is a sensitive indicator of the leukemic cell mass. The only chance of cure for

From: *Methods in Molecular Medicine, Vol. 125: Myeloid Leukemia: Methods and Protocols*
Edited by: H. Iland, M. Hertzberg, and P. Marlton © Humana Press Inc., Totowa, NJ

selected patients is an allogeneic transplant; however, the recent introduction of the highly successful Bcr-Abl kinase inhibitor imatinib mesylate (Glivec, Novartis Pharmaceuticals, Basel, Switzerland) has substantially improved treatment response. In patients with a complete cytogenetic remission, residual leukemic cells expressing *BCR-ABL* mRNA are usually detectable by the polymerase chain reaction (PCR) technique. Qualitative PCR provides limited information of treatment response, whereas serial monitoring of *BCR-ABL* levels by real-time quantitative reverse transcription (RT) PCR (RQ-PCR) can identify patients in need of therapeutic intervention before the onset of overt relapse.

The reliability of RQ-PCR techniques is very dependent on careful experimental design and appropriate validation of all aspects of the procedure (reviewed in **refs. 3,4**). The technique is based on the generation of a fluorescent signal coupled with instrumentation for the amplification, detection, and quantification of gene expression. There are now a number of probe systems and instruments for RQ-PCR (reviewed in **ref. 5**). The method described here uses TaqMan® fluorescence hybridization probes on the 7700 Sequence Detection System (Applied Biosystems, Foster City, CA). The probe consists of an oligonucleotide with both a fluorescent reporter and a quencher dye attached. When the probe is intact, the proximity of the reporter dye to the quencher dye results in suppression of the reporter fluorescence, primarily by fluorescence resonance energy transfer (FRET). The probe is cleaved by the 5′ to 3′ nuclease activity of AmpliTaq DNA polymerase during the extension phase of the PCR cycle, which results in an increase of reporter fluorescence signal. The increase in fluorescence is proportional to the amount of accumulated product, and the SDS software is used to determine the starting copy number relative to a series of standards (**Fig. 1**). A control gene is quantitated to control for variation in the efficiency of the RT step and for variation in the degree of degradation of the RNA. The quantitative results of the target gene are reported relative to the control gene, which is the normal *BCR* gene in our assay. The assay performance is monitored by quality control samples that are performed with every RQ-PCR assay.

RQ-PCR for monitoring the level of *BCR-ABL* transcripts is sensitive and reliable, and enables a high-throughput analysis (*6–9*). Rising levels of *BCR-ABL* are strongly predictive of cytogenetic and hematological relapse after an allogeneic transplant (*10–12*). Monitoring imatinib-treated CML patients by quantitative RT-PCR has proven effective for defining patient response. Early reduction of *BCR-ABL* can predict a subsequent cytogenetic response (*13–16*). The level of *BCR-ABL* predicts for disease-free survival (*17,18*) and clinical outcome (*15,19*), while the proportional reduction in *BCR-ABL* is closely correlated with the level of cytogenetic response (*19*).

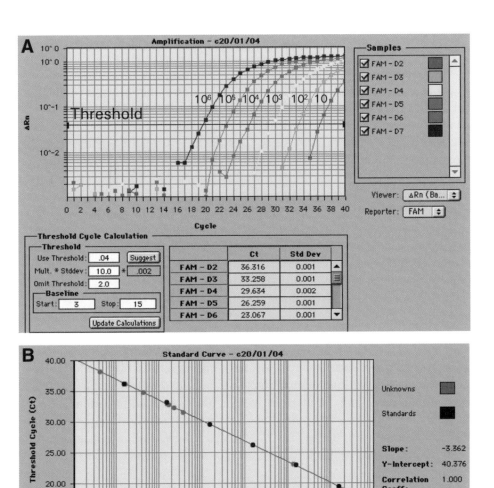

Fig. 1. Amplification plot and standard curve generated by real-time quantitative reverse-transcription polymerase chain reaction of *BCR-ABL*. Ten-fold serial dilutions of plasmids for each gene are analyzed in every real-time quantitative reverse-transcription polymerase chain reaction (RQ-PCR) analysis to generate a standard curve for quantitative analysis. (**A**) PCR amplification plots of the 10-fold serial dilutions of the b3a2 *BCR-ABL* standard with known starting copy number of approx 10^6 to 10 copies. The accumulation of fluorescence occurs at each cycle. The 7700 software calculates the fractional cycle number (cycle threshold [Ct]) where the amplification plot crosses a defined fluorescence threshold. The Ct values are used to generate a standard curve (**B**). The correlation coefficient should be between 0.997 and 1.0, and the slope value for the plasmid standards lies between –3.3 and –3.59. The Ct values of the unknown samples are calculated from the standard curve.

The majority of CML patients have breakpoints that result in a fusion mRNA in which either *BCR* exon 13 (known as b2 for its location within the major breakpoint cluster region of the *BCR* gene) or exon 14 (b3) is fused to *ABL* exon a2 to form the b2a2 and b3a2 transcripts. The resultant fusion protein encoded by *BCR-ABL* is 210 kd (p210). However, a small number of patients have breakpoints outside of the standard region and various *BCR* exons may be fused to either *ABL* exon 2 or 3 (reviewed in **ref. 20**). The resultant atypical fusion proteins vary in size but maintain an activated tyrosine kinase. Rare cases of CML involve the e1a2 transcript, which is more commonly seen in patients with acute lymphoblastic leukemia, and the e19a2 transcript, which may be associated with chronic neutrophilic leukemia *(21,22)*. Aberrant fusion transcripts have been described that involve the insertion of intronic sequences *(23–25)* and breakpoints within coding regions *(26)*. When using a quantitative PCR technique to monitor treatment response in CML it is necessary to charac-terize the *BCR-ABL* breakpoint to exclude false-negative results. Our RQ-PCR technique evaluates the b2a2 and b3a2 transcripts only. Therefore, an investi-gation for an atypical transcript is undertaken by a qualitative PCR technique if a newly diagnosed patient with CML has a negative *BCR-ABL* value by RQ-PCR. The PCR technique uses primers that span *BCR* exon 1 and *ABL* exon 3. Amplification products of atypical lengths are sequenced to characterise the *BCR-ABL* breakpoint. This procedure is particularly relevant for patients with Philadelphia chromosome-negative CML. In these cases the presence of a *BCR-ABL* transcript must be demonstrated in order for the patient to receive imatinib therapy.

2. Materials

2.1. RNA Extraction

1. Lysis buffer: 0.144 M NH$_4$Cl and 0.01 M NH$_4$HCO$_3$. Autoclave and store at room temperature. Stable for 6 mo. The lysis buffer is prepared from stock solutions of 1.44 M NH$_4$Cl (autoclave) and 1.0 M NH$_4$HCO$_3$ (avoid inhaling fumes during preparation and do not autoclave because the fumes are overpowering if auto-claved). Stable for 12 mo at room temperature.
2. Sterile 50-mL tubes (Becton Dickinson).
3. Sterile mixing cannula.
4. RNAse- and DNAse-free 1.5-mL and 2.0-mL microcentrifuge tubes (Quantum Scientific).
5. 18-gauge blunt needles (Becton Dickinson) and 3-mL syringes.
6. Barrier or filter pipet tips.
7. Trizol RNA isolation solution (Invitrogen). Store at 2–8°C. Trizol is used in a laminar-flow hood. Use gloves and eye protection. If skin contact occurs, apply glycerol to the site immediately.

8. RNAse- and DNAse-free water. Deionized water treated with 0.001% diethylpyrocarbonate (DEPC) filtered through a 0.2-μm filter and autoclaved (ICN Biochemicals). Aliquot into 250-μL lots in 1.5-mL RNAse- and DNAse-free microcentrifuge tubes. Store at room temperature. DEPC is a suspected carcinogen and should be treated with care.
9. Chloroform. Use a fresh 10-mL aliquot for each batch of extractions. Use in the fume hood.
10. Isopropanol. Use a fresh 10-mL aliquot for each batch of extractions. Store at –20°C until required.
11. 30 mL of 75% ethanol solution, prepared in DEPC water on the day of the extraction run.
12. PCR cabinet with ultraviolet (UV) light.

2.2. cDNA Synthesis

1. Sterile 0.2-mL capped PCR tubes (Interpath Services).
2. 500-μL single-use lots of autoclaved MiliQ water. Store at room temperature in 1.5-mL microcentrifuge tubes.
3. 250 μM stock solution of Random Hexamers (Geneworks). Supplied as a 100-μg lyophilized triethylammonium salt, which is dissolved by the addition of 200 μL DEPC-treated water. Store in 100-μL lots at –20°C.
4. SuperScript II RNase H⁻ Reverse Transcriptase (Invitrogen). Supplied with 0.1 M dithiothreitol (DTT) and 5X First Strand Buffer. Store at –20°C.
5. 10 mM stock of deoxynucleotide triphosphates (dNTPs) (Amersham Biosciences). Store at –20°C in 100-μL lots.
6. Thermal cycler (Bio-Rad).

2.3. Plasmid Standards

1. Primer Express software (Applied Biosystems).
2. PCR primers. All primers are ordered as a 50 μM solution and stored in 30-μL lots at –20°C.
3. 1.5-mL screw-top caps with O-ring.
4. 25 mM MgCl₂ (Applied Biosystems). Store at –20°C.
5. 10X PCR buffer (Applied Biosystems). Store at –20°C.
6. AmpliTaq Gold (Applied Biosystems). Store at –20°C.
7. 10 mM stock of dNTPs (Amersham Biosciences). Store at –20°C in 100-μL lots.
8. Agarose, molecular biology grade (Progen). Store at room temperature.
9. Gel loading buffer: 50 mg bromophenol blue, 50 mg xylene cyanol, and 30 mL glycerol made up to 100 mL with sterile water.
10. Puc*19*/Hpa*1* DNA molecular-weight marker (Geneworks). Store at –20°C.
11. UltraClean PCR Clean-up DNA purification kit (Mo Bio Laboratories). Store at room temperature.
12. pGEM-T Easy Vector System II (Promega). Includes JM109 Competent Cells. Store at –20°C.
13. LB medium: 1% w/v bacto-tryptone, 0.5% w/v yeast extract, and 1% w/v NaCl.

14. Ampicillin: 25 mg/mL in sterile water. Filter sterilize through a 0.22-μm filter.
15. LB-ampicillin agar plates: Add 4 g of bacto-agar to 200 mL Luria-Bertani (LB) medium, autoclave, and cool to 55°C. Add 0.3 mL of ampicillin and pour into Petri dishes. Store the plates at 4°C after allowing to set.
16. 0.1 M isopropyl-β-thio-galactoside (IPTG). Filter sterilize through a 0.22-μm filter.
17. 50 mg/mL X-gal (Promega).
18. Plasmid midi kit (Qiagen). Store at room temperature.
19. Sca1 restriction enzyme (New England Biolabs).
20. Plasmid diluent: 1 mM Tris-HCl (pH 8.0), 0.1 mM ethylenediamine tetraacetic acid (EDTA), and 50 μg/mL salmon sperm DNA. Store at 4°C.

2.4. Quality Control Samples

1. Trizol RNA isolation solution (Invitrogen).
2. RNAse- and DNAse-free 2.0-mL microcentrifuge tubes (Quantum Scientific).
3. BCR-ABL-positive cell lines.
4. BCR-ABL-negative cell line.
5. Tissue-culture media and reagents—RPMI-1640, Dulbecco's modified Eagle's medium (DMEM), phosphate-buffered saline, trypsin, L-glutamine, penicillin/streptomycin, fetal calf serum (CSL).
6. Tissue-culture flasks (Cellstar).

2.5. Real-Time Quantitative RT-PCR

1. Primer Express software (Applied Biosystems).
2. TaqMan fluorescent hybridization probes (Applied Biosystems). Probes are prepared with a 5' FAM reporter dye and a 3' 6-carboxytetramethylrhodamine (TAMRA) quencher dye. Reconstitute the lyophilized material in the appropriate amount of sterile water to give a concentration of 10 μM. The probe is supplied with a pmol concentration; therefore, divide the pmol value by 10 to calculate the volume to add to the probe. Store in 30-μL lots at –20°C. Do not freeze and thaw more than five times.
3. PCR primers. All primers are ordered as a 50 μM solution and stored in 30-μL lots at –20°C.
4. TaqMan Universal PCR Master Mix (Applied Biosystems).
5. MicroAmp Optical 96-well Reaction Plate (Applied Biosystems).
6. MicroAmp Optical Cap (Applied Biosystems).
7. ABI Prism 7700 Sequence Detection System (Applied Biosystems).
8. ABI Prism SDS software (Applied Biosystems).
9. QC Reporter 2.0 software program (Chiron Healthcare).

2.6. Qualitative PCR for Atypical BCR-ABL Transcripts

1. PCR primers. All primers are ordered as a 50 μM solution and stored in 30-μL lots at –20°C.
2. 10 mM stock of dNTPs (Amersham Biosciences). Store at –20°C in 100-μL lots.
3. 25 mM MgCl$_2$ (Applied Biosystems). Store at –20°C.

4. Expand Long Template PCR System (Roche). Store at –20°C.
5. Agarose, molecular-biology grade (Progen). Store at room temperature.
6. SPP1/*Eco*R1 DNA molecular-weight marker (Geneworks). Store at –20°C.

2.7. Qualitative PCR for p210 BCR-ABL

1. Primer Express software (Applied Biosystems).
2. PCR primers. All primers are ordered as a 50 μ*M* solution and stored in 30-μL lots at –20°C.
3. 10 m*M* stock of dNTPs (Amersham Biosciences). Store at –20°C in 100-μL lots.
4. 25 m*M* MgCl$_2$ (Applied Biosystems). Store at –20°C.
5. 10X PCR buffer (Applied Biosystems). Store at –20°C.
6. AmpliTaq Gold (Applied Biosystems). Store at –20°C.
7. Agarose, molecular-biology grade (Progen). Store at room temperature.
8. Puc*19*/Hpa*II* DNA molecular-weight marker (Geneworks). Store at –20°C.

3. Methods
3.1. RNA Extraction

1. Isolate the white cells from 10 to 20 mL of peripheral blood. Pour the whole blood into a 50-mL tube. Aliquot 70 mL of lysis buffer into a clean UV-irradiated beaker (use a clean beaker for every patient). Pour lysis buffer into the 50-mL tube from the beaker to a volume of 50 mL and mix or stand for 10 min. Centrifuge for 10 min at 2000*g* to pellet the white cells.
2. Carefully remove the supernatant by using a waste vacuum system and a sterile mixing cannula, without disturbing the white cell pellet. Remove as much of the lysed cells as possible without disturbing the white cell pellet. If processing more than one patient sample, rinse the vacuum waste system inlet with water and replace the cannula for each sample. Add 20 mL lysis buffer and resuspend the white cells with a sterile transfer pipet. Mix or stand for 5 min and repeat the centrifugation. Remove the supernatant, leaving the white cell pellet.
3. As a general rule for white cells derived from 20 mL of blood, 3.2 mL of Trizol reagent is sufficient to stabilize the RNA. For patients at diagnosis or at relapse, large white cell pellets may require either reduction of the pellet or addition of extra Trizol. The extra Trizol reagent must be sufficient to completely dissolve the white cells. We have successfully adopted these guidelines to determine the amount of Trizol rather than basing the volume on the white cell concentration, which is not practical to measure in our laboratory. Add the appropriate amount of Trizol to the 50-mL tube and draw the solution up and down six times into a blunt 18-gauge needle attached to a 3-mL syringe (a blunt needle avoids the risk of needle-stick injury). This will lyse the white cells and shear the DNA, which reduces the risk of DNA contamination during the RNA extraction procedure. If white cells are still present after mixing, add extra Trizol and mix until the white cells are lysed. If the Trizol mixture is extremely viscous, add extra Trizol until the viscosity is reduced.

4. Transfer 1.6 mL of the Trizol homogenate into RNAse/DNAse-free 2-mL tubes labeled with the appropriate patient identification. The homogenate may be stored at –80°C before continuation of the RNA extraction procedure.

5. We extract the RNA from up to 20 frozen Trizol homogenates in one batch. Every effort is made to prevent sample contamination or carry-over during this procedure. Fresh protective bench paper is applied to all work areas, and pipets and racks are UV irradiated before use. Barrier tips are used and replaced at each step, and the procedure is performed in a laminar fume hood.

6. Thaw the homogenates at room temperature or place in a 37°C heating block for 5 min to permit the complete dissociation of nucleoprotein complexes.

7. The extraction procedure is performed essentially according to the manufacturer's instructions, with the exception that an increased volume of chloroform is added to allow better separation of the phase layers.

8. Add 350 µL of chloroform to the Trizol homogenate and shake vigorously for 15 s (do not vortex). Place on ice for 3 min.

9. Centrifuge at $12,000g$ for 15 min. This procedure separates the phases. The RNA is located in the upper phase and should be clear and distinctly separated from the interphase, which contains DNA and protein. If the upper phase is not clear, additional chloroform may be added and the centrifugation repeated.

10. Transfer approx 350 µL of the upper phase to an RNAse/DNAse-free 1.5-mL tube. To avoid DNA contamination, do not disturb the interphase. If the interphase is drawn into the pipet tip, repeat the centrifugation step.

11. Add 350 µL of cold isopropanol. Invert the tubes and check for DNA contamination, which may be visible as white strands. Remove with a pipet tip if present. Incubate on ice for 10 min. If necessary, the tubes can be stored refrigerated overnight. Centrifuge at $12,000g$ for 10 min. Remove the supernatant.

12. Wash the RNA pellet with 1 mL of 75% ethanol. Vortex for 10 s and centrifuge at $7500g$ for 5 min. Discard the supernatant. Pellets can be stored at –80°C for future use. In that case, add 1 mL of 75% ethanol for storage.

13. Centrifuge the tubes again briefly and remove the final traces of ethanol.

14. Air dry the pellet for 10–20 min in the PCR cabinet. Do not over-dry the pellet, as it will be hard to dissolve.

15. Add 40 µL of DEPC water and allow to dissolve for 15 min at 55°C. The volume of water may be reduced for very small RNA pellets.

16. The concentration of RNA is determined by assessing the absorbance at 260 nm and 280 nm. RNA is stored at –80°C.

3.2. cDNA Synthesis

cDNA synthesis is performed using the SuperScript II method according to the manufacturer's procedure. A batch of 24 samples is prepared, which includes two positive and two negative controls. RNA is added in a PCR cabinet, which is located in a separate laboratory from the PCR set-up area. PCR cycling is performed in a separate laboratory from the RNA preparation and the PCR set-up laboratories. The reverse transcription procedure is performed in duplicate for each patient RNA.

1. To a sterile 0.2-mL tube add 2 μL of random hexamers (25 μ*M* final concentration) and a volume of DEPC water to give a total volume of 2 μg of RNA in 9 μL of DEPC water.
2. In the PCR cabinet, add 2 μg of RNA and mix by drawing repeatedly into the pipet tip. Transfer the tubes to the thermal cycler and heat the mixture to 70°C for 10 min. Quick-chill on ice and return the tubes to the PCR cabinet.
3. Prepare a master mix of the SuperScript II reagent components. For each sample, add 4 μL of 5X First Strand Buffer, 2 μL of 0.1 *M* DTT, and 1 μL dNTP mix (10 m*M* each).
4. Add 7 μL of the master mix to each sample and mix by drawing into the pipet tip. Briefly centrifuge the tubes at 12,000*g* to collect the reactants in the bottom of the tube.
5. Transfer the tubes to the thermal cycler and incubate at 42°C for 2 min. Pause the reaction and return the tubes to the PCR cabinet.
6. Remove the SuperScript II from the freezer. Mix and centrifuge briefly at 12,000*g* to collect the solution at the bottom of the tube. Place the SuperScript II on ice.
7. Add 2 μL of SuperScript II to each tube in the PCR cabinet. Mix well by drawing into the pipet tip. Briefly centrifuge the tubes at 12,000*g* and transfer the samples into the thermal cycler.
8. Continue the reaction at 25°C for 10 min, 42°C for 50 min, 70°C for 15 min, and hold at 4°C.
9. After completion of the reaction, the samples may be stored at –20°C until required.

3.3. Plasmid Standards

Plasmids containing a cDNA fragment of the genes under analysis are prepared by PCR cloning. The plasmids are used to construct standard curves for quantitation of each of the target and control genes. In our quantitative PCR assay, we prepared plasmids for the quantitation of the b2a2 *BCR-ABL* transcript and the *BCR* control gene from a cell line expressing the b2a2 *BCR-ABL* transcript (KCL22). A plasmid for the quantitation of the b3a2 *BCR-ABL* transcript was prepared by N. Cross *(27)*. This plasmid contains a modified b3a2 *BCR-ABL* transcript derived from the K562 cell line. Approx 200 bases are removed from *ABL* exons 2 and 3, and 100 bases of a different sequence ligated in that region. The plasmid contains an intact sequence in the region of the sequence used for quantitation of the b3a2 transcript in our assay. However, a standard for the b3a2 *BCR-ABL* transcript can be prepared if required by following the same procedure as for the b2a2 *BCR-ABL* transcript and using a b3a2 *BCR-ABL* expressing cell line.

3.3.1. PCR

1. Using the Primer Express software, primers were designed to amplify a region flanking the primers that are used in the quantitative assay. These primers produce a PCR fragment that is larger than that used for the quantitative assays and includes the same sequence.
   Primers for the *BCR* standard:
   Forward primer: 5′ tca cca aga gag aga ggt cca a
   Reverse primer: 5′ gtc tga aag agc gat gcc ct
   Primers for the b2a2 standard:
   Forward primer: 5′ aga agc ttc tcc ctg aca tc
   Reverse primer: 5′ aga tgc tac tgg ccg ctg aa
2. Extract RNA from the b2a2 expressing cell line and prepare cDNA using the procedures outlined under **Subheadings 3.1.** and **3.2.**
3. Add 2.5 µL of cDNA to a 0.2-mL tube containing 2.5 µL of 10X PCR buffer, 5 µL of 25 m*M* MgCl$_2$, 0.5 µL of 10 m*M* dNTP mix, 0.1 µL of 50 µ*M* forward and reverse primers, and 0.5 µL of 5 U/µL of AmpliTaq gold. Add sterile water to 25 µL.
4. Transfer the reactions to the thermal cycler and amplify with the following conditions:
   a. 1 cycle at 95°C for 12 min.
   b. 30 cycles at 95°C for 30 s, 60°C for 30 s, 72°C for 30 s.
   c. 1 cycle at 72°C for 7 min.
5. Assess the size of each amplification product by electrophoresis of 5 µL mixed with 1 µL gel loading buffer on a 2.0% agarose gel using the *Puc*19 size marker. The b2a2 fragment is 127 bp and the *BCR* fragment is 293 bp.

3.3.2. Cloning

1. Purify the remaining PCR product using the UltraClean PCR Clean-up DNA purification kit according to the manufacturer's instructions.
2. 100 ng of the purified PCR product is cloned using the pGEM-T Easy Vector System II kit according to the manufacturer's instructions.
3. Prepare the plasmid DNA using the Qiagen Plasmid midi kit according to the manufacturer's instructions.
4. The presence of the cloned insert is determined by PCR amplification as under **Subheading 3.3.1.**, followed by sequencing to confirm the correct sequence.
5. Linearize the plasmid by digestion with *Sca*1 restriction enzyme.
6. Determine the concentration of the plasmid DNA by assessing absorbance at 260 nm and 280 nm. The copy number of the plasmid is calculated from the concentration and size of the plasmid (vector size + insert size [bp]), and using Avogadro's number of 6.02336×10^{23} molecules in 1 mole of template (6.02336×10^{14} molecules in 1 nmole). Using the b2a2 plasmid as an example:
   a. Calculate the molecular weight of the plasmid by multiplying the size by 660 (average molecular weight of double stranded DNA) = $3129 \times 660 = 2,065,140$.
   b. Therefore, 1 mole of template = 2,065,140 g and 1 m mole of template = 2,065,140 ng.

    c. Determine the nmole concentration of the plasmid in 1 ng using the formula 1/molecular weight of the plasmid (ng) = 4.84228×10^{-7} nmoles.

    d. 1 ng = $4.84228 \times 10^{-7} \times 6.02336 \times 10^{14}$ molecules = 2.917×10^{8} molecules.

    e. We use 2.5 μL of plasmid in the quantitative PCR; therefore, 2.5 μL of plasmid = 2.5×59 (59 = plasmid concentration ng/μL) $\times 2.917 \times 10^{8} = 4.3 \times 10^{10}$ molecules.

3.3.3. Preparation of Plasmid Dilutions

A 10-fold dilution series in the range of approx 10^{6} to 10 copies is prepared for the *BCR-ABL* standards and in the range of approx 10^{6} to 10^{3} copies for the *BCR* standards. All plasmids and dilutions are prepared in separate areas from the patient samples to avoid the possibility of contamination (*see* **Note 1**). All pipets are calibrated every 3 mo to optimize the accuracy of the volume dispensed.

1. Allow the standard diluent to equilibrate to room temperature.
2. A preliminary dilution of the plasmids in the standard diluent may be performed to give a solution of approx 1×10^{10} molecules per 2.5 μL.
3. Ten-fold serial dilutions in the desired range are prepared in 1800 μL of standard diluent. Mix each solution well before proceeding with the next dilution. Each dilution series is analyzed by the quantitative PCR method as outlined under **Subheading 3.6.** to ensure the standard curve is valid. Run each standard in triplicate for the curve validation. The correlation coefficient of the standard curve should be between 0.997 and 1.0 and the slope between −3.3 and −3.59. The dilution series will need to be re-diluted if the correlation coefficient and slope are outside the limits.
4. After validation of the standard curve, the dilutions in the desired range are aliquoted into 100-μL lots in 1.5-mL screw-top tubes with O-ring and stored at −80°C. One tube of each dilution is further aliquoted into 14-μL lots. One of each of these tubes is stored at −20°C and is used five times. This limits the number of times each standard is thawed and frozen. The remainder of the plasmid and high-copy-number dilutions are stored at −80°C and can be used for the preparation of further dilutions when required.

3.4. Quality Control Samples

Quality control samples are analyzed in every RQ-PCR run to monitor assay performance. Low and high levels of the control are prepared by diluting two *BCR-ABL*-positive cell lines and one -negative cell line that were grown using standard tissue-culture techniques. In our laboratory, we use the K562 cell line, containing the b3a2 *BCR-ABL* transcript, and the Molm-1 cell line, containing the b2a2 *BCR-ABL* transcript. We selected the HeLa cell line as a negative control because the expression level of the *BCR* control gene in this cell line was at a similar level to that found in peripheral blood. By mixing each of the cell lines together, only two controls are required to monitor both the b2a2 and b3a2 assays.

1. Using standard tissue-culture techniques, the cells are grown until there are enough cells to provide an adequate supply of control material to last several years.
2. The low control is prepared by diluting the cells at a ratio of: 5×10^2 K562 cells : 5×10^2 Molm-1 cells : 5×10^6 Hela cells.
3. The high control is prepared by diluting the cells at a ratio of: 4×10^5 K562 cells : 6×10^5 Molm-1 cells : 4×10^6 Hela cells.
4. The diluted cell mixture is centrifuged at 2000g to pellet the cells, which are then washed twice in phosphate-buffered saline.
5. Dissolve the pellet in an adequate volume of Trizol solution to give approx 5×10^6 cells in 1.6 mL. Draw the solution through an 18-gauge blunt needle repeatedly to shear the DNA.
6. Add 1.6 mL of the solution to 2-mL tubes and store at –80°C.
7. The Hela cells are also used as a negative control. Aliquots of 2×10^6 Hela cells are stored at –80°C in 1.6 mL of Trizol.
8. As required, a tube of each control is removed from the freezer and the RNA is extracted as outlined under **Subheading 3.1.**, and cDNA is prepared as outlined under **Subheading 3.2.**

3.5. Real-Time Quantitative RT-PCR

Three separate RQ-PCR reactions are prepared for the b2a2 *BCR-ABL* transcript, the b3a2 *BCR-ABL* transcript, and the *BCR* control gene. The results are reported as a ratio of *BCR-ABL/BCR%*, which compensates for variations in the quality of the RNA sample and for differences in the efficiency of the RT (*see* **Note 2**). The probes and primers were selected using the Primer Express software following the manufacturer's guidelines (*see* **Note 3**). The probes are labeled with a 5′ FAM reporter dye and a 3′ TAMRA quencher dye. The three assays are processed in the same 96-well reaction plate, because the same PCR reaction conditions are used for each. Each patient cDNA duplicate sample is processed once within two separate quantitative runs. Therefore, the samples are processed in duplicate and the results of the two RQ-PCR analyses are averaged. The standards, controls, and no-template control are processed once within each run, except for the lowest standards for the b2a2 and b3a2 *BCR-ABL* transcripts (representing approx 10 copies per 2.5 µL). These standards are run in duplicate due to the wider variability of the assay at low copy number (*see* **Note 4**). The preparation of the PCR reactions and the addition of the cDNA are performed in separate laboratories. An Excel spreadsheet is prepared for each assay, and the cells within the spreadsheet correspond to the 96-well reaction plate. The location of each standard, patient sample, and control within the plate is marked, and the spreadsheet is printed and used during PCR preparation to guide the loading of the wells. The TaqMan analysis uses fluorescent probes; therefore, powder-free gloves must be used during all steps of the procedure and the tubes or plates must not be marked with a fluorescent marking pen.

1. The sequence of the primers and probes are:
   b2a2 *BCR-ABL*:
   Forward primer: 5′ atc cgt gga gct gca gat g
   Reverse primer: 5′ cgc tga agg gct tct tcc tt
   TaqMan probe: 5′ cca act cgt gtg tga aac tcc aga ctg tcc
   Amplicon length 96 bp
   b3a2 *BCR-ABL*:
   Forward primer: 5′ ggg ctc tat ggg ttt ctg aat g
   Reverse primer: 5′ cgc tga agg gct ttt gaa ct
   TaqMan probe: 5′ cat cgt cca ctc agc cac tgg att taa gc
   Amplicon length 74 bp
   BCR:
   Forward primer: 5′ cct tcg acg tca ata aca agg at
   Reverse primer: 5′ cct gcg atg gcg ttc ac
   TaqMan probe: 5′ tcc atc tcg ctc atc atc acc gac a
   Amplicon length 67 bp
2. The probes and primers are thawed and mixed thoroughly before use. Centrifuge briefly to collect the material at the bottom of the tube.
3. Prepare master mixes for each transcript by adding the following to a 1.5-mL tube for each patient sample + 2 positive controls + 2 negative controls + 1: 12.5 µL 2X TaqMan universal master mix, the forward and reverse primers at a final concentration of 0.2 μM, the probe at a final concentration of 0.1 μM and sterile water to a total volume of 22.5 µL. A no-template control is included for each mix.
4. Mix the tubes thoroughly and centrifuge briefly to collect the mix at the bottom of the tube.
5. Pipet 22.5 µL of each master mix into the appropriate wells of the 96-well plate.
6. In a separate laboratory, thaw the standards. Mix and centrifuge briefly to collect the standard at the bottom of the tube.
7. In the PCR cabinet, add 2.5 µL of each standard, patient sample, and control into the appropriate wells.
8. Cap the wells with strips of optical caps.
9. Centrifuge the 96-well plate briefly to collect the mix at the bottom of the wells.
10. Load the PCR plate into the 7700 Sequence Detector System. Refer to the manufacturer's user manual for instructions for use of the instrument.
11. A template is prepared on the analyzer for the set-up of the RQ-PCR that has the positions and concentrations of the standards already indicated. The reaction volume and thermal cycler conditions are preprogrammed. The template is copied for each new run, and the position and identification of the patient samples, controls, and no-template controls are entered. Once the template copy is programmed, the run is started.
12. The thermal cycling conditions for each reaction are:

    a. 1 cycle at 50°C for 2 min.
    b. 1 cycle at 95°C for 10 min.
    c. 40 cycles at 95°C for 15 s, 60°C for 1 min.
13. The PCR is completed in approx 2 h. Following completion, save the run. Check each well of the reaction plate to ensure that evaporation has not occurred and then discard the plate.
14. The SDS software is used to analyze the PCR results. The standard curves are calculated and the patient and control results are printed on an experiment report (*see* **Note 4**).
15. Results are reported as a percentage ratio of *BCR-ABL/BCR%*. The quality control values are accepted according to Westgard Quality Control rules *(28)* (*see* **Note 5**).
16. The level of *BCR* transcript determines the quality of RNA. Values greater than 30,000 transcripts are adequate and produce appropriate *BCR-ABL/BCR%* results.

3.6. Qualitative PCR for Atypical BCR-ABL Transcripts

For patients with CML where the usual p210 transcripts are not detected, we perform a qualitative PCR that amplifies a region spanning *BCR* exon 1 and *ABL* exon 3 in order to identify atypical *BCR-ABL* transcripts. As quality control material, the RNA of patients with the p210 and p190 *BCR-ABL* transcripts are used. The preparation of the PCR reactions and the addition of the cDNA are performed in separate laboratories.

1. The primers used in the PCR are:
    Forward Primer: 5′ acc gca tgt tcc ggg aca aaa g
    Reverse Primer: 5′ tgt tga ctg gcg tga tgt agt tgc ttg g *(29)*.
2. The patient RNA is extracted as outlined under **Subheading 3.1.**, and cDNA is prepared as outlined under **Subheading 3.2.**
3. The quality of the cDNA is confirmed by quantitation of the *BCR* control gene by RQ-PCR analysis as outlined under **Subheading 3.5.** Samples with *BCR* values less than 30,000 transcripts are not of sufficient quality for analysis.
4. Thaw the PCR reagents and primers and mix thoroughly before use (except for the enzyme, which is stored at –20°C until added to the master mix). Centrifuge briefly to collect the material at the bottom of the tube.
5. Prepare a master mix on ice by adding the following into a 1.5-mL tube for each patient sample + 2 positive controls + 1 no-template control + 1: 1.5 μL $MgCl_2$, 2.5 μL dNTP (10 m*M* mix); 5 μL 10X Expand long template Buffer 3; the forward and reverse primers at a final concentration of 0.3 μ*M*, 0.75 μL of 5 U/μL Expand long template enzyme mix and sterile water to a total volume of 47 μL.
6. Mix the tubes thoroughly and centrifuge briefly to collect the mix at the bottom of the tube.
7. Pipet 47 μL of the master mix into 0.2-mL tubes.
8. In a separate laboratory, add 3 μL of the cDNA, mix thoroughly, and centrifuge briefly to collect the mix at the bottom of the tube.

9. Transfer the reactions to the thermal cycler and amplify with the following conditions:
   a. 1 cycle at 94°C for 2 min.
   b. 10 cycles at 94°C for 10 s, 65°C for 30 s, 68°C for 2 min.
   c. 20 cycles at 94°C for 10 s, 65°C for 30 s, 68°C for 2 min—increase the 68°C step by 20 s at each cycle.
   d. 1 cycle at 68°C for 7 min.
10. After completion of the PCR, assess the size of each amplification product by electrophoresis of 5 µL of the PCR product mixed with 1 µL gel loading buffer on a 2.0% agarose gel, using the SPP1 size marker.
11. The size of the b2a2 *BCR-ABL* product is 1886 bp, the b3a2 *BCR-ABL* product is 1961 bp, and the e1a2 *BCR-ABL* product is 483 bp. The presence of other sized bands is indicative of an atypical *BCR-ABL* transcript. Sequence the atypical band to determine the transcript type. Sequences of unknown origin that are present within the *BCR-ABL* transcript may by derived from intronic sequences. An inverted intronic sequence has been described that was inserted due to the introduction of cryptic splice sites *(23)*.

3.7. Qualitative PCR for p210 BCR-ABL

Our laboratory uses the quantitative PCR and atypical *BCR-ABL* PCR methods to assess all CML patients. However, a qualitative nested PCR method has been designed in our laboratory to specifically amplify the p210 *BCR-ABL* transcript, and the method is presented here. The primers will amplify only the b2a2 or b3a2 *BCR-ABL* transcripts and will not amplify atypical *BCR-ABL* transcripts. We use a sample that is known to contain both the b2a2 and b3a2 *BCR-ABL* transcripts as a quality control.

1. Primers were designed using Primer Express software. The sequence of the primers are:
   First-step forward primer: 5′ tgc aga tgc tga cca act cgt
   First-step reverse primer: 5′ cca ctg gcc aca aaa tca tac ag
   Second-step forward primer: 5′ tga aac tcc aga ctg tcc aca
   Second-step reverse primer: 5′ ggt cca gca gga agg ttt t
2. The patient RNA is extracted as outlined under **Subheading 3.1.**, and cDNA is prepared as outlined under **Subheading 3.2.**
3. Thaw the PCR reagents and primers and mix thoroughly before use (except for the enzyme, which is stored at −20°C until added to the master mix). Centrifuge briefly to collect the material at the bottom of the tube.
4. Prepare a master mix for the first and second-step PCR by adding the following to a 1.5-mL tube for each patient sample + 1 positive control + 1 no-template control + 1: 2 µL MgCl$_2$, 2.5 µL of 10X PCR buffer, 0.625 µL dNTP (10 m*M* mix), the forward and reverse primers at a final concentration of 0.5 µ*M*, 0.25 µL of 5 U/µL of AmpliTaq gold, and sterile water, to a total volume of 22.5 µL for the first-step mix and 23 µL for the second-step mix. Mix the tubes thoroughly and centrifuge briefly to collect the mix at the bottom of the tube.

5. Pipet 22.5 µL of the first-step master mix and 23 µL of the second-step master mix into 0.2-mL tubes. Store the second-step tubes at 4°C until completion of the first-step PCR.

6. In a separate laboratory, add 2.5 µL of the cDNA to the first-step mix, mix thoroughly, and centrifuge briefly to collect the mix at the bottom of the tube.

7. Transfer the reactions to the thermal cycler and amplify with the following conditions:
   a. 1 cycle at 95°C for 10 min.
   b. 30 cycles at 95°C for 30 s, 60°C for 30 s, 72°C for 30 min.
   c. 1 cycle at 72°C for 7 min.

8. The following steps are performed in a separate area from the PCR master mix setup and the cDNA addition. After completion of the first-step PCR, dilute the PCR products 1 in 100 in sterile water. Mix the tubes thoroughly and centrifuge briefly to collect the mix at the bottom of the tube.

9. Add 2 µL of the 1 in 100 dilution to the second-step mix. Mix the tubes thoroughly and centrifuge briefly to collect the mix at the bottom of the tube.

10. Transfer the reactions to the thermal cycler and amplify with the same conditions as under **Subheading 3.7.7.**

11. After completion of the PCR, assess the size of each amplification product by electrophoresis of 5 µL of the PCR product mixed with 1 µL gel loading buffer on a 2.0% agarose gel, using the Puc19 size marker.

12. The size of the first-step b2a2 *BCR-ABL* product is 220 bp, and the b3a2 *BCR-ABL* product is 295 bp. The size of the second-step b2a2 *BCR-ABL* product is 142 bp, and the b3a2 *BCR-ABL* product is 217 bp. An unusual PCR artifact fragment may be present when the patient has both the b2a2 and b3a2 *BCR-ABL* transcripts (*see* **Note 6**).

13. The sensitivity of the second-step PCR is one K562 cell diluted in 10^6 *BCR-ABL* negative cells.

4. Notes

1. Measures are in place throughout every step to prevent cross-contamination of plasmid or patient samples as well as contamination with PCR product. The majority of patients undergoing analysis have minimal residual disease or undetectable *BCR-ABL* levels, and it is therefore essential for patient management that false-positive results do not occur. The main area of concern is in the preparation and dilution of high-copy-number plasmids. This is done in a separate laboratory from the RNA extraction and PCR setup laboratories, using separate dedicated equipment. Other measures include the use of sterile barrier tips, UV-irradiated pipets, RNAse- and DNAse-free tubes, and dedicated equipment for each procedure. The RNA extraction, PCR setup, PCR, and the post-PCR manipulation (if required) are performed in separate laboratories. To reduce the possibility of RNA degradation, the samples are processed into Trizol solution as soon after collection as possible and usually within 24 h. All samples are stored at room temperature before the addition of Trizol. We have found that storage at

4°C will rapidly degrade the *BCR-ABL* mRNA.

2. The selection of an appropriate control gene constitutes one of the most important aspects for accurate RQ-PCR. For example, GAPDH is frequently used as a control for RQ-PCR assays. However, there is overwhelming evidence suggesting that its use is inappropriate (reviewed in **refs. *3,4***). The control should ideally have a similar expression level to the target and degrade at a similar rate to compensate for variations in the quality of the RNA between samples. We have chosen the normal *BCR* gene, as it has a similar expression level to *BCR-ABL* and it degrades at a similar rate *(14)*. To compensate for differences in the efficiency of each RT reaction, the control gene and the *BCR-ABL* gene are reverse transcribed in the same reaction. Calculating a ratio of *BCR-ABL* to *BCR* compensates for the variations.

3. The primers and probes were designed using Primer Express software and specifically amplify RNA. One of the primers hybridizes at the junction of an exon boundary. The amplicon sizes for the three transcripts are all less than 100 bp, which allows a sensitive detection system. One K562 cell is detectable in a background of 10^5 *BCR-ABL*-negative cells. During the development of the TaqMan assay, we validated the *BCR-ABL* quantitative values by correlation with the percentage of the Philadelphia chromosome as assessed by cytogenetic analysis. A good correlation was found, except that a small percentage of patients with the b2a2 *BCR-ABL* transcript had lower quantitative values than expected. By sequence analysis of the PCR amplicon of these patients, it was found that they all had a polymorphism located at the hybridization site of the sixth base from the 3′ end of the reverse primer. The efficiency of primer annealing was reduced in the patients with the polymorphism, which resulted in an approx 10-fold lower quantitative value. The problem was overcome by redesigning the primer, which avoided the polymorphic site (*see* **Fig. 2**). These data highlight the importance of avoiding polymorphisms when designing probes and primers, although the position of these sites is not always known, as in our case.

4. We routinely analyze the three separate PCR reactions that are required for the quantitation of *BCR-ABL* on the same 96-well plate, which contains the three different standard curves. The SDS software will analyze only one standard curve per reaction, and therefore each set of data for the three transcripts must be saved into a separate file for analysis. This is done by copying the original file into three separate files and assigning all of the wells, except for those to be analyzed for a particular transcript, as "not in use." The three files are analyzed separately. We set a threshold of 0.04 and a baseline reading between 3 and 15, which is usually sufficient to ensure that the threshold is above the background fluorescence readings and within the linear portion of the curves. The threshold may need to be increased on the very rare occasion that the linear portion is not reached. The standard curve is analyzed and accepted if the slope value is between −3.3 and −3.59 and the correlation coefficient is between 0.997 and 1.0. If any point on the standard curve is an obvious outlier it can be removed and the standard curve reanalyzed. We have not found it necessary to run the standard

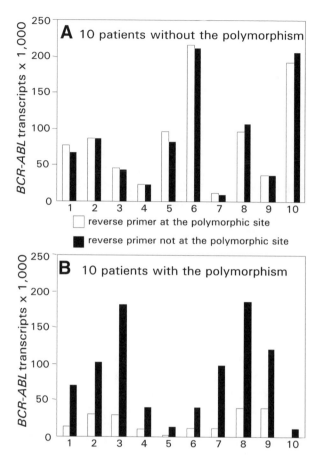

Fig. 2. Impact of a polymorphism at the reverse primer binding site on quantitation of *BCR-ABL* transcript levels. In a subset of patients with the b2a2 *BCR-ABL* transcript, the initial quantitative levels were up to 10-fold lower than expected. Sequencing revealed a polymorphism located at the reverse primer hybridization site. The single base mismatch significantly affected the binding of the primer to the template and thus the accuracy of quantitation. Re-designing the primer to avoid the polymorphism significantly improved the results. **A** represents the b2a2 *BCR-ABL* transcript level of 10 patients who did not have the polymorphism. The white columns represent the value using the original primer that hybridized at the polymorphic site, and the shaded columns represent the value using the re-designed primer that did not hybridize at the polymorphic site. There was no difference in the results with either primer. **B** represents the b2a2 *BCR-ABL* transcript level of 10 patients who did have the polymorphism. There was up to a 10-fold lower quantitative value when the original primer was used. In patient 10, the value was falsely negative. The graphs demonstrate that the accuracy of quantitation may be compromised when there is a single base mismatch at a primer site.

Table 1
The Inter-Assay Variation of Threshold Cycle (Ct) Values for the Six b3a2 *BCR-ABL* Standards Measured Over 2 Yr ($n =$ 134) and Using a Threshold of 0.04

Copy number of standards	Mean standard Ct value	2 standard deviation range	Coefficient of variation (%)
15	36.45	35.36–37.54	1.50%
1.5×10^2	33.01	32.35–33.67	1.00%
1.5×10^3	29.53	28.90–30.16	1.06%
1.5×10^4	26.12	25.61–26.63	0.98%
1.5×10^5	22.75	22.20–23.30	1.21%
1.5×10^6	19.37	18.96–19.78	1.05%

samples in duplicate apart from the lowest standard, as a result of the wider variability at high threshold cycle (Ct) levels. The inter-assay reproducibility of the standard values is usually within 1.3 Ct, except for the lowest standard (*see* **Table 1**). The 2 standard deviation range provides an estimate of measurement reliability of the Ct values at approx the 95% level of confidence. The patient and control results are calculated from the standard curve and printed on the experiment report. Before accepting the results, the fluorescent curve of each control and patient sample must be viewed to ensure that the curve is linear and therefore acceptable. For some patients with *BCR-ABL* values that are not detectable, the background fluorescence may "creep" above the threshold. If this occurs, the quantitative value will be calculated from the fractional Ct value at the point it crosses the threshold. Therefore, a very high quantitative value will be assigned instead of a negative value. These samples must be noted and the correct value assigned on the experiment report. The HeLa negative control does on occasion produce a positive value that is less than 10 copies, in which case it is assigned as not detected. Patient values that are below this level are also assigned as not detected. If the negative control is greater than 10 copies, contamination may have occurred, and the samples are repeated. If the contamination represents only a very small number of copies, it will not influence the result of patients with values that are greater than 2 logs higher, and these samples need not be repeated. We have identified what appears to be a software error for the no-template control result. If these samples are assigned as "NTC" during sample setup, the result will always be printed as zero on the experiment report even for positive values (*see* arrows in **Fig. 3**). Therefore, the no-template control fluorescence data must be viewed to ensure that it is actually negative. The *BCR* control transcript value provides an indication of the quality of the RNA. Values range from 30,000 to greater than 300,000 transcripts per 2.5 μL of cDNA for acceptable quality. Below 30,000 transcripts, the RNA is considered degraded and a repeat sample is requested. The RQ-PCR procedure, including processing the RNA extraction batch, the reverse transcription PCR,

Applied Biosystems

File Name : c20/01/04   **Plate Type** : 7700 Single Reporter
User :   **PCR Volume** : 25   **Exp. Time** : 25
Date : Fri, Mar 19, 2004
Comments :

Thermal Cycle Conditions

Cycle	Temperature	Time	Repeat	Ramp Time	Auto Increment
Hold	50.00	2:00		Auto	
Hold	95.00	10:00		Auto	
Cycle	95.00	0:15	40	Auto	
	60.00	1:00		Auto	

Standard Curve

Slope : −3.36	**Threshold** : 0.04
Intercept : 40.38	**Baseline Range** : (3 , 15)
Fit R : 1.00	

Sample Information

Well	Type	Sample Name	Replicate	Ct	Quantity	Std. Dev.	Mean
D2	STND	B3A2		36.32	1.5e+01	0.00	15.00
D3	STND	B3A2		33.26	1.5e+02	0.00	150.00
D4	STND	B3A2		29.63	1.5e+03	0.00	1500.00
D5	STND	B3A2		26.26	1.5e+04	0.00	15000.00
D6	STND	B3A2		23.07	1.5e+05	0.00	150000.0
D7	STND	B3A2		19.57	1.5e+06	0.00	1500000.
D10	UNKN	Patient 1		34.88	4.3e+01	0.00	43.09
D12	UNKN	Patient 2		40.00		0.00	0.00
E3	UNKN	Patient 3		31.73	3.7e+02	0.00	373.19
E4	UNKN	Patient 4		32.46	2.3e+02	0.00	226.07
E9	UNKN	Hela c20.1.04		40.00		0.00	0.00
E10	UNKN	Low control c20.1.04		32.89	1.7e+02	0.00	168.69
E11	UNKN	High control c20.1.04		23.19	1.3e+05	0.00	129349.4
D8	NTC ←		NTC	22.43 ←		0.00	0.00 ←
E12	NTC		NTC	40.00		0.00	0.00

Fig. 3. Caution is required when reviewing the experimental report for samples designated as no-template controls (NTC). For samples assigned as NTC during sample set-up, the result will always be printed as zero on the experiment report, even for positive values. The experiment report highlights a sample that has been assigned as an NTC. The arrows indicate that despite the very high threshold cycle (Ct) value of 22.43, the result is calculated as 0 instead of the actual value of greater than 150,000 transcripts. Therefore, during analysis of the real-time quantitative reverse-transcription polymerase chain reaction results, careful evaluation of the NTC Ct values and amplification curves must be undertaken to ensure that there is no contamination.

Table 2
The Estimate of Measurement Reliability of the *BCR-ABL/BCR*%
Values at Approximately the 95% Level of Confidence Was
Determined Using Two Levels of Quality Control

	Mean *BCR-ABL/ BCR*%	2 Standard deviation range	Coefficient of variation (%)
Low control	0.072	0.036–0.108	25.0%
High control	77	57–97	13.0%

the quantitative PCR, and the result analysis takes approx 1.5 d. The complete RQ-PCR procedure is performed in duplicate; therefore, the final patient results are available at 4 d after the start of analysis.

5. Analyzing quality control samples at two different *BCR-ABL* expression levels within each run assesses the performance of the TaqMan assay. The dynamic range of the assay is greater than 4 logs and the control sample *BCR-ABL* expression differs by approx 3 logs, and therefore monitors high and low expression. The positive and negative control samples undergo RNA extraction and reverse transcription with the patient samples. A mean and 2 standard deviation range is calculated for each control by repeated analysis and this range is used to verify and accept the results of each RQ-PCR analysis. The rules for acceptance or rejection of the control values are based on those proposed by Westgard *(28)*: (1) the values are accepted if they are within 2 standard deviations of the mean value; (2) the values are accepted if one value is between 2 and 3 standard deviations; (3) the values are rejected if the same control value is between 2 and 3 standard deviations in the next analysis; and (4) the values are rejected if one value is greater than 3 standard deviations from the mean value. QC Reporter II software is used to record and monitor the controls. If rule 3 or 4 is applicable, the analysis must be repeated after an investigation of the cause of the shift in results. For every RQ-PCR analysis, the lot number of each reagent, the preparation date of the standards, and the receipt date of each primer and probe is recorded. The dates that the reagents and aliquots of the standards, probes, and primers are first in use, are also recorded. This allows us to troubleshoot the system by relating the shift in results to a change in a reagent lot. The analysis is repeated with replacement of the appropriate reagents and accepted if the quality control results are within range. **Table 2** shows the estimate of measurement reliability at approx the 95% level of confidence for the control samples. There is a wider variability at very low levels; however, we have determined that a twofold change in *BCR-ABL/BCR*% can reliably be detected for most samples. This was determined by performing a mixed model analysis of variance in which the samples with an increase in gene expression were fixed effects and duplicates within a low level control sample were random effects. The test confirmed that a twofold change in expression level was statistically different, $p = 0.003$ (F value 9.31).

6. When the qualitative nested PCR method is used to identify the p210 *BCR-ABL* transcripts as outlined under **Subheading 3.7.**, a PCR artifact may be visualized on the agarose gel. In patients who have both the b2a2 and b3a2 *BCR-ABL* transcripts, a fragment of approx 300 bp may be amplified in addition to the b2a2 fragment of 142 bp and the b3a2 fragment of 217 bp. Sequencing has revealed that the 300-bp fragment is an unusual PCR artifact caused by recombination of the sequences that share homology between the 217- and 142-bp fragments.

Acknowledgments

The authors thank Dr Barney Rudzki, Rebecca Lawrence, and Chani Field for assistance in the preparation of the manuscript.

References

1. Daley, G. Q., Van Etten, R. A., and Baltimore, D. (1990) Induction of chronic myelogenous leukemia in mice by the P210bcr/abl gene of the Philadelphia chromosome. *Science* **247,** 824–830.
2. Heisterkamp, N., Jenster, G., ten Hoeve, J., Zovich, D., Pattengale, P. K., and Groffen, J. (1990) Acute leukaemia in bcr/abl transgenic mice. *Nature* **344,** 251–253.
3. Bustin, S. A. (2000) Absolute quantification of mRNA using real-time reverse transcription polymerase chain reaction assays. *J. Mol. Endocrinol.* **25,** 169–193.
4. Bustin, S. A. (2002) Quantification of mRNA using real-time reverse transcription PCR (RT-PCR): trends and problems. *J. Mol. Endocrinol.* **29,** 23–39.
5. van der Velden, V. H., Hochhaus, A., Cazzaniga, G., Szczepanski, T., Gabert, J., and van Dongen, J. J. (2003) Detection of minimal residual disease in hematologic malignancies by real-time quantitative PCR: principles, approaches, and laboratory aspects. *Leukemia* **17,** 1013–1034.
6. Branford, S., Hughes, T. P., and Rudzki, Z. (1999) Monitoring chronic myeloid leukaemia therapy by real-time quantitative PCR in blood is a reliable alternative to bone marrow cytogenetics. *Br. J. Haematol.* **107,** 587–599.
7. Stentoft, J., Pallisgaard, N., Kjeldsen, E., Holm, M. S., Nielsen, J. L., and Hokland, P. (2001) Kinetics of BCR-ABL fusion transcript levels in chronic myeloid leukemia patients treated with STI571 measured by quantitative real-time polymerase chain reaction. *Eur. J. Haematol.* **67,** 302–308.
8. Emig, M., Saussele, S., Wittor, H., et al. (1999) Accurate and rapid analysis of residual disease in patients with CML using specific fluorescent hybridization probes for real time quantitative RT-PCR. *Leukemia* **13,** 1825–1832.
9. Mensink, E., van de Locht, A., Schattenberg, A., et al. (1998) Quantitation of minimal residual disease in Philadelphia chromosome positive chronic myeloid leukaemia patients using real-time quantitative RT-PCR. *Br. J. Haematol.* **102,** 768–774.
10. Lin, F., van Rhee, F., Goldman, J. M., and Cross, N. C. (1996) Kinetics of increasing BCR-ABL transcript numbers in chronic myeloid leukemia patients who relapse after bone marrow transplantation. *Blood* **87,** 4473–4478.

11. Olavarria, E., Kanfer, E., Szydlo, R., et al. (2001) Early detection of BCR-ABL transcripts by quantitative reverse transcriptase-polymerase chain reaction predicts outcome after allogeneic stem cell transplantation for chronic myeloid leukemia. *Blood* **97,** 1560–1565.

12. Radich, J. P., Gooley, T., Bryant, E., et al. (2001) The significance of bcr-abl molecular detection in chronic myeloid leukemia patients "late," 18 months or more after transplantation. *Blood* **98,** 1701–1707.

13. Merx, K., Muller, M. C., Kreil, S., et al. (2002) Early reduction of BCR-ABL mRNA transcript levels predicts cytogenetic response in chronic phase CML patients treated with imatinib after failure of interferon alpha. *Leukemia* **16,** 1579–1583.

14. Hughes, T. and Branford, S. (2003) Molecular monitoring of chronic myeloid leukemia. *Semin. Hematol.* **40,** 62–68.

15. Wang, L., Pearson, K., Ferguson, J. E., and Clark, R. E. (2003) The early molecular response to imatinib predicts cytogenetic and clinical outcome in chronic myeloid leukaemia. *Br. J. Haematol.* **120,** 990–999.

16. Muller, M. C., Gattermann, N., Lahaye, T., et al. (2003) Dynamics of BCR-ABL mRNA expression in first-line therapy of chronic myelogenous leukemia patients with imatinib or interferon alpha/ara-C. *Leukemia* **17,** 2392–2400.

17. Hughes, T. P., Kaeda, J., Branford, S., et al. (2003) Frequency of major molecular responses to imatinib or interferon alfa plus cytarabine in newly diagnosed chronic myeloid leukemia. *N. Engl. J. Med.* **349,** 1423–1432.

18. Paschka, P., Muller, M. C., Merx, K., et al. (2003) Molecular monitoring of response to imatinib (Glivec) in CML patients pretreated with interferon alpha. Low levels of residual disease are associated with continuous remission. *Leukemia* **17,** 1687–1694.

19. Branford, S., Rudzki, Z., Harper, A., et al. (2003) Imatinib produces significantly superior molecular responses compared to interferon alfa plus cytarabine in patients with newly diagnosed chronic myeloid leukemia in chronic phase. *Leukemia* **17,** 2401–2409.

20. Melo, J. V. (1997) BCR-ABL gene variants. *Baillieres Clin. Haematol.* **10,** 203–222.

21. Saglio, G., Guerrasio, A., Rosso, C., et al. (1990) New type of Bcr/Abl junction in Philadelphia chromosome-positive chronic myelogenous leukemia. *Blood* **76,** 1819–1824.

22. Pane, F., Frigeri, F., Sindona, M., et al. (1996) Neutrophilic-chronic myeloid leukemia: a distinct disease with a specific molecular marker (BCR/ABL with C3/A2 junction). *Blood* **88,** 2410–2414.

23. Branford, S., Rudzki, Z., and Hughes, T. P. (2000) A novel BCR-ABL transcript (e8a2) with the insertion of an inverted sequence of ABL intron 1b in a patient with Philadelphia-positive chronic myeloid leukaemia. *Br. J. Haematol.* **109,** 635–637.

24. Okamoto, K., Karasawa, M., Sakai, H., Ogura, H., Morita, K., and Naruse, T. (1997) A novel acute lymphoid leukaemia type BCR/ABL transcript in chronic myelogenous leukaemia. *Br. J. Haematol.* **96,** 611–613.

25. Rubinstein, R. and Purves, L. R. (1998) A novel BCR-ABL rearrangement in a Philadelphia chromosome-positive chronic myelogenous leukaemia variant with thrombocythaemia. *Leukemia* **12**, 230–232.
26. How, G. F., Lim, L. C., Kulkarni, S., Tan, L. T., Tan, P., and Cross, N. C. (1999) Two patients with novel BCR/ABL fusion transcripts (e8/a2 and e13/a2) resulting from translocation breakpoints within BCR exons. *Br. J. Haematol.* **105**, 434–436.
27. Cross, N. C., Feng, L., Chase, A., Bungey, J., Hughes, T. P., and Goldman, J. M. (1993) Competitive polymerase chain reaction to estimate the number of BCR-ABL transcripts in chronic myeloid leukemia patients after bone marrow transplantation. *Blood* **82**, 1929–1936.
28. Westgard, J. O., Barry, P. L., Hunt, M. R., and Groth, T. (1981) A multi-rule Shewhart chart for quality control in clinical chemistry. *Clin. Chem.* **27**, 493–501.
29. Cross, N. C., Hughes, T. P., Feng, L., et al. (1993) Minimal residual disease after allogeneic bone marrow transplantation for chronic myeloid leukaemia in first chronic phase: correlations with acute graft-versus-host disease and relapse. *Br. J. Haematol.* **84**, 67–74.

5

Detection of *BCR-ABL* Mutations and Resistance to Imatinib Mesylate

Susan Branford and Timothy Hughes

Summary

The major mechanism of imatinib resistance for patients with chronic myeloid leukemia (CML) is clonal expansion of leukemic cells with mutations in the Bcr-Abl fusion tyrosine kinase that reduce the capacity of imatinib to inhibit kinase activity. The early detection of such mutations may allow timely treatment intervention to prevent or overcome resistance. Direct sequencing of the *BCR-ABL* kinase domain is relatively rapid and allows detection of emerging mutations at a sensitivity of approx 20%. Mutations have been detected over a range of 242 amino acids, which spans the entire kinase domain. For optimal sensitivity, the kinase domain of the abnormal gene should be isolated by reverse-transcription (RT) polymerase chain reaction (PCR) amplification using primers that hybridize to the *BCR* and *ABL* genes. The quality of the RNA is assessed by real-time quantitative PCR prior to analysis, and *BCR-ABL* levels are determined. Only RNA of adequate quality is used to ensure accurate and reproducible mutation analysis. Depending on the level of *BCR-ABL* transcripts, a one- or two-step PCR is required to amplify the kinase domain. Direct sequencing with dye terminator chemistry is performed using PCR-purified products. The sequence is compared to an *ABL* kinase domain reference sequence using sequencing analysis software, which aligns the sequences and highlights single or multiple mutations.

Key Words: Chronic myeloid leukemia; *BCR-ABL*; imatinib mesylate; mutation; kinase domain; real-time quantitative PCR; direct sequencing.

1. Introduction

Chronic myeloid leukemia (CML) is characterized by the Philadelphia chromosome translocation (t(9;22)). The resultant *BCR-ABL* fusion gene encodes a protein with constitutive tyrosine kinase activity that is causally associated with CML *(1–3)*. The level of *BCR-ABL* mRNA can be used as a sensitive marker of disease progress. CML progresses from a relatively benign chronic phase to an accelerated phase that is characterized by increasing numbers of hematopoietic cells and additional chromosomal abnormalities. The disease terminates in the

From: *Methods in Molecular Medicine, Vol. 125: Myeloid Leukemia: Methods and Protocols*
Edited by: H. Iland, M. Hertzberg, and P. Marlton © Humana Press Inc., Totowa, NJ

blast crisis, which is distinguished by large numbers of immature blast cells that populate the bone marrow and peripheral blood. The only chance of cure for selected patients is an allogeneic transplant, which is most successful if performed early after diagnosis while the patient is still in the chronic phase. However, the procedure is associated with considerable morbidity and mortality. Treatment options for patients with CML have been substantially improved in recent years by the use of the specific tyrosine kinase inhibitor imatinib mesylate (Glivec, Novartis Pharmaceuticals, Basel, Switzerland) (4–9). The inhibitor binds to the Bcr-Abl protein in the inactive conformation by binding to amino acids in the ATP binding pocket of the ABL kinase domain and blocking ATP binding (10,11). The downstream signal transduction pathways are thereby blocked, because the transfer of phosphate from ATP is prevented. Phosphorylation of proteins in the signal transduction pathways has a critical role in a range of biological processes, including cell growth, differentiation, and apoptosis. Imatinib therapy leads to growth arrest or apoptosis of BCR-ABL-expressing cells (4,12,13).

Despite the efficacy and safety of imatinib therapy, relapse and resistance occurs in a number of patients, particularly those in the accelerated phase or blast crisis. Relapse occurs in almost all patients treated in the blast crisis, while approx 15 to 20% of chronic-phase patients also relapse within the first 2–3 yr of therapy. The majority of patients who acquire resistance after an initial response have evidence of activated Bcr-Abl tyrosine kinase (14). The major mechanism of activation is now recognized as point mutation within the BCR-ABL kinase domain (14–16), and 36 different point mutations within this region have been identified to date (refs. 15–22 and Branford, unpublished data) (Fig. 1). It is believed that the mutations emerge under the selective pressure of imatinib therapy, and it is likely that further mutations will be detected. In a recent comprehensive survey of amino acid substitutions that confer resistance using an in-vitro screen of randomly mutated BCR-ABL, numerous substitutions were identified in addition to those reported in patients (23). Mutations within the kinase domain can prevent imatinib from binding either by interrupting critical contact points between imatinib and the protein or by inducing a conformation to which imatinib is unable to bind. Biochemical and cellular assays have demonstrated that the different BCR-ABL mutations result in varying levels of resistance (15,17,18,24,25), and clinical studies have shown that the location of the mutation may impact on the disease outcome. Mutations located in a region of the kinase domain known as the P-loop confer a worse prognosis (16,20,26). The different mutations may therefore require differing strategies to overcome resistance, such as dose escalation for those that confer moderate resistance, and combination therapy or transplant for highly resistant mutations. In some cases, cessation of imatinib may be advantageous.

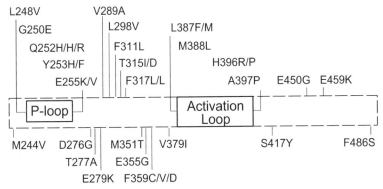

Fig. 1. Linear representation of the ABL kinase domain, showing the relative location of the point mutations identified in imatinib-treated patients to date. A number of nucleotide substitutions resulted in the replacement of the same amino acid. For example, mutation at nucleotides 756 and 757 both resulted in the Q252H mutation (nucleotides numbered according to GenBank accession number M14752). In our series of 279 imatinib-treated patients who are monitored for mutations at least every 6 mo, we have detected mutations in 66 patients (24%). These patients represent all phases of the disease, and virtually all mutations lead to loss of imatinib response *(16)*. Multiple mutations have been detected in 23% of the patients with mutations, and the most frequently detected mutations in our patients are M351T, E255K, F359V, and T315I.

It is therefore important that emerging mutations be detected early to allow timely treatment intervention before overt relapse.

A number of procedures have been described for the detection of kinase domain mutations that involve polymerase chain reaction (PCR) amplification of either the *BCR-ABL* kinase domain or the *ABL* kinase domain (reviewed in **ref.** *27*). Amplification of the *ABL* kinase domain does not distinguish the *BCR-ABL* allele and is therefore less sensitive because the *BCR-ABL* target sequence is diluted by the normal *ABL* sequence. Various primer combinations have been used that either amplify the entire kinase domain *(28)* or restrict the amplification to exclude the region of the kinase domain beyond the activation loop *(14,17–19)*. Mutation detection usually involves either direct sequencing of the amplified product or subcloning of the PCR product and sequence analysis of multiple clones. Subcloning is a time-consuming technique and is thus less suitable for widespread testing compared to direct sequencing.

Our method involves RT-PCR amplification of the entire kinase domain of the *BCR-ABL* allele using a 5′ *BCR* primer and a 3′ *ABL* primer. A second-step PCR using *ABL* primers may be necessary for samples with low *BCR-ABL* transcript levels. A number of mutations have been described in the region beyond the activation loop, and it is therefore essential to amplify the entire kinase domain. The PCR product is directly sequenced in the forward and reverse directions using dye terminator chemistry and a 3700 DNA Sequencer (Applied Biosystems, Foster City, CA, USA) *(16,28)*. Mutation Surveyor software (SoftGenetics, LLC, State College, PA) is used to analyze the sequence. RNA extracted from peripheral blood or bone marrow is suitable for analysis. The technique is also applicable for imatinib-treated patients with Philadelphia chromosome-positive acute lymphoblastic leukemia (ALL). These patients may have a *BCR-ABL* transcript that is the same as that present in most patients with CML (b2a2 or b3a2 *BCR-ABL*), or the transcript may involve the fusion of *BCR* exon 1 to *ABL* exon 2 (e1a2 *BCR-ABL*). For patients with the e1a2 transcript, an alternate 5′ PCR primer is required.

The ability to detect mutations is very dependent on the quality of the RNA, which is assessed prior to mutation analysis by measurement of the level of normal *BCR* mRNA using real-time quantitative PCR *(29)*. A cutoff level based on the number of detectable *BCR* transcripts in the sample was established as an indicator of degraded RNA. Samples with *BCR* levels below the cutoff are not assessed for mutations. This technique permits the detection of single or multiple mutations in patients with disease status ranging from a complete cytogenetic response (Philadelphia chromosome negative) to overt relapse, at a sensitivity of 20%. To date, we have detected 24 different point mutations, spanning the entire kinase domain and ranging from amino acid 244 to 486 (GenBank accession number M14752). Identification of these mutations is of clinical significance, because virtually all CML patients with detectable mutations acquire resistance to imatinib *(16,22)*.

2. Materials

2.1. Semi-Nested PCR Reaction

1. Sterile 0.2-mL capped PCR tubes (Interpath Services).
2. Sterile 1.5-mL capped PCR tubes (Interpath Services).
3. 500-µL single-use lots of autoclaved MiliQ water. Store at room temperature in 1.5-mL tubes.
4. PCR primers. All primers are ordered as a 50 µ*M* solution and stored in 30-µL lots at 20°C. Primers were designed using Primer Express software (Applied Biosystems).
5. 15 m*M* stock of dNTPs (Amersham Biosciences). Store at –20°C in 100-µL lots.
6. 25 m*M* MgCl$_2$ (Applied Biosystems). Store at –20°C.
7. Expand Long Template PCR System (Roche). Store at –20°C.
8. PCR cabinet with ultraviolet light.
9. UltraClean PCR Clean-up DNA purification kit (Mo Bio Laboratories). Store at room temperature.
10. Agarose, molecular-biology grade (Progen). Store at room temperature.
11. SPP1/*Eco*R1 DNA molecular-weight marker (Geneworks). Store at –20°C.

2.2. Sequencing Reaction

1. Sterile 0.2-mL capped PCR tubes (Interpath Services).
2. Sterile 1.5-mL capped PCR tubes (Interpath Services).
3. ABI Prism Dye terminator cycle sequencing ready reaction kit (Big Dye 3) (Applied Biosystems). Aliquot into 30-μL lots and wrap in foil to protect from the light. Store at –20°C.
4. PCR primers. All primers are ordered as a 50 μ*M* solution and stored in 30-μL lots at –20°C.
5. 75% isopropanol that is prepared at least weekly.
6. Glycogen, molecular-biology grade (Roche Diagnostics).
7. Mutation Surveyor software (SoftGenetics).

3. Methods
3.1. Semi-Nested PCR Reaction

Full details of methods for peripheral blood or bone marrow sample preparation, RNA extraction, cDNA synthesis, and real-time quantitative PCR analysis of *BCR-ABL* and *BCR* appear in Chapter 4. These procedures are performed prior to mutation analysis and determine the quality and suitability of the sample (*see* **Note 1**).

1. Primers were designed using Primer Express software. The sequence of the primers for CML and ALL patients with the b2a2 or b3a2 *BCR-ABL* transcripts are:
   First-step forward primer: 5′ tga cca act cgt gtg tga aac tc
   First-step reverse primer: 5′ tcc act tcg tct gag ata ctg gat t
   Second-step forward primer: 5′ cgc aac aag ccc act gtc t
   The second-step reverse primer is the same reverse primer that is used for the first-step PCR. The first-step forward primer hybridizes in *BCR* exon b2 (b2 may alternatively be referred to as *BCR* exon 13).
   In the case of ALL patients who have a *BCR-ABL* transcript that involves the fusion of *BCR* exon 1 to *ABL* exon 2 (e1a2 *BCR-ABL* transcript), an alternative first-step forward primer is used that hybridizes to *BCR* exon 1:
   e1a2 transcript: First-step forward primer: 5′ acc gca tgt tcc ggg aca aaa g
   The reverse primer and the second-step forward primer are the same primers that are listed above for b2a2 and b3a2 transcripts.
2. Thaw the PCR reagents and first-step primers and mix thoroughly before use (except for the enzyme, which is stored at –20°C until added to the master mix). Centrifuge briefly to collect the material at the bottom of the tube.
3. Prepare a master mix on ice. The amount of master mix prepared is dependent on the level of *BCR-ABL* transcripts, and two separate master mixes may be required (*see* **Note 1**). For samples with low *BCR-ABL* levels that require the addition of 3 μL of cDNA (150 ng), pipet the following into a 1.5-mL tube for each patient sample + 1 positive control + 1 no-template control + 1: 0.75 μL MgCl$_2$, 1.25 μL dNTP (15 m*M* mix), 2.5 μL 10X Expand long template Buffer 3, 0.15 μL of the forward

and reverse primers (final concentration of 0.3 μ*M* each), 0.375 μL of 5 U/μL Expand long template enzyme mix, and sterile water to a total volume of 22 μL (Mix 1). For samples requiring the addition of 2 μL of cDNA (100 ng), prepare a mix containing the same reagent volumes as above but adjust the volume of water to 23 μL (Mix 2). The most appropriate positive control to use is a previously analyzed patient sample of adequate RNA quality with a mid-range *BCR-ABL* transcript level (*see* **Note 2**).

4. Mix the tubes thoroughly and centrifuge briefly to collect the mix at the bottom of the tube.
5. Pipet 22 μL of Mix 1 into 0.2-mL tubes for samples requiring 3 μL of cDNA and 23 μL of Mix 2 for samples requiring 2 μL of cDNA into 0.2-mL tubes.
6. In a separate laboratory, thaw the cDNA, mix, and centrifuge briefly. Add 2 μL or 3 μL of the cDNA to the appropriate 0.2-mL tubes, mix thoroughly, and centrifuge briefly to collect the mix at the bottom of the tube.
7. Transfer the reactions to the thermal cycler and amplify with the following conditions:
   1 cycle at 94°C for 2 min.
   10 cycles at 94°C for 10 s, 60°C for 30 s, 68°C for 2 min.
   20 cycles at 94°C for 10 s, 60°C for 30 s, 68°C for 2 min—increase the 68°C step by 20 s at each cycle.
   1 cycle at 68°C for 7 min.
8. After completion of the PCR, assess the size of each amplification product by electrophoresis of 5 μL of the PCR product mixed with 1 μL gel loading buffer on a 2.0% agarose gel, using the SPP1 size marker. The no-template control sample should not contain an amplified product. If it does, the PCR should be repeated. The positive control should have a detectable product, otherwise the PCR should be repeated (*see* **Note 2**). If a product is present of the correct size (1504 bp for b2a2, 1579 bp for b3a2, and 1641 bp for e1a2), purify the PCR product using the UltraClean Purification kit according to the manufacturer's instructions.
9. If a faint product of the correct size is visible or if no product is present, the second-step PCR is required. Purify the PCR product using the UltraClean Purification kit according to the manufacturer's instructions. Do not purify the no-template control.
10. Thaw the PCR reagents and second-step primers (the second-step reverse primer is the same as the first-step reverse primer) and mix thoroughly before use (except for the enzyme, which is stored at −20°C until added to the master mix). Centrifuge briefly to collect the material at the bottom of the tube.
11. Prepare a master mix on ice by adding the following to a 1.5-mL tube for each patient sample + 1 positive control + 1 no-template control + 1: 0.75 μL MgCl$_2$, 1.25 μL dNTP (15 m*M* mix), 2.5 μL 10X Expand long template Buffer 3, 0.15 μL of the forward and reverse primers (final concentration of 0.3 μ*M* each), 0.375 μL of 5 U/μL Expand long template enzyme mix, and sterile water to a total volume of 23 μL.
12. Mix the tubes thoroughly and centrifuge briefly to collect the mix at the bottom

of the tube.
13. Pipet 23 μL of the master mix into 0.2-mL tubes.
14. In a laboratory that is separate from the PCR setup and cDNA addition laboratories, add 2 μL of the purified PCR products that require the second-step PCR and 2 μL of the first-step no-template control to the 0.2-mL tubes. Mix thoroughly and centrifuge briefly to collect the mix at the bottom of the tube.
15. Transfer the reactions to the thermal cycler and amplify with the following conditions:
   1 cycle at 94°C for 2 min.
   10 cycles at 94°C for 10 s, 60°C for 30 s, 68°C for 2 min.
   30 cycles at 94°C for 10 s, 60°C for 30 s, 68°C for 2 min—increase the 68°C step by 20 s at each cycle.
   1 cycle at 68°C for 7 min.
16. After completion of the PCR, assess the size of each amplification product by electrophoresis of 5 μL of the PCR product mixed with 1 μL gel loading buffer on a 2.0% agarose gel, using the SPP1 size marker. The no-template control sample should not contain an amplified product, but if it does, the PCR should be repeated. If a product of the correct size (863 bp) is obtained from the patient samples, purify the PCR product using the UltraClean Purification kit according to the manufacturer's instructions. Additional bands may be present on the gel that may or may not interfere with the sequencing reaction (*see* **Note 3**).
17. The samples are ready for the sequencing reaction and are stored at 4°C after completion.

3.2. Sequencing Reaction

Sequencing reactions are performed in the forward and reverse directions. The primers used are the second-step forward primer and the first-step reverse primer. The primers will allow sequencing of a region that encompasses the entire *BCR-ABL* kinase domain. The amount of purified product added to the sequencing reaction may be varied if required (*see* **Note 4**).

1. Thaw the Big Dye 3 sequencing reagent on ice, while protecting from the light. Thaw the primers, mix, and centrifuge briefly to collect the material at the bottom of the tube.
2. Prepare two master mixes on ice for the forward and reverse sequencing reactions, one containing the forward primer and one containing the reverse primer. For each mix, pipet the following into a 1.5-mL tube for each sample + 1: 4 μL of Big Dye 3 sequencing reagent, 0.3 μL primer (final concentration of 0.75 μ*M*), and sterile water to a total volume of 18 μL. The volume of master mix prepared may need to be adjusted for samples that produce faint amplified products (*see* **Note 4**).
3. Mix the tubes thoroughly and centrifuge briefly to collect the mix at the bottom of the tube.
4. Pipet 18 μL (*see* **Note 4**) of each master mix into 0.2-mL tubes.
5. In a laboratory that is separate from the PCR setup and cDNA addition laborato-

ries, add 2 μL of the purified PCR product (*see* **Note 4**) to the two tubes containing the forward and reverse mixes. Mix thoroughly and centrifuge briefly to collect the mix at the bottom of the tube.

6. Transfer the reactions to the thermal cycler and amplify with the following conditions:
1 cycle at 96°C for 10 s.
25 cycles at 50°C for 5 s, 60°C for 4 min.
Hold at 4°C.
7. After completion of the reaction, the reaction product is purified. The tubes may be stored at 4°C before purification but must be protected from the light by covering with foil.
8. Add 80 μL of 75% isopropanol to the reaction product and mix by drawing into the pipet tip several times.
9. Add the mix to a 1.5-mL tube that contains 1 μL of glycogen.
10. Vortex thoroughly and leave at room temperature for 15 min.
11. Centrifuge at 12,000*g* for 20 min to pellet the DNA. Place the tubes with the hinge of the lid facing outwards to ensure that the location of the pellet is standardized after centrifugation. This will help to avoid contact with the pellet during removal of the supernatant.
12. Immediately after the centrifuge has stopped, carefully remove the supernatant without disturbing the pellet. If there is any delay between centrifugation and removal of the supernatant, re-centrifuge the tubes for a further 2 min to ensure that the pellet does not redissolve.
13. Add 250 μL of 75% isopropanol and vortex thoroughly. Centrifuge for 5 min at 12,000*g*. Place the tubes with the hinge of the lid facing outwards as before.
14. Immediately after the centrifuge has stopped, carefully remove the supernatant without disturbing the pellet. If there is any delay between centrifugation and removal of the supernatant, re-centrifuge the tubes for a further 2 min to ensure that the pellet does not redissolve.
15. Centrifuge again briefly and remove all traces of the isopropanol.
16. Place the tubes with the lid open into a 55°C heating block for 1 to 2 min until all the isopropanol has evaporated. Ensure that the pellet is still visible and has not been inadvertently removed during the purification procedure.
17. The pellets are stored at −20°C until analysis on the sequencer.
18. The sequencing files are analyzed using Mutation Surveyor software (*see* **Note 5**).

4. Notes

1. The reliability of the procedure to detect mutations is very dependent on the quality of the RNA. Poor quality samples are excluded from analysis for this reason. Procedures have been adopted to minimize RNA degradation, and include processing the samples into Trizol RNA stabilization solution (Invitrogen Life Technologies, Carlsbad, CA) within hours of collection. Samples are stored at room temperature if there is a delay in processing. We have found that storage at 4°C will rapidly degrade the *BCR-ABL* mRNA. Samples collected at other sites are stored in Trizol at −80°C before delivery to the laboratory on dry ice. The quality

of the RNA is assessed prior to sequencing using real-time quantitative PCR to determine the levels of *BCR-ABL* mRNA and a control mRNA. A cutoff level based on the number of detectable *BCR* control transcripts in the sample was established as an indicator of degraded RNA. When samples that did not comply with these cutoff values are used for mutation analysis, unreliable results may be obtained, as evidenced by conflicting results between repeat analyses. The cutoff value varies depending on the level of the *BCR-ABL* transcripts. For patients with very low *BCR-ABL* levels it is particularly important that the sample is of high quality; otherwise, the sample will not amplify in the two-step PCR. The indicators used in our analysis are: *BCR* values of >100,000 transcripts if the BCR-*ABL/BCR* ratio is <0.1% (patients with very low *BCR-ABL* levels), *BCR* values of >50,000 transcripts if the *BCR-ABL/BCR* ratio is 0.1% to 1.0%, and *BCR* values >7,000 transcripts if the *BCR-ABL/BCR* ratio is >1.0%. Individual laboratories will need to determine an appropriate method to indicate adequate quality RNA if the real-time technique is not available. To allow amplification of samples with very low *BCR-ABL* values in the second-step PCR, the amount of cDNA added to the first-step PCR is increased. For patients with *BCR-ABL/BCR* ratios of less than 1.0%, 3µL of cDNA (150 ng) is added. These patients usually have a complete cytogenetic response to imatinib and a lower incidence of acquired resistance. However, we have detected mutations in some patients with this level of response, and it is therefore important that the mutation technique be optimized to allow analysis in these patients *(16)*. For patients with higher *BCR-ABL* levels, 2µL of cDNA (100 ng) is usually adequate to amplify a suitable product in the first-step PCR. The amount of master mix and cDNA added for each patient is therefore tailored to the *BCR-ABL* level.

2. The accuracy of mutation detection is also dependent on the efficiency of the PCR reaction. For this reason a quality control sample that has a mid-range *BCR-ABL* level (approx 1.0–8.0% *BCR-ABL/BCR*%) is used to monitor the PCR. This level of *BCR-ABL* is within the range of values that is equivalent to a partial cytogenetic response (Philadelphia chromosome level 1–35%). As an indication of adequate efficiency of PCR amplification, the positive control should amplify in the first-step PCR. We have found that failure to amplify correctly in the first-step PCR may lead to inaccuracy of mutation analysis, and low-abundance mutations may not be detectable if the second-step PCR proceeds. For this reason, the first-step PCR is repeated if the quality control sample fails to produce a band of the correct size on the agarose gel.

3. On occasion, additional bands are visualized on the agarose gel after PCR amplification that may interfere with the sequencing analysis. In the second-step PCR, a product of approx 1600 bp is sometimes present in addition to the correct band of 863 bp. The larger band is the first-round product and will not interfere with the sequencing reaction. However, bands of a smaller size than 863 bp represent artifact amplification and will interfere with the sequencing reaction. During method optimization it was found that alternative transcription occurred in some samples and produced a PCR product with ABL exon 7 spliced out. When the

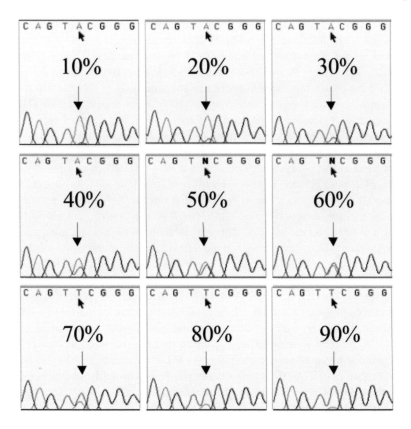

Fig. 2. Determination of the sensitivity of mutation analysis. The sensitivity of the mutation analysis was determined by preparing a dilution series of a *BCR-ABL*-expressing cell line that contained the Y253F mutation into a cell line containing the wild-type *BCR-ABL* sequence, in 10% increments. The wild-type sequence contains an adenine at the nucleotide indicated by an arrow. The mutant sequence contains a thymine at this position. The mutant was first reliably detected at a level of 20% and became the predominant nucleotide at 70%. The N indicates that approximately equal amounts of mutant and wild type were detected at a concentration of 50% and 60%.

PCR for these samples was repeated, the correct product was amplified. When products are present after amplification of a smaller than expected size, the PCR reaction should be repeated.

4. We have not found it necessary to calculate the concentration of the purified PCR product before addition to the sequencing reaction. Visual analysis of the intensity of the product on an agarose gel is adequate to determine the volume to add to the reaction. The Big Dye sequencing chemistry is suitable for a broad range of concentrations and 2 µL of product produces good quality sequencing for most

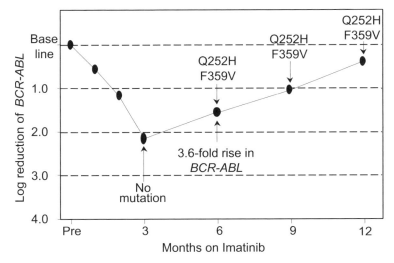

Fig. 3. Acquisition of mutations is associated with resistance to imatinib, as shown by rising levels of *BCR-ABL* transcripts. The graph represents the log reduction of *BCR-ABL* transcripts from the baseline level in a newly diagnosed chronic-phase patient treated with imatinib. The patient achieved a complete cytogenetic response by 3 mo of imatinib therapy, after which there was a steady increase in the *BCR-ABL* level and loss of a major cytogenetic response (defined as Philadelphia chromosome present in 0–35% of metaphases). Two kinase-domain mutations became detectable at the time of the *BCR-ABL* increase, which corresponded with the loss of imatinib response.

samples. The volume of product may be increased successfully by up to 8 µL for samples producing very faint bands on an agarose gel. The volume of water added to the reaction is adjusted accordingly.

5. Analysis of the sequence is performed using software that aligns the forward and reverse sequences against a reference sequence of the *ABL* kinase domain. Any variation from the reference sequence is highlighted. The sequence we use is GenBank accession number M14752. However, we have found that this sequence has a number of nucleotides within the kinase domain that differ from other ABL sequences in GenBank, including mRNA sequence X16416 and the DNA sequence U07563 as well as the sequence found in patients. The discrepant nucleotides are 894 A>G, 1062 A>G, 1334 G>T, 1335 T>G, 1375 A>G (the first nucleotides are those published in M14752). It is therefore important that a correct reference sequence be used to determine true nucleotide substitutions. The entire chromatogram is carefully inspected to ensure that the sequencing is of adequate quality to allow true mutations to be detected. Poor quality sequencing may have high background levels that interfere with analysis. In this situation, the sequencing reaction should be repeated. When mutations are detected in patients for the first time, the whole procedure, including RT-PCR and quantitative PCR, is repeated using a second RNA sample from the same time-point if available, or

from the same RNA if a second sample is not available. Detection of the mutation is considered confirmed only if the same mutation is detected in the repeat analysis. The PCR procedures can be performed within 2 d. To determine the sensitivity of the assay, a *BCR-ABL*-expressing cell line containing the Y253F mutation was mixed with wild-type *BCR-ABL*-expressing cells from 10% to 90% in 10% increments. RNA was extracted from each sample using the Trizol procedure and mutation analysis was performed in duplicate. The *BCR-ABL* mutant was clearly detected at a dilution ratio of 20% (**Fig. 2**). The patients in our center are monitored for mutations approximately every 6 mo, and more frequently if mutations are already present. There is a strong correlation between an increase in the *BCR-ABL* level as monitored by real-time quantitative PCR and the detection of mutations. For this reason, the frequency of mutation analysis is increased when the *BCR-ABL* level increases (**Fig. 3**).

Acknowledgments

The authors thank Dr Barney Rudzki, Rebecca Lawrence, and Chani Field for assistance in the preparation of the manuscript.

References

1. Daley, G. Q., Van Etten, R. A., and Baltimore, D. (1990) Induction of chronic myelogenous leukemia in mice by the P210bcr/abl gene of the Philadelphia chromosome. *Science* **247,** 824–830.
2. Heisterkamp, N., Jenster, G., ten Hoeve, J., Zovich, D., Pattengale, P. K., and Groffen, J. (1990) Acute leukaemia in bcr/abl transgenic mice. *Nature* **344,** 251–253.
3. Elefanty, A. G., Hariharan, I. K., and Cory, S. (1990) bcr-abl, the hallmark of chronic myeloid leukaemia in man, induces multiple haemopoietic neoplasms in mice. *EMBO J.* **9,** 1069–1078.
4. Druker, B. J., Talpaz, M., Resta, D. J., et al. (2001) Efficacy and safety of a specific inhibitor of the BCR-ABL tyrosine kinase in chronic myeloid leukemia. *N. Engl. J. Med.* **344,** 1031–1037.
5. Druker, B. J., Sawyers, C. L., Kantarjian, H., et al. (2001) Activity of a specific inhibitor of the BCR-ABL tyrosine kinase in the blast crisis of chronic myeloid leukemia and acute lymphoblastic leukemia with the Philadelphia chromosome. *N. Engl. J. Med.* **344,** 1038–1042.
6. Talpaz, M., Silver, R. T., Druker, B. J., et al. (2002) Imatinib induces durable hematologic and cytogenetic responses in patients with accelerated phase chronic myeloid leukemia: results of a phase 2 study. *Blood* **99,** 1928–1937.
7. Kantarjian, H., Sawyers, C., Hochhaus, A., et al. (2002) Hematologic and cytogenetic responses to imatinib mesylate in chronic myelogenous leukemia. *N. Engl. J. Med.* **346,** 645–652.
8. O'Brien, S. G., Guilhot, F., Larson, R. A., et al. (2003) Imatinib compared with interferon and low-dose cytarabine for newly diagnosed chronic-phase chronic myeloid leukemia. *N. Engl. J. Med.* **348,** 994–1004.
9. Sawyers, C. L., Hochhaus, A., Feldman, E., et al. (2002) Imatinib induces hema-

tologic and cytogenetic responses in patients with chronic myelogenous leukemia in myeloid blast crisis: results of a phase II study. *Blood* **99**, 3530–3539.

10. Schindler, T., Bornmann, W., Pellicena, P., Miller, W. T., Clarkson, B. and Kuriyan, J. (2000) Structural mechanism for STI-571 inhibition of abelson tyrosine kinase. *Science* **289**, 1938–1942.

11. Nagar, B., Bornmann, W. G., Pellicena, P., et al. (2002) Crystal structures of the kinase domain of c-Abl in complex with the small molecule inhibitors PD173955 and imatinib (STI-571). *Cancer Res.* **62**, 4236–4243.

12. Gambacorti-Passerini, C., le Coutre, P., Mologni, L., et al. (1997) Inhibition of the ABL kinase activity blocks the proliferation of BCR/ABL+ leukemic cells and induces apoptosis. *Blood Cells Mol. Dis.* **23**, 380–394.

13. Deininger, M. W., Goldman, J. M., Lydon, N., and Melo, J. V. (1997) The tyrosine kinase inhibitor CGP57148B selectively inhibits the growth of BCR-ABL-positive cells. *Blood* **90**, 3691–3698.

14. Gorre, M. E., Mohammed, M., Ellwood, K., et al. (2001) Clinical resistance to STI-571 cancer therapy caused by BCR-ABL gene mutation or amplification. *Science* **293**, 876–880.

15. Shah, N. P., Nicoll, J. M., Nagar, B., et al. (2002) Multiple BCR-ABL kinase domain mutations confer polyclonal resistance to the tyrosine kinase inhibitor imatinib (STI571) in chronic phase and blast crisis chronic myeloid leukemia. *Cancer Cell* **2**, 117–125.

16. Branford, S., Rudzki, Z., Walsh, S., et al. (2003) Detection of BCR-ABL mutations in patients with CML treated with imatinib is virtually always accompanied by clinical resistance, and mutations in the ATP phosphate-binding loop (P-loop) are associated with a poor prognosis. *Blood* **102**, 276–283.

17. Hochhaus, A., Kreil, S., Corbin, A. S., et al. (2002) Molecular and chromosomal mechanisms of resistance to imatinib (STI571) therapy. *Leukemia* **16**, 2190–2196.

18. von Bubnoff, N., Schneller, F., Peschel, C., and Duyster, J. (2002) BCR-ABL gene mutations in relation to clinical resistance of Philadelphia-chromosome-positive leukaemia to STI571: a prospective study. *Lancet* **359**, 487–491.

19. Roche-Lestienne, C., Soenen-Cornu, V., Grardel-Duflos, N., et al. (2002) Several types of mutations of the Abl gene can be found in chronic myeloid leukemia patients resistant to STI571, and they can pre-exist to the onset of treatment. *Blood* **100**, 1014–1018.

20. Kreill, S., Mueller, M., Hanfstein, B., et al. (2003) Management and clinical outcome of CML patients after imatinib resistance associated with ABL kinase domain mutations [abstract]. *Blood* **102**, 71a.

21. Al-Ali, H. K., Heinrich, M. C., Lange, T., et al. (2004) High incidence of BCR-ABL kinase domain mutations and absence of mutations of the PDGFR and KIT activation loops in CML patients with secondary resistance to imatinib. *Hematol. J.* **5**, 55–60.

22. Gambacorti-Passerini, C. B., Gunby, R. H., Piazza, R., Galietta, A., Rostagno, R., and Scapozza, L. (2003) Molecular mechanisms of resistance to imatinib in Philadelphia-chromosome-positive leukaemias. *Lancet Oncol.* **4**, 75–85.

23. Azam, M., Latek, R. R., and Daley, G. Q. (2003) Mechanisms of autoinhibition

and STI-571/imatinib resistance revealed by mutagenesis of BCR-ABL. *Cell* **112**, 831–843.

24. Corbin, A. S., Buchdunger, E., Pascal, F., and Druker, B. J. (2002) Analysis of the structural basis of specificity of inhibition of the Abl kinase by STI571. *J. Biol. Chem.* **277**, 32,214–32,219.

25. Corbin, A. S., La Rosee, P., Stoffregen, E. P., Druker, B. J., and Deininger, M. W. (2003) Several Bcr-Abl kinase domain mutants associated with imatinib mesylate resistance remain sensitive to imatinib. *Blood* **101**, 4611–4614.

26. Branford, S., Rudzki, Z., Miller, B., et al. (2003) Mutations in the catalytic core (P-loop) of the BCR-ABL kinase domain of imatinib-treated chronic myeloid leukemia patients in chronic phase are strongly associated with imminent progression to blast crisis [abstract]. *Blood* **102**, 71a.

27. Shah, N. P. and Sawyers, C. L. (2003) Mechanisms of resistance to STI571 in Philadelphia chromosome-associated leukemias. *Oncogene* **22**, 7389–7395.

28. Branford, S., Rudzki, Z., Walsh, S., et al. (2002) High frequency of point mutations clustered within the adenosine triphosphate-binding region of BCR/ABL in patients with chronic myeloid leukemia or Ph-positive acute lymphoblastic leukemia who develop imatinib (STI571) resistance. *Blood* **99**, 3472–3475.

29. Branford, S., Hughes, T. P. and Rudzki, Z. (1999) Monitoring chronic myeloid leukaemia therapy by real-time quantitative PCR in blood is a reliable alternative to bone marrow cytogenetics. *Br. J. Haematol.* **107**, 587–599.

6

Deletion of the Derivative Chromosome 9 in Chronic Myeloid Leukemia

Lynda J. Campbell

Summary

With the development of fluorescence *in situ* hybridization (FISH), it was possible to detect the *BCR-ABL* fusion signal in both metaphase spreads and interphase cells of patients with chronic myeloid leukemia (CML). However, the use of FISH to detect residual disease in patients with CML post therapy was limited by the false positive rate using the early single fusion probes. Therefore, dual fusion probes that created a fusion signal on the derivative chromosome 9 in addition to the fusion sifnal on the Philadelphia chromosome or derivative chromosome 22 were developed. Using these second-generation probes, it was discovered that a significant proportion of CML cases has a sub-microscopic deletion at the site of the *ABL-BCR* fusion. This chapter outlines a testing strategy to identify deleltions of the derivative chromosome 9 and to use combinations of probes to identify residual disease in these cases.

Key Words: Cytogenetic; karyotype; interstitial deletion; fluorescence *in situ* hybridization; *BCR*; *ABL*; derivative chromosome.

1. Introduction

The hallmark discoveries of the genetics of chronic myeloid leukemia (CML) have mirrored the evolution of the fields of cytogenetics and molecular genetics. CML was first recognized as a distinct entity in 1845, but it was not until 1960, when Nowell and Hungerford identified a small marker chromosome (known as the Philadelphia chromosome) in the blood of patients with CML, that cancer cytogenetics was born. The abnormality was identified as a reciprocal translocation between chromosomes 9 and 22 by Janet Rowley in 1973. Subsequently, the underlying genetic events were described in the 1980s, with the translocation found to produce a fusion gene, *BCR-ABL*, at the site of the breakpoint on the derivative chromosome 22, der(22) *(1)*. It was also established that the single translocation event produced two fusion genes, a *BCR-*

From: *Methods in Molecular Medicine, Vol. 125: Myeloid Leukemia: Methods and Protocols*
Edited by: H. Iland, M. Hertzberg, and P. Marlton © Humana Press Inc., Totowa, NJ

ABL fusion on der(22) and an *ABL-BCR* fusion on the derivative chromosome 9, der(9).

The development of fluorescence *in situ* hybridization (FISH) and probes to detect the presence of the *ABL* and *BCR* genes enabled the *BCR-ABL* fusion to be visualized as co-localization of signals that could be identified in both metaphase chromosome spreads and also in nondividing interphase cells. Being able to detect a *BCR-ABL* fusion in interphase cells also opened up the possibility of detecting minimal residual disease (MRD) via FISH in patients after therapy or stem cell transplantation. However, the first *BCR/ABL* probes available suffered from a relatively high false-positive rate, with accidental co-localization of signals observed in approx 5% of interphase cells on normal control slides *(2)*. A second generation of probes was developed, so that either an extra signal remained on the der(9) proximal to the breakpoint or a second fusion signal was generated on the der(9) in the presence of the t(9;22)(q34;q11·2) *(3)*.

Study of CML cases using second-generation probes identified a subset of patients with CML who appeared to have a sub-microscopic interstitial deletion of the der(9) in the region of the *ABL-BCR* fusion. Approximately 15% of patients with the standard t(9;22)(q34;q11·2) and a higher percentage of patients with complex translocations showed evidence of an interstitial deletion that involved both 9q and 22q sequences on the der(9) (*see* **Fig. 1**). In some cases, these deletions appeared to extend for megabases on either side of the 9q34;22q11·2 breakpoint. It was also determined that the deletion had occurred at the time of translocation and was either present or absent in all cells containing the t(9;22) *(4–7)*.

Importantly, a der(9) deletion appeared to influence prognosis. Patients with der(9) deletions were shown to have an inferior outcome compared with those who showed no evidence of a deletion. In a study by Sinclair et al. *(4)*, the median survival of CML patients with a der(9) deletion was 36 mo vs >90 mo for patients with no deletion. The deletion status was independent of either the Sokal or the Hasford/European prognostic scoring systems. Deletion status appeared to predict outcome in patients treated with hydroxyurea or interferon or, preliminary evidence suggested, stem cell transplantation.

The mechanism by which the deletion confers an inferior outcome has remained uncertain. Patients with a deletion failed to express the *ABL-BCR* transcript, but the effect on prognosis appeared to be independent of *ABL-BCR* expression *(8,9)*. The most likely explanation for the effect on outcome appears to be that the deletion removed an as yet unidentified tumor suppressor gene or genes. When a third chromosome has been involved in a complex 9;22 translocation, the deletion has been shown to involve the third derivative chromosome as well. Anelli et al. described a t(9;22;11) with loss of 9q34, 22q11·2,

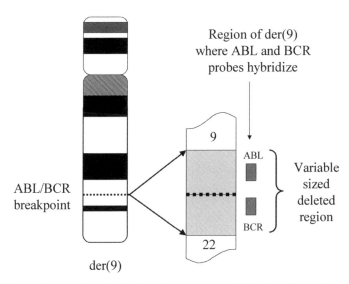

Fig. 1. The region on the derivative chromosome 9 that is affected by interstitial deletions. Deletion of the derivative chromosome 9 at the *ABL/BCR* breakpoint usually results in loss of both chromosome 9 and chromosome 22 sequences on either side of the breakpoint.

and 11q13 sequences, causing deletion of genes known to be involved in apoptosis and cell proliferation control *(10)*.

The studies identifying the inferior outcome of patients with der(9) deletions were, for the most part, retrospective and performed in the pre-imatinib era. Whether the adverse prognosis associated with these deletions still persisted for patients treated with imatinib was an important question. Initial studies have suggested that the poor prognosis may be at least partly abrogated by imatinib therapy *(11)*. Huntly et al. showed no difference in overall survival between patients with and without deletions in a large cohort of patients treated with imatinib. However, they did show the time to disease progression was considerably shorter and both hematological and cytogenetic response rates lower in patients with a deletion. The follow-up period of this study was 48 mo and 49 mo, respectively, for patients with and without deletions. It will be interesting to observe whether differences in overall survival emerge over time.

Despite the unanswered question regarding the prognostic implication of identifying the deletion, it is regarded as good practice to test all new cases of CML with FISH to ascertain whether a deletion has occurred. There are a number of probes available to detect *BCR-ABL* fusion signals. Not all will identify a deletion. Moreover, once a deletion has been identified, few of the currently available probes are suitable for detection of MRD in those cases. **Figure 2** illustrates some of the most commonly used probes. The probe shown in **Fig.**

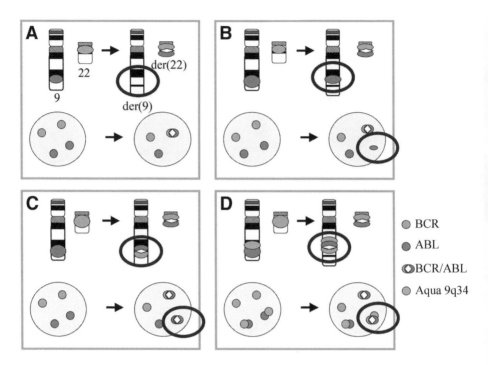

Fig. 2. Fluorescent signal patterns seen with *BCR/ABL* probes. Depending on the probe strategy employed, several fluorescent signal patterns can be seen with *BCR/ABL* probes (signals that are lost when the der(9) is deleted are circled): (A) single fusion *BCR/ABL* probe results in a fusion signal only on the der(22) with no signal on the der(9) and so no ability to detect deletion of the der(9); (B) extra signal or ES probe with a single fusion on the der(22) and a small extra red signal generated on the der(9) will detect deletions involving chromosome 9 but not chromosome 22 sequences on the der(9); (C) dual fusion probe generating an *ABL/BCR* fusion signal on the der(9) and a *BCR/ABL* signal on the der(22); (D) dual fusion probe with an added aqua-labeled 9q34 probe.

2A, a single fusion probe, cannot identify der(9) deletions. Probes shown in **Fig. 2B,C** can be used to identify deletions. However, their use in MRD detection requires the addition of an aqua-labeled 9q34 probe, as illustrated in **Fig. 2D**, where an aqua-labeled 9q34 probe has been added to the dual fusion probe shown in **Fig. 2C**. It has been common practice in our laboratory to monitor patients with demonstrated deletions using a cocktail of dual fusion *BCR/ABL* probes with an aqua-labeled 9q34 probe added. This approach was recently validated by Smoley et al., who confirmed that the mixture effectively discriminated between cells with overlapping *BCR* and *ABL* signals and those with a true *BCR/ABL* fusion, allowing quantification of MRD *(12)*.

The following method is based on the FISH method described in Chapter 2, with particular reference to its use in CML cases.

2. Materials

1. Chromosome suspension produced according to the protocol outlined in Chapter 2. A cell suspension derived from any of the three cultures described would be suitable for FISH (*see* **Note 1**).
2. *BCR/ABL* dual color dual fusion translocation probe (*see* **Note 2**).
3. 9q34 aqua-labeled probe (*see* **Note 2**).
4. Reagents outlined in Chapter 2 for use in FISH studies.

3. Methods

In all newly diagnosed cases of CML, FISH should be performed following the method outlined in Chapter 2, using a *BCR/ABL* dual-color dual-fusion translocation probe (*see* **Note 3**).

When FISH slides are prepared for analysis, at least 10 metaphase spreads and/or 50 interphase cells should be scored (*see* **Note 4**). All FISH slides should be scored by two individuals and representative images captured via an image analysis system or photographed and stored.

A deletion of the der(9) is indicated by the presence of only one fusion signal per cell, located on the der(22) or Philadelphia chromosome. The second fusion signal that would normally be found on the der(9) is not present. The karyotype should be expressed according to the FISH nomenclature outlined in ISCN (1995) *(13)* (*see* **Note 5**).

To use FISH to look for MRD in a case with a demonstrated deletion of the der(9), add a 9q34 aqua-labeled probe to the probe/hybridization buffer mixture (*see* Subheading 3.3., step 4 in Chapter 2). The combined probe/buffer mixture consists of: 1 µL *BCR/ABL* dual fusion probe/1 µL 9q34 probe/1 µL purified H_2O/7 µL hybridization buffer (*see* **Note 6**).

Proceed through the subsequent FISH steps according to the protocol in Chapter 2.

Cells should be scored, looking specifically for *BCR/ABL* (red/green) fusion signals. When assessing MRD, it is preferable to score at least 200 to 300 interphase cells. Only when a *BCR/ABL* fusion signal is identified, is it necessary to score the additional aqua 9q34 probe. If the cell contains a true fusion signal (instead of an incidental co-localization of *ABL* and *BCR* signals), the deletion of the der(9) that has resulted in only one fusion signal being seen will also result in the deletion of one aqua 9q34 signal. Thus, a cell containing the t(9;22) will contain one fusion signal/one red (*ABL*) signal/one green (*BCR*) signal/one aqua (9q34) signal, whereas a false-positive cell will contain one fusion signal/one red (*ABL*) signal/one green (*BCR*) signal/*two* aqua (9q34) signals (*see* **Note 7**).

4. Notes

1. The diagnostic marrow or blood sample for all new CML cases should have two cultures established for conventional cytogenetic analysis; at the Victorian Cancer Cytogenetics Service (VCCS), two synchronized cultures are set up, one inoculated with less sample than the other. A marrow or blood sample from a patient with untreated CML may grow so aggressively in culture that as little as one drop of marrow added to a 10-mL culture is sufficient to produce several milliliters of suspension. CML cells are relatively robust, and a successful cytogenetic result may be obtained from a specimen taken 2 to 3 d before cultures are initiated.
2. The quantities of probe and hybridization buffer described are recommended for Vysis® probes. When using probes from other suppliers, check the product insert for exact quantities.
3. There are a number of probes available that produce signals to identify the presence of both the *BCR/ABL* fusion on der(22) and the *ABL/BCR* fusion on der(9). The use of a dual fusion probe is preferred, because it will identify the cases with loss of only chromosome 9 or chromosome 22 sequences on the der(9). Most cases show loss of both 9 and 22 sequences, indicating that an extensive deletion has occurred (*see* **Fig. 1**).
4. Ideally, metaphase spreads should be identified and the location of the fusion signals confirmed on the der(22) and der(9). In patients with a deletion of the der(9), only the der(22) *BCR/ABL* fusion signal will be observed, together with signals identifying the normal copies of *ABL* and *BCR* on chromosomes 9 and 22, respectively. However, if metaphases cannot be located, the pattern of two fusion signals/one red (*ABL*) signal/one green (*BCR*) signal indicates the presence of the t(9;22) without a deletion of the der(9); the pattern of one fusion signal/one red (*ABL*) signal/one green (*BCR*) signal indicates the presence of the t(9;22) with a deletion of the der(9). The latter pattern of signals in interphase may also reflect a false-positive cell with incidental co-localization of one red and one green signal to simulate a fusion signal. Thus, this pattern is useful only in confirming the presence of the t(9;22) when it is seen in 10% or more of interphase cells *(2)*.
5. The standard karyotype for an individual with chronic myeloid leukemia as assessed by conventional cytogenetics is 46,XX or XY,t(9;22)(q34;q11·2). When metaphase FISH with a dual fusion probe is added, the karyotype becomes 46,XX,t(9;22)(q34;q11·2).ish t(9;22)(*ABL*+,*BCR*+;*BCR*+,*ABL*+), indicating that there are positive fluorescent signals for both *ABL* and *BCR* on the der(9) and the der(22). When a deletion has been identified, the karyotype becomes 46,XX,t(9;22)(q34;q11).ish t(9;22)(*ABL*–,*BCR*–;*BCR*+,*ABL*+), showing that the expected *ABL* and *BCR* signals on the der(9) are missing. There is considerable controversy surrounding the interpretation of the FISH nomenclature guidelines *(13)*. However, any changes must await the next edition of the International System for Human Cytogenetic Nomenclature (ISCN).
6. If a deletion has been identified, studies performed after therapy to assess response to therapy cannot be reliably interpreted using any of the dual-color dual-fusion or extra signal probes, unless an additional probe is added to the probe mixture (*see* **Fig. 2**).

7. As the added 9q34 probe is labeled with an aqua fluorescent signal, it may be difficult to visualize against the pale blue 4′,6′-diamidino-2-phenylindole (DAPI) counterstain if the DAPI stain is strong. Further dilution of DAPI with extra antifade solution is advised.

References

1. Goldman, J. M. and Melo, J. V. (2003) Chronic myeloid leukemia—advances in biology and new approaches to treatment. *N. Engl. J. Med.* **349,** 1451–1464.
2. Chase, A., Grand, F., Zhang, J. G., Blackett, N., Goldman, J., and Gordon, M. (1997) Factors influencing the false positive and negative rates of BCR-ABL fluorescence in situ hybridization. *Genes Chrom Cancer* **18,** 246–253.
3. Dewald, G. W., Wyatt, W. A., Juneau, A. L., et al. (1998) Highly sensitive fluorescence in situ hybridization method to detect double BCR/ABL fusion and monitor response to therapy in chronic myeloid leukemia. *Blood* **91,** 3357–3365.
4. Sinclair, P. B., Nacheva, E. P., Leversha, M., et al. (2000) Large deletions at the t(9;22) breakpoint are common and may identify a poor-prognosis subgroup of patients with chronic myeloid leukemia. *Blood* **95,** 738–744.
5. Herens, C., Tassin, F., Lemaire, V., et al. (2000) Deletion of the 5′-ABL region: a recurrent anomaly detected by fluorescence in situ hybridization in about 10% of Philadelphia-positive chronic myeloid leukemia patients. *Br. J. Haematol.* **110,** 214–216.
6. Huntly, B. J. P., Reid, A. G., Bench, A. J., et al. (2001) Deletions of the derivative chromosome 9 occur at the time of the Philadelphia translocation and provide a powerful and independent prognostic indicator in chronic myeloid leukemia. *Blood* **98,** 1732–1738.
7. Kolomietz, E., Al-Maghrabi, J., Brennan, S., et al. (2001) Primary chromosomal rearrangements of leukemia are frequently accompanied by extensive submicroscopic deletions and may lead to altered prognosis. *Blood* **97,** 3581–3588.
8. de la Fuente, J., Merx, K., Steer, E. J., et al. (2001) ABL-BCR expression does not correlate with deletions on the derivative chromosome 9 or survival in chronic myeloid leukemia. *Blood* **98,** 2879–2880.
9. Huntly, B. J. P., Bench, A. J., Delabesse, E., et al. (2002) Derivative chromosome 9 deletions in chronic myeloid leukemia: poor prognosis is not associated with loss of ABL-BCR expression, elevated BCR-ABL levels, or karyotypic instability. *Blood* **99,** 4547–53.
10. Anelli, L., Albano, F., Zagaria, A., et al. (2004) A chronic myelocytic leukemia case bearing deletions on the three chromosomes involved in a variant t(9;22;11). *Cancer Genet. Cytogenet.* **148,** 137–140.
11. Huntly, B. J. P., Guilhot, F., Reid, A. G., et al. (2003) Imatinib improves but may not fully reverse the poor prognosis of patients with CML with derivative chromosome 9 deletions. *Blood* **102,** 2205–2212.
12. Smoley, S. A., Brockman, S. R., Paternoster, S. F., Meyer, R. G., and Dewald, G. W. (2004) A novel tricolor dual-fusion fluorescence in situ hybridisation method to detect BCR/ABL fusion in cells with t(9;22)(q34;q11.2) associated with dele-

tion of DNA on the derivative chromosome 9 in chronic myelocytic leukemia. *Cancer Genet. Cytogenet.* **148,** 1–6.

13. Mitelman, F. (ed) (1995) *An International System for Human Cytogenetic Nomenclature.* S. Karger, Basel.

7

Diagnosis and Monitoring of *PML-RARA*-Positive Acute Promyelocytic Leukemia by Qualitative RT-PCR

Vincenzo Rossi, Laura Levati, and Andrea Biondi

Summary

The t(15;17) is the diagnostic hallmark of acute promyelocytic leukemia (APL). As a result, the RARA and the promyelocytic leukemia (PML) genes are fused. The use of reverse-transcription polymerase chain reaction (RT-PCR) for the detection of the *PML-RARA* and *RARA-PML* fusion genes is the only technique that defines the PML breakpoint type and that allows the definition of a correct strategy for subsequent minimal residual disease (MRD) monitoring. Standardized conditions for RT-PCR analysis of fusion transcripts from chromosome aberrations in acute leukemia, including APL, have recently been reported in the context of the Biomed-1 Concerted Action, and are described in detail in this chapter.

Key Words: Acute promyelocytic leukemia; RT-PCR; t(15;17); fusion transcript; minimal residual disease.

1. Introduction

The t(15;17) is the diagnostic hallmark of acute promyelocytic leukemia (APL) and initially had been considered to be present in all patients with this condition *(1,2)*. Conventional cytogenetics and, more recently, fluorescence *in situ* hybridization (FISH) enable the identification of both derivative chromosomes 15q and 17q, both in the "classic" and variant APL forms *(3)*. At the molecular level, the *RARA* locus is fused with the N-terminal of *PML* (reviewed in **ref. 4**) on chromosome 15q21. The breakpoint on the *RARA* locus occurs invariably in the 17-kb-long intron 2, whereas three different breakpoint regions in the *PML* locus have been defined: intron 6 (breakpoint bcr1, occurring in 55% of the cases), exon 6 (bcr2, 5%), and intron 3 (bcr3, 40%) (**Fig. 1**). Accordingly, three different isoforms of the *PML-RARA* chimeric transcript can be generated, and are named Long (L or bcr1), Variant (V or bcr2), and Short (S or bcr3).

From: *Methods in Molecular Medicine, Vol. 125: Myeloid Leukemia: Methods and Protocols*
Edited by: H. Iland, M. Hertzberg, and P. Marlton © Humana Press Inc., Totowa, NJ

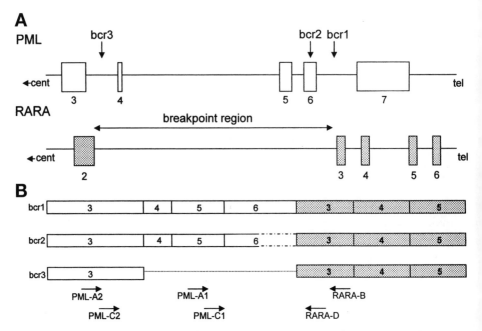

Fig. 1. Schematic diagram of (**A**) exon/intron structure of *PML* and *RARA* genes, and (**B**) the three types of *PML/RARA* fusion transcripts. The arrows indicate the relative primer positions

In addition to *PML*, different partners of *RARA* have been described, including promyelocytic leukemia zinc finger (*PLZF*) on chromosome 11q23 (*5*), nucleolar phosphoprotein nucleophosmin (*NPM*) on chromosome 5q31 (*6*), and nuclear mitotic apparatus protein (*NUMA*) on chromosome 11q13 (*7*). Recently, the *STAT5b* gene, located at 17q21, has been identified as a new *RARA* partner in an APL case associated with a der(17) (*8*).

Reverse-transcription polymerase chain reaction (RT-PCR) for the detection of the *PML-RARA* and *RARA-PML* fusion genes is the only technique that defines the PML breakpoint type and that allows the definition of a correct strategy for subsequent minimal residual disease (MRD) monitoring. The observation that *RARA-PML* transcripts are present in most but not all APL cases has favored the use of *PML-RARA* transcripts as the preferred PCR target for the detection of APL at diagnosis and during monitoring. The advantage of routinely using this assay at diagnosis to better address treatment has been subsequently validated in prospective multicenter trials (reviewed in **refs. *9–11***).

Standardized conditions for RT-PCR analysis of fusion transcripts from chromosome aberrations in acute leukemia, including APL, have been reported in the context of the Biomed-1 Concerted Action (*12*), and are

Table 1
**Primers for Reverse-Transcription Polymerase Chain
Reaction Analysis of *PML-RARA* Fusion Gene**

Primer code	Size	Sequence (5'–3')
PML-A1	21	CAGTGTACGCCTTCTCCATCA
PML-A2	18	CTGCTGGAGGCTGTGGAC
RARA-B	20	GCTTGTAGATGCGGGGTAGA
PML-C1	21	TCAAGATGGAGTCTGAGGAGG
PML-C2	19	AGCGCGACTACGAGGAGAT
RARA-D	20	CTGCTGCTCTGGGTCTCAAT

Table 2
**Size of Polymerase Chain Reaction (PCR) Products for Each of the *PML-RARA*
Primer Sets**

	First-round PCR		Nested PCR	
Primer sets	PML A1–RARA B	PML A2–RARA B	PML C1–RARA D	PML C2–RARA D
bcr 1	381		214	
bcr 2	345*		178*	
bcr 3		376		289

*The size of the bcr2 +ve products is variable as a result of variable breakpoint location within exon 6 of the *PML* gene.

here described in detail. In dilution experiments, a sensitivity of 10^{-2} to 10^{-3} has been reached in first-round PCR, and 10^{-3} to 10^{-4} in nested PCR. The sensitivity is at least one log better for bcr3 than for bcr1/2. **Table 1** shows the sequence of the primers, whereas **Table 2** shows the size of PCR fragments generated as a result of different breakpoint regions in the *PML* locus, and/or the presence of alternative splicing of *PML* transcripts *(4)*. In the case of bcr2 breakpoints, the sizes of PCR fragments are different due to the variability of the breakpoint location within *PML* exon 6.

With respect to the original method we described *(13)*, the Biomed-1 proto-col includes several advantages: (1) a common PCR protocol (annealing tem-perature, MgCl₂ concentration, number of cycles, and so on) can be used for the screening of different translocations in the same group of patients; (2) a standardized method was validated for multicenter studies both for molecular diagnosis and monitoring of leukemia patients. According to most investiga-tors, high-quality RNA and efficient RT are the crucial determinants for suc-cessful RT-PCR of *PML-RARA*. Because of frequent leukopenia and the associated coagulopathy, the yield and quality of RNA from diagnostic samples are frequently poor (*see* **Note 1**).

Several studies have attempted to correlate the type of *PML-RARA* transcript either with clinico-biological features at diagnosis, or with treatment response and outcome (reviewed in **ref. 9**). Because bcr2 and bcr1 are located in PML exon 6 and intron 6, respectively, sequencing of all apparent L transcript cases would be needed to clearly distinguish these two isoforms. Such distinction is usually not reported in clinical studies with a large number of patients. Accordingly, the vast majority of analyzed series have compared the two major *PML-RARA* isoforms (i.e., bcr1 plus bcr2 cases vs bcr3 cases). At diagnosis, no correlation was found with respect to sex, platelet count, presence of coagulopathy, or retinoic acid syndrome, when comparing patients with L-type or S-type *PML-RARA* transcripts. However, patients with S-type transcripts had significantly higher white blood cell counts and more frequently M3v morphology. Although S-type transcripts correlated with established adverse prognostic features (i.e., hyperleukocytosis, M3v), this association did not translate into poorer outcome when compared to patients with L-type transcripts in the context of combined all-trans retinoic acid (ATRA) and chemotherapy treatment *(9–11)*.

Among the different methods (conventional karyotyping, FISH, *PML* immunostaining with specific antibodies, and RT-PCR detection of the *PML-RARA* fusion gene), RT-PCR appears to be the most suitable for MRD detection. For a variety of reasons and because of the relatively low sensitivity of RT-PCR for *PML-RARA*, diagnosis and monitoring of bone marrow (BM) samples is preferred to the use of peripheral blood (PB), especially when the circulating blast cell (or leukemic promyelocyte) count is low. The recently introduced real-time quantitative RT-PCR (RQ-PCR) can also be applied for MRD monitoring.

Overall, there is general agreement that a positive *PML-RARA* test after consolidation is a strong predictor of subsequent hematological relapse, whereas repeatedly negative results are associated with long survival in the majority of patients *(9–11)*. On that basis, positivity at two consecutive tests was suggested to be sufficient for clinical intervention even before clinical relapse occurs *(14)*. However, these correlations are not absolute, as cases have been reported who either remain PCR-positive in long-term remission or, more frequently, ultimately relapse after negative tests *(10,11)*.

2. Materials

2.1. RNA Extraction

1. Guanidinium-isothiocyanate solution (GTC): 4 M guanidinium-isothiocyanate, 0.5% N-lauroylsarcosine, 25 mM Na citrate (pH 7.0), and 0.1 M β-mercaptoethanol.

2. 2.0 M Na acetate, pH 4.0.
3. Acid phenol, pH 4.3.
4. Chloroform-isoamyl alcohol, 49:1.
5. Isopropanol.
6. 75% ethanol kept at –20°C.

2.2. cDNA Synthesis

1. Random hexamers, 5 μM.
2. Diethylpyrocarbonate (DEPC)-treated water or double-distilled water for clinical use.
3. 5X RT buffer: 20 mM Tris-HCl, 50 mM KCl, pH 8.3.
4. dNTP mixture of 10 mM each nucleotide.
5. 0.1 M dithiothreitol (DTT).
6. RNase inhibitor (40 U/μL).
7. Reverse transcriptase enzyme: Superscript II 200 U/μL (Invitrogen, Carlsbad, CA).

2.3. Polymerase Chain Reaction

2.3.1. First-Round PCR Mixture

1. 0.2-mL plastic tube with cap.
2. 16.4 μL of water.
3. 2.5 μL of 10X reaction buffer: 200 mM Tris-HCl (pH 8.4), 500 mM KCl, final concentration 1X.
4. 1.5 μL of 25 mM MgCl$_2$, final concentration 1.5 mM.
5. 0.5 μL of dNTP mix (10 mM each nucleotide), final concentration 0.2 mM.
6. 1.0 μL of 10 μM PML-A1 primer for bcr1/2 or PML-A2 primer for bcr3, final concentration 0.4 μM.
7. 1.0 μL of 10 μM RARA-B primer (for both breakpoints), final concentration 0.4 μM (*see* **Table 1** for sequences).
8. 0.1 μL of Taq DNA polymerase (5 U/μL), final concentration 0.5 U/25 μL.
9. 2.0 μL of cDNA (100 ng of RNA equivalent).
   Final reaction volume 25 μL.

2.3.2. Nested PCR Mixture

1. 17.4 μL of water.
2. 1.0 μL of first-round PCR product (in place of cDNA).
3. Use the same final volume and the same reagents as for the first-round PCR, with the following exception: use PML-C1 for bcr1/2, or PML-C2 for bcr3 as the forward primers, and use RARA-C as the reverse primer for both breakpoints.

2.4. Gel Electrophoresis

1. 5X Tris-borate electrophoresis buffer (TBE): 54 g Tris-base, 27.55 g boric acid, 20 mL of 0.5 M ethylenediamine tetraacetic acid (EDTA). Make up to 1 L and store at room temperature.

2. Ethidium bromide 10 mg/mL; NB: ethidium bromide is carcinogenic; always wear gloves!
3. Loading buffer: 0.25% bromophenol blue, 0.25% xylene cyanide, 25% Ficoll 400.

3. Methods

Always use gloves, sterile tubes, and filter tips for RNA manipulation and RT-PCR to avoid RNA degradation and sample contamination.

3.1. RNA Isolation (see Notes 2 and 3)

If total RNA is extracted using the Chomczynski-Sacchi guanidinium thiocyanate-phenol-chloroform method *(15)*, proceed as follows:

1. Add to the guanidinium thiocyanate cell lysate solution one-tenth volume of 2 *M* NaAc, an equal volume of acid phenol, and one-fifth volume of chloroform-isoamyl alcohol (49:1); vortex and place on ice for 10 min.
2. Spin at 14,000*g* for 10 min at 4°C.
3. Transfer the supernatant into a new tube and add an equal volume of isopropanol; mix well and place at room temperature for 10 min, for precipitation.
4. Spin at 14,000*g* for 15 min at 4°C and remove the supernatant.
5. Wash the pellet with 500 µL of 75% cold ethanol. Spin 3 min at 14,000*g* at 4°C; remove the supernatant.
6. Repeat **step 5**.
7. Dry the pellet in speed-vac for 5 min, then dissolve it in 10–20 µL DEPC-treated water; store at –70°C.
8. Determine the RNA concentration by spectrophotometer at 260 nm, and the integrity by gel electrophoresis (*see* **Note 4**).

3.2. cDNA Synthesis

1. In a 0.5-mL microfuge tube, mix 1 µL of random hexamers and 8 µL of DEPC-treated water.
2. Add 2 µL of total RNA 0.5 µg/µL (*see* **Note 5**).
3. Mix and incubate at 70°C for 3 min.
4. Put on ice, spin briefly and add: 4 µL of 5X RT buffer, 1 µL of 10m*M* mixed dNTP, 2 µ of 0.1 *M* DTT, 1 µL RNase inhibitor, and 1 µL reverse transcriptase; mix very well and place at room temperature for 10 min.
5. Incubate at 42°C for 45 min, at 99°C for 5 min, and at 4°C for 5 min.
6. Store the cDNA at –20°C.

An aliquot of 2 µL of cDNA (equivalent to 100 ng of total RNA) is usually used for the PCR reaction (*see* **Note 6**). The quality of the RNA and the efficiency of the reverse transcriptase reaction should be assessed (*see* **Notes 4** and **7–9**).

3.3. First-Round and Nested PCR Conditions (see Notes 10–13)

1. Initial DNA melting denaturation and Taq polymerase activation: 95°C for 2 min (the time depends on the kind of polymerase that is used).
2. PCR cycles: 94°C for 30 s (melting), 65°C for 30 s (annealing), 72°C for 30 s (extension), for a total of 35 cycles. No final extension is needed.

3.4. Gel Electrophoresis

1. A 1% gel is made by boiling 1 g agarose in 100 mL 1X TBE.
2. Cool to approx 50°C and add 2 μL of ethidium bromide; NB: ethidium bromide is carcinogenic; always wear gloves!
3. Pour the agarose into an appropriate casting tray.
4. At the end of PCR, electrophorese 10 μL of reaction product plus 2 μL of loading buffer for 1 h at 80–90 volts.
5. Examine the results by ultraviolet lamp transilluminator. In positive samples from patients at diagnosis, single bands are usually visualized in first-round PCR analysis. However, multiple PCR bands, caused by alternative splicing of PML exons, can appear in bcr1/2-positive samples when amplified using primers for bcr3 breakpoint identification (*13*) (*see* **Note 14**).

4. Notes

1. The sensitivity of *PML-RARA* fusion gene detection by RT-PCR is lower in comparison with the detection of other fusion genes, such as *BCR-ABL*. It is likely that such a difference is due either to different levels of expression or to greater instability of the *PML-RARA* fusion transcripts. *PML-RARA* mRNA undergoes rapid degradation. We have observed a one-third to one-half log reduction for every 24 h that a BM sample is left at room temperature, as shown in **Fig. 2**. This problem is usually not relevant at diagnosis, but can be crucial for the assessment of MRD during follow-up. As a consequence, analysis can result in a false-negative result, or in the appearance of faint bands in agarose gel electrophoresis despite the presence of appropriate bands for the control genes (*ABL* or *RARA*) that are normally used to assess the quality of the cDNA. Accordingly, the quality of RNA is an essential step in the procedure. **Notes 2–14** reflect several years' experience as the referral diagnostic laboratory in Italy for both adult and childhood APL patients (*9*).
2. *Analysis of BM samples.* Owing to the several critical parameters that we listed, and to the relatively low sensitivity of the RT-PCR, diagnosis and monitoring of BM samples must be preferred to PB, where the blast cells count could be low.
3. *Rapid processing of the bone marrow (BM) sample.* Perform Ficoll-Paque density gradient centrifugation to obtain mononuclear cells (MNC); lyse the sample immediately in GTC, RNAzol, or Trizol; and freeze at –20°C or –70°C. When processed in this way, the sample can be preserved indefinitely. The use of dry pellets of MNC without lysing solution has been suggested by some groups. How-

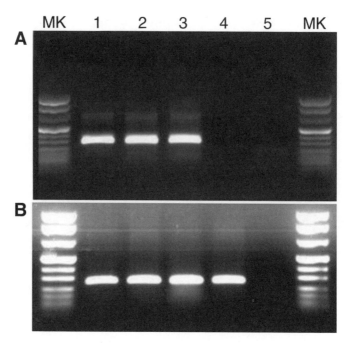

Fig. 2. Ethidium bromide-stained agarose gel showing instability of *PML-RARA* transcripts. The gel shows bcr3 +ve nested polymerase chain reaction (PCR) products. (**A**) 1 = positive control, 2 = BM sample of patient at diagnosis, 3 = follow-up bone marrow (BM) sample that has been processed immediately, 4 = the same follow-up BM sample processed after 24 h and analyzed after 48 h, 5 = negative control (water only, no cDNA template), MK = marker. (**B**) Amplification of Abl-1 control gene for the same samples.

ever, that approach can cause rapid degradation of RNA during the process of freezing and thawing. In our experience, even the immediate lysis of BM samples without Ficoll density separation does not result in RNA samples of good quality for further analysis. Samples that cannot be processed immediately should be kept at 4°C, but not frozen, for not longer than 24 h. If the sample is delivered to a referral laboratory, it should be sent at 4°C. Ficoll density separation should be performed immediately upon receipt of the BM sample, and in any case no later than 24 h following sample collection. The use of nucleic acid preservative reagents has been shown to be useful for increasing RNA stability in PB samples *(16)*, but less effective in BM, and accordingly is not applicable to APL samples.

4. *Integrity of RNA*. An aliquot of RNA is run on 1% agarose gel electrophoresis, and a partial assessment of RNA integrity is based on the presence and quality of RNA ribosomal bands.

5. If necessary, increase the amount of RNA to be retro-transcribed in vitro (2–5 µg instead of the routinely used 1 µg).

6. If necessary, increase the amount of cDNA to be amplified (3–4 µL of cDNA instead of the usual 2 µL).

7. *Improvement of RNA extraction and cDNA synthesis.* As an alternative to the standard Chomczynski-Sacchi guanidinium thiocyanate-phenol-chloroform method, several commercial kits are now available for RNA extraction. RNA and cDNA can now be obtained from a limited number of cells either manually or automatically. For cDNA synthesis, the use of random hexamers instead of oligo-dT results in a better yield, even in the presence of partially degraded RNA. In our hands, the use of random nonamers as cDNA primers does not significantly increase the sensitivity of the test.

8. *Assessment of the efficiency of the reverse transcription reaction.* Perform a PCR to amplify a properly selected control gene using the same cDNA that is being tested for the presence of *PML-RARA* transcripts. The selection of the control gene should take into account several factors; in particular, its rate of degradation should be similar to that of *PML-RARA (17)*. We prefer the use of *ABL* to *RARA* as a control, because the latter is normally more stable and accordingly its expression may give a false impression regarding the integrity of the RNA that is being tested.

9. *Control of the quality of the RNA through RQ-PCR.* Unlike RT-PCR, RQ-PCR allows monitoring of the rate of accumulation of the amplification products, the course of the reaction (real-time analysis), and the "threshold cycle" (Ct) of the chimeric and control genes. If the Ct value for the control gene is extremely high (e.g., above 29–30), this indicates poor quality of the tested sample (as a result of either RNA degradation or low efficiency of the cDNA synthesis), and accordingly it renders the sample nonevaluable *(18,19)*.

10. Participate in inter-laboratory quality control on blinded diagnostic and follow-up samples.

11. Positive and negative controls are to be used in each PCR experiment in order to verify the efficiency of the reaction and to check for possible contamination.

12. Check the test sensitivity periodically by performing PCR dilution experiments on a positive cDNA. This is mandatory any time a newly synthesized primer set is introduced.

13. Perform a nested PCR analysis to increase the test sensitivity and specificity even with diagnostic samples. This strategy helps avoid false-negative results in samples that have not been analyzed immediately or have not been preserved properly.

14. In follow-up samples during treatment, it is not unusual to detect the presence of amplified nonspecific products, which appear as single or multiple bands in the electrophoresis gel, even when the primers and PCR protocols are used according to the Biomed-1 Concerted Action Report *(12)*. The problem is more frequently encountered when a bcr3 breakpoint is amplified. The nonspecific products usually differ in size from the expected band, but it may happen that the observed amplified band(s) is(are) in the same range as those seen in a positive case. **Figure 3** shows some representative cases. These results should be interpreted conservatively, especially in a patient who has been persistently negative

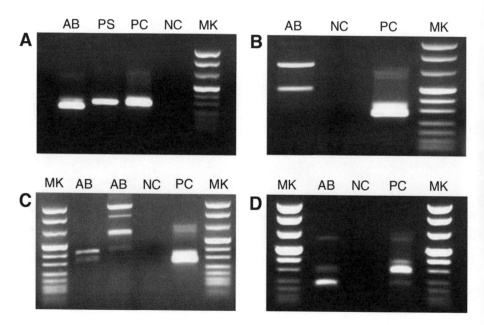

Fig. 3. Ethidium bromide-stained agarose gel demonstrating nonspecific bcr3 +ve (**A–C**) and bcr1 +ve (**D**) nested polymerase chain reaction products in tests for negative patients. AB = nonspecific bands in negative samples, PS = positive samples, PC = positive controls, NC = negative controls, MK = markers.

in previous tests. Before issuing a final positive result it is reasonable to proceed as follows:

a. Repeat the PCR: the amplified abnormal products may be the result of a random event, and accordingly it is unlikely they will recur.

b. Use a 2–3% agarose gel to obtain a better separation of the amplified products.

c. Repeat the analysis by starting from a new RNA aliquot that has been properly preserved.

d. Use Hot Start Taq polymerase; in Hot Start PCR, the preliminary activation of the enzyme at high temperature reduces the annealing of primers to nonspecific target sequences, and consequently reduces the formation of nonspecific amplified products.

e. If the result is confirmed after all the above-mentioned procedures, a positive test is considered likely. The suggestion to repeat BM evaluation promptly (e.g., 1 mo) should be made in order to confirm the diagnosis of molecular (and impending hematological) relapse.

References

1. Larson, R. A., Kondo, K., Vardiman, J. W., Butler A. E., Golomb, H. M., and Rowley, J. D. (1984) Evidence for a 15;17 translocation in every patient with acute promyelocytic leukemia. *Am. J. Med.* **76,** 827–841.

2. Rambaldi, A. and Biondi, A. (2002) Acute promyelocytic leukaemia, in *Leukemia* (Henderson, E. S., Lister, T. A., Greaves, M. F., eds.), Saunders, Philadelphia, pp. 529–543.

3. Grimwade, D., Biondi, A., Mozziconacci, M. J., et al. (2000) Characterization of acute promyelocytic leukemia cases lacking the classic t(15;17): results of the European Working Party. Groupe Francais de Cytogenetique Hematologique, Groupe de Francais d'Hematologie Cellulaire, UK Cancer Cytogenetics Group and BIOMED 1 European Community-Concerted Action "Molecular Cytogenetic Diagnosis in Haematological Malignancies." *Blood* **96,**1297–1308.

4. Grignani, F., Fagioli, M., Alcalay, M., et al. (1994) Acute promyelocytic leukemia: from genetics to treatment. *Blood* **83,** 10–25.

5. Chen, Z., Brand, N. J., Chen, A., et al. (1993) Fusion between a novel Kruppel-like zinc finger gene and the retinoic acid receptor-alpha locus due to a variant t(11;17) translocation associated with acute promyelocytic leukaemia. *EMBO J.* **12,** 1161–1167.

6. Redner, R. L., Rush, E. A., Faas, S., Rudert, W. A., and Corey, S. J. (1996) The t(5;17) variant of acute promyelocytic leukemia expresses a nucleophosmin-retinoic acid receptor fusion. *Blood* **87,** 882–886.

7. Wells, R. A., Catzavelos,]ô., and Kamel-Reid, S. (1997) Fusion of retinoic acid receptor alpha to NuMA, the nuclear mitotic apparatus protein, by a variant translocation in acute promyelocytic leukaemia. *Nat. Genet.* **17,** 109–113.

8. Arnould, C., Philippe, C., Bourdon, V., Grégoire, M. J., Berger, R., and Jonveaux, P. (1999) The signal transducer and activator of transcription STAT5b gene is a new partner of retinoic acid receptor alpha in acute promyelocytic-like leukaemia. *Hum. Mol. Genet.* **8,** 1741–1749.

9. Lo Coco, F., Diverio, D., Falini, B., Biondi, A., Nervi, C., and Pelicci, P. G. (1999) Genetic diagnosis and molecular monitoring in the management of acute promyelocytic leukemia. *Blood* **94,**12–22.

10. Lo Coco, F., Breccia, M., and Diverio, D. (2003) The importance of molecular monitoring in acute promyelocytic leukaemia. *Best Pract. Res. Clin. Haematol.* **16,** 503–520. Review.

11. Reiter, A., Lengfelder, E., and Grimwade, D. (2004) Pathogenesis, diagnosis and monitoring of residual disease in acute promyelocytic leukaemia. *Acta Haematol.* **112,** 55–67. Review.

12. van Dongen, J. J., Macintyre, E. A., Gabert, J. A., et al. (1999) Standardized RT-PCR analysis of fusion gene transcripts from chromosome aberrations in acute leukemia for detection of minimal residual disease. Report of the BIOMED-1 Concerted Action: investigation of minimal residual disease in acute leukemia. *Leukemia* **13,** 1901–1928.

13. Biondi, A., Rambaldi, A., Pandolfi, P. P., et al. (1992) Molecular monitoring of the myl/retinoic acid receptor-α fusion gene in acute promyelocytic leukemia by polymerase chain reaction. *Blood* **80,** 492–497.

14. Lo Coco, F., Diverio, D., Avvisati, G., et al. (1999) Therapy of molecular relapse in acute promyelocytic leucemia. *Blood* **94,** 2225–2229.

15. Chomczynski, P. and Sacchi, N. (1987) Single step method of RNA isolation by guanidium thiocyanate-phenol-chloroform extraction. *Anal. Biochem.* **162,** 156–159.

16. Müller, M. C., Merx, K., Weisser, A., Lahaye, T., Hehlmann, R., and Hochhaus, A. (2002) Improvement of molecular monitoring of residual disease in leukemias by bedside RNA stabilization. *Leukemia* **16,** 2395–2399.
17. van der Velde, V. H. J., Boeckx, N., Gonzalez, M., et al. (2004) Differential stability of control gene and fusion gene transcripts over time may hamper accurate quantification of minimal residual disease- a study within the Europe Against Cancer Program. *Leukemia* **18,** 884–886.
18. Gabert, J., Beillard, E., van der Velden, V. H. J., et al. (2003) Standardization and quality control studies of "real-time" quantitative reverse transcriptase polymerase chain reaction of fusion gene transcripts for residual disease detection in leukemia—A Europe Against Cancer Program. *Leukemia* **17,** 2318–2357.
19. Beillard, E., Pallisgaard, N., van der Velde, V. H. J., et al. (2003) Evaluation of candidate control genes for diagnosis and residual disease detection in leukemic patients using "real-time" quantitative reverse-transcriptase polymerase chain reaction (RQ-PCR)—a Europe against cancer program. *Leukemia* **17,** 2474–2486.

8

Diagnosis and Monitoring of *PML-RARα*-Positive Acute Promyelocytic Leukemia by Quantitative RT-PCR

Elisa Mokany, Alison V. Todd, Caroline J. Fuery, and Tanya L. Applegate

Summary

The last 15 yr have produced dramatic improvements in the survival rate of patients with acute promyelocytic leukemia (APL). These improvements have been due mainly to the introduction of targeted therapies and improved methods for diagnosing and monitoring this disease. The underlying molecular lesion in APL involves a t(15:17) translocation which leads to the generation of *PML-RARα* fusion transcripts and proteins. The *PML-RARα* fusion transcripts have been shown to be useful markers for establishing the diagnosis and for monitoring the response to treatment.

This manuscript describes the application of QZyme™ reverse-transcription polymerase chain reaction (RT-PCR) to the quantification of *PML-RARα* transcripts as a marker of APL. QZyme™ is a method for real time detection and quantification of target genes or transcripts. The principle of QZyme analysis is similar to other quantitative PCR systems; however, the mechanism is quite different. QZyme exploits the catalytic activity of DNAzymes (deoxyribozymes), which are oligonucleotides that can bind and cleave nucleic acid substrates. The approach is well suited to monitoring minimal residual disease (MRD) in patients with APL, as a result of its ability to detect low numbers of transcripts and accurately measure differences in concentration over a broad dynamic range. Further, its capacity for duplex analysis has multiple advantages for analysis of clinical specimens.

Protocols for duplex, single-tube QZyme RT-PCR assays, which allow simultaneous quantification of *PML-RARα* fusion transcripts (either L-type and V-type, or S-type) and the internal control *BCR* transcript, are provided. These protocols can be used for analyzing patient RNA specimens and are suitable for clinical trial monitoring. For this type of work, it is recommended that investigators validate the assays to ensure reproducible, accurate, and specific results on the equipment in their own laboratories. Assay validation is critical for real-time quantitative RT-PCR (RQ-PCR) and is often overlooked. A guide to the steps involved in validation and recommendations for acceptance criteria is included in this chapter.

From: *Methods in Molecular Medicine, Vol. 125: Myeloid Leukemia: Methods and Protocols*
Edited by: H. Iland, M. Hertzberg, and P. Marlton © Humana Press Inc., Totowa, NJ

Key Words: QZyme™ PCR; duplex reaction; RQ-PCR; single tube; acute promyelocytic leukemia; real time quantitative RT-PCR; molecular monitoring; minimal residual disease; *PML-RARα*; fusion gene; validation; limit of detection; limit of quantitation; reproducibility.

1. Introduction

1.1. Acute Promyelocytic Leukemia

The clinical course of acute promyelocytic leukemia (APL) has dramatically improved over the last 15 yr, from one that was almost invariably fatal to one of the more curable types of cancer. This has been achieved through the introduction of therapies, including all-*trans* retinoic acid (ATRA) and arsenic trioxide (As_2O_3), which target the fundamental underlying molecular lesion. Ninety-nine percent of APL patients have a rearrangement of the promyelocytic leukemia (PML) and retinoic acid receptor α (*RARα*) genes, located on chromosomes 15 and 17, respectively, leading to the generation of *PML-RARα* fusion transcripts and proteins. In most cases these rearrangements are the result of a t(15→17) reciprocal chromosomal translocation. While the breakpoint is always within intron 2 of the *RARα* gene, the breakpoints within the *PML* gene can occur either within intron 6 (the long L-type or *BCR* 1 form), within exon 6 (the variable V-type or *BCR* 2 isoform), or within intron 3 (the short S-type or *BCR* 3 isoform) *(1,2)*.

Treatment of *PML-RARα*-positive patients with ATRA combined with chemotherapy induces long-term remission and apparent cure in approx 70% of patients. Fortunately for those 30% who ultimately relapse, most can obtain a second remission following salvage treatment with further ATRA or As_2O_3 *(3)*. These improved outcomes have been achieved through the dedication of clinicians in testing and refining therapeutic regimens within the context of large clinical trials throughout the world, including Europe, North America, Eastern Asia, and Australasia. Coinciding with advances in therapy, new tools for diagnosing and monitoring APL have been developed *(4)*. Molecular techniques are a boon for clinicians, because individual patient outcomes are difficult to predict on the basis of classic hematological parameters alone. Further, molecular approaches such as polymerase chain reaction (PCR) enable detection of leukemic cells below the threshold of cytomorphology or karyotyping. PCR is faster than traditional methods, thus expediting accurate diagnosis of this rapidly fatal disease. Early administration of targeted therapy is critical to successfully induce remission in APL patients. Because of the advantages outlined above, qualitative reverse-transcription (RT)-PCR detection of *PML-RARα* is now routinely used in many laboratories as a diagnostic marker for APL.

Early studies, which examined the use of qualitative RT-PCR for longitudinal APL monitoring, established that molecular detection of minimal residual disease (MRD) could serve as an independent prognostic indicator *(5)*. Detection of *PML-RARα* transcripts at the conclusion of consolidation therapy, or subsequent recurrence of detectable transcripts (molecular relapse), was predictive of imminent clinical relapse. This observation translated into immediate clinical benefit, because pre-emptive therapy at the point of molecular relapse, rather than hematological relapse, improved the long-term survival for individual patients *(6)*. However, qualitative PCR fails to detect MRD in a subgroup of patients that ultimately relapse. Such false negatives are likely to reflect poor specimen RNA quality, which remains difficult to accurately determine with qualitative methods. Recent studies indicate quantitative real-time PCR will be a more powerful tool for monitoring APL *(7–11)*. These studies suggest that quantification of fusion transcripts may further improve prediction of patient relapse and help tailor therapy to individuals. As a consequence, molecular monitoring is already being incorporated into protocols for current multi-center therapeutic trials *(12)*.

1.2. Real-Time Quantitative PCR Using QZyme™

QZyme™ PCR (BD Biosciences Clontech) is a novel method that allows real-time detection and quantification of genomic DNA, cDNA, or mRNA targets. The protocol is well suited to assessment of MRD because of its capacity to accurately measure differences in target concentration over a broad dynamic range, typically extending over five orders of magnitude *(13)*. Further, the method can detect low numbers of copies of a target transcript, giving a clinician the best chance of detecting the earliest stages of molecular relapse. Finally, QZyme PCR is readily amenable to duplex analysis, which has multiple advantages for analysis of clinical specimens *(14)*. Duplex analysis allows the investigator to maximize the amount of information obtained from each clinical specimen, increasing sample throughput and reducing the cost per data point. Most importantly, duplex reactions allow the inclusion of an internal as opposed to a parallel control. The internal control enables a more accurate and reliable measurement of RNA integrity and its ability to be amplified. The inclusion of a quantitative internal control helps to minimize false-negative results resulting from poor-quality specimens, which pose a serious risk in the management of leukemia patients during remission.

1.3. The QZyme Strategy: Analysis of APL Specific Fusion Transcripts

Two duplex, single-tube QZyme RT-PCR assays were developed to simultaneously quantify *PML-RARα* fusion transcripts (either L-type and most V-type [*see* **Note 1**], or S-type) together with an internal control transcript, *BCR*. Our reasons for choosing *BCR* as the control have been discussed previously *(15)*. These QZyme assays are suitable for quantifying fusion transcripts in total RNA extracted from bone marrow or peripheral blood specimens from patients with APL.

The general principle of QZyme analysis is similar to those of other quantitative PCR systems; however, the mechanism is quite different. The protocol exploits the catalytic activity of DNAzymes (deoxyribozymes), which are DNA enzymes that have a conserved catalytic core and variable hybridizing arms. The arms bind complementary nucleic acid substrates and cleave them at specific phosphodiester bonds. The strategy of QZyme, as specifically applied to single-tube, duplex RT-PCR of *PML-RARα* and *BCR* transcripts, is illustrated in **Fig. 1**. In the first step, 3′ primers specific to *RARα* exon 3 and *BCR* exon 15 are extended by reverse transcriptase to make cDNA copies of the two transcripts. This cDNA is then amplified by PCR using the same two 3′ primers and two 5′ QZyme primers included in the mix. The 5′ QZyme primer for *PML-RARα* has a 3′ terminus, complementary to either *PML* exon 3 (for S-type transcripts) or exon 6 (for V-type or L-type transcripts), and a 5′ tag of the inactive antisense of DNAzyme B. Similarly, the 5′ QZyme primer for *BCR* has a 3′ terminus complementary to *BCR* exon 14, and a 5′ tag of the inactive antisense of a second DNAzyme D. During PCR, amplicons are produced which contain either *PML-RARα* or *BCR* sequence joined to catalytically active DNAzymes. Two DNAzyme substrates are also present in the reaction mix: (1) the B-FAM substrate, cleaved by B DNAzymes on the termini of *PML-RARα* amplicons, and (2) the D-CAL Orange substrate, cleaved by D DNAzymes on the termini of *BCR* amplicons. Cleavage of the substrates results in separation of the fluorophore and quencher dye pairs on each substrate. Real-time monitoring of the resulting increase in fluorescence from FAM and CAL Orange allows quantification of *PML-RARα* and *BCR* transcripts, respectively.

2. Materials

2.1. Calibrators and Controls

1. Plasmid L-type *PML-RARα* (8194 bp) contains full-length L-type *PML-RARα* cDNA (2888 bp), containing *PML* exons 1–6 and *RARα* exons 3–9 cloned into the pTL2 expression vector between the restriction enzymes *Bgl*II and *Eco*RI. This L-type plasmid was derived with permission from the plasmid MyP-RARα *(16)* kindly provided by Prof. P. Chambon, Université Louis Pasteur, Paris, France.

2. Plasmid S-type *PML-RARα* (7725 bp) contains full-length S-type *PML-RARα* cDNA (2420 bp), containing *PML* exons 1–3 and *RARα* exons 3–9 derived from patient material and cloned into the pTL2 expression vector between the restriction enzymes *Bgl*II and *Eco*RI. This S-type plasmid was derived from the L-type *PML-RARα* described in **step 1**.

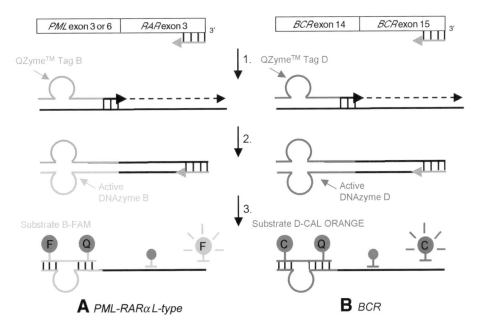

Fig. 1. Strategy for duplex single-tube reverse-transcription polymerase chain reaction (PCR) for *PML-RARα* and *BCR*. Sequential reactions in single-tube duplex reaction are: (1) reverse transcription of each transcript with 3′ primer making cDNA copy, inactivation of reverse transcription, and activation of polymerase; (2) PCR with 5′ QZyme™ primer and 3′ primer to generate amplicons containing active DNAzymes; (3) real-time quantitation of transcripts.

3. The human cell line Meg-01 (DSMZ No ACC 364) was expanded in culture according to conditions recommended by the supplier. Total RNA from this cell line was used as a negative control for *PML-RARα* transcripts and construction of calibrators.
4. Nuclease-free water (Ambion, Inc., Part No. AM-9930) is used at all stages of this protocol to prevent RNA degradation.

2.2. Extraction and Quantification of Total RNA

1. TRIzol reagents (Life Technologies, Part No. 15596–026).
2. QIAamp RNA Blood Mini Kit (50) (Qiagen, Part No. 52304).
3. 10X MULTI-CORE™ Buffer (Promega, Part No. R9991).
4. RQ1 RNase-Free DNase (Promega, Part No. M6101, 1 U/μL).
5. RNasin® Ribonuclease Inhibitor (Recombinant), 40 U/μL (Promega, Part No. N2515).
6. MgCl$_2$, 25 mM (Applied Biosystems, Part No. N808–0130).

2.3. Duplex Single-Tube Real-Time Quantitative RT-PCR

1. BD QTaq™ DNA polymerase mix (BD Biosciences Clontech, Part No. 639651); includes BD QTaq DNA polymerase (with built-in, hot start antibody), reaction buffer, dNTPs, and $MgCl_2$.
2. Moloney murine leukemia virus (M-MLV) Reverse Transcriptase (RNase H minus), 200U/µL (Promega Part No. M5301).
3. 50X BD QZyme™ Gene-Specific Primers (D-tag; 5' and 3' *BCR* primers) (BD QZyme Quantitative PCR reagent Part No. 638294, BD Biosciences Clontech; *see* **Note 2**).
4. 50X BD QZyme Gene-Specific Primers (B-tag; 5' and 3' S-type *PML-RARα* primers) (BD QZyme Quantitative PCR reagent Part No. 638292, BD Biosciences Clontech; *see* **Note 2**).
5. 50X BD QZyme Gene-Specific Primers (B-tag; 5' and 3' L-type/V-type *PML-RARα* primers) (BD QZyme Quantitative PCR reagent, Part No. 638293, BD Biosciences Clontech; *see* **Note 2**).
6. 100X BD QZyme Substrate D (CAL ORANGE).
7. 100X BD QZyme Substrate B (FAM).
8. Calibrators and patient RNA samples as prepared under **Subheading 3.**
9. MicroAmp® optical 96-well plate (Applied Biosystems, Part No. N-801–0560).
10. PCR cooler (Eppendorf, cat. no. 3881 000.023). This should be stored in the –20°C freezer until required.
11. MicroAmp optical caps (Applied Biosystems, Part No. N801–0935).
12. MicroAmp cap installing tool (Applied Biosystems, Part No. N801–0438).
13. ABI PRISM® 7700 Sequence Detection System and Sequence Detection Software 1.9.1 (Applied Biosystems) and computer (*see* **Note 3**).

3. Methods

The single-tube RT-PCR method presented in this chapter displays features that provide advantages compared to other published real-time methods. The majority of real-time PCR methods utilize plasmids as calibrators from which to estimate the number of mRNA transcripts in patient samples (*see* **Note 4**). This method exploits the advantages of both types of calibrators (plasmid and total RNA) with two calibration curves. Dilutions of the plasmid containing the full-length fusion target cDNA allow the estimation of copy number (*PML-RARα* calibration curve), whereas dilutions of total RNA allow estimation of endogenous *BCR* mRNA expression and controls for the activity of the reverse transcriptase. Both the target and endogenous control mRNA transcripts are amplified simultaneously from patient samples. The combination of calibrators chosen in this chapter are designed to mimic the complex milieu of the patient samples being tested while simultaneously allowing an estimation of the exact copy number of the target (not achievable from mRNA transcripts in total RNA) (*see* **Note 4**).

3.1. Calibration Curves for PML-RARα

Calibration curves for quantifying either *PML-RARα* L-type/V-type transcripts (*see* **Note 5**), or *PML-RARα* S-type transcripts, are constructed using the appropriate *PML-RARα* plasmids (*see* **Subheading 2.1.**, **steps 1** and **2**) diluted in a background of total RNA from Meg-01 (*see* **Subheading 2.1.**, **step 3**). The following instructions will refer to a generic "plasmid," applicable to the plasmid suitable for the breakpoint occurring in the patient cohort being tested.

Calibrator 1 is stored frozen in single-use aliquots, from which all other calibrators are made (by serial dilution as discussed later) on the day of the experiment (*see* **Note 6**). It is recommended that concentrations of total RNA <100 ng/μL should not be stored at −80°C for more than 1 mo. All solutions of plasmid or RNA should be mixed thoroughly before each individual pipetting step. Solutions should be aspirated below the meniscus, and the pipet tip should be rinsed in the solution five times by aspirating and ejecting the same volume that was originally dispensed.

1. In a separate room (*see* **Note 7**), thaw the concentrated *PML-RARα* plasmid solutions appropriate for the patients to be tested (i.e., plasmid L-type *PML-RARα* or plasmid S-type *PML-RARα*), and Meg-01 total RNA on ice.
2. Dilute the plasmid stocks to 1×10^6 *PML-RARα* copies/μL and store multiple aliquots at −20°C.
3. To construct a series of plasmid dilutions for the *PML-RARα* calibrator curves, make a stock of 111 ng/μL Meg-01 total RNA, which will be used to prepare Calibrator 1, and make up multiple aliquots of 120 μL of 100 ng/μL Meg-01 total RNA, which will be used to prepare calibrators 2–5. Store these aliquots at −80°C (*see* **Note 6**).
4. To make up Calibrator 1, dilute plasmid (1×10^6 copies/μL) 1 in 10 in a background of Meg-01 total RNA (111 ng/μL) and store in single-use 20-μL aliquots at −80°C.
5. Thaw a 20-μL aliquot of Calibrator 1 (containing 100,000 copies/μL in 100 ng/μL of Meg-01 total RNA) and a 120-μL aliquot of 100 ng/μL Meg-01 total RNA. Calibrators 2–5 are made by performing fourfold serial dilutions of Calibrator 1 as follows:
    a. For Calibrator 2 (25,000 copies/μL): add 5 μL of Calibrator 1 to 15 μL of 100 ng/μL Meg-01 total RNA.
    b. For Calibrator 3 (6250 copies/μL): add 5 μL of Calibrator 2 to 15 μL of 100 ng/μL Meg-01 total RNA.
    c. For Calibrator 4 (1563 copies/μL): add 5 μL of Calibrator 3 to 15 μL of 100 ng/ μL Meg-01 total RNA.
    d. For Calibrator 5 (391 copies/μL): add 5 μL of Calibrator 4 to 15 μL of 100 ng/μL Meg-01 total RNA.

3.2. Calibration Curves for BCR

Calibration curves for quantifying *BCR* transcripts are constructed by diluting Meg-01 total RNA in Nuclease-free water.

1. Make up multiple aliquots of 120 μL of 100 ng/μL Meg-01 total RNA and store frozen as Calibrator 1 for *BCR* curve. Calibrators 2–5 are made by performing fourfold serial dilutions of Calibrator 1 as follows:
   a. For Calibrator 2 (25,000 pg Meg-01 total RNA/μL): add 5 μL of Calibrator 1 to 15 μL of nuclease-free water.
   b. For Calibrator 3 (6250 pg Meg-01 total RNA/μL): add 5 μL of Calibrator 2 to 15 μL of nuclease-free water.
   c. For Calibrator 4 (1563 pg Meg-01 total RNA/μL): add 5 μL of Calibrator 3 to 15 μL of nuclease-free water.
   d. For Calibrator 5 (391 pg Meg-01 total RNA/μL): add 5 μL of Calibrator 4 to 15 μL of nuclease-free water.

3.3. Extraction and Quantitation of Total RNA

All RNA extractions are performed in a biohazard-protection hood (*see* **Note 7**). Two different methods are described to extract total RNA: (1) from patient samples, and (2) from cultured cells.

3.3.1. Extraction of RNA From Patient Specimens

1. For the extraction of RNA from patient specimens, use TRIzol reagent (Life Technologies) according to the manufacturer's recommendations. Be sure to work quickly and keep patient samples ice-cold to minimize degradation.
2. To measure concentration of total RNA, centrifuge at 10,000*g* for 15 s and return to ice. Measure the absorbance of a sample of the concentrated stock at 260 nm on the ultraviolet spectrophotometer (following manufacturer's instructions for use). Calculate the concentration of the RNA solution using the following formula:

$$\text{Concentration } (\mu g/mL) = 40 \times A_{260} \times \text{dilution factor}$$

3. Where possible, dilute diagnostic RNA samples (pretreatment) to 10 ng/μL and follow-up samples (posttreatment) to 100 ng/μL in nuclease-free water. Aliquot at least two 12-μL single-use samples (allows 5-μL duplicates to be analyzed per experiment and repeated) to avoid freeze thawing of samples (*see* **Note 8**).
4. Keep concentrated stocks of total RNA on dry ice at all times and return to –80°C storage when completed. Smaller aliquots of the concentrated stock can be made where possible to avoid freeze thawing of the entire sample for further analysis of other transcripts of interest.

3.3.2. Extraction of Total RNA From Cultured Cells

For extraction of total RNA from cultured cells, follow the instructions of "QIAamp RNA mini protocol" ("QIAamp RNA blood mini handbook" from

Qiagen) using the protocol "for pelleted cells." Use 600 μL of buffer RLT and 1 mL buffer RPE for every 5×10^6 cells (*see* **Note 9**). Place the eluted RNA immediately onto ice at the end of the protocol. Digest potential contaminating DNA as follows:

1. To make up digestion mix for 1×50 μL of RNA solution, add 7 μL of MULTI-CORE Buffer (10X solution), 5 μL of RQ1 RNase-Free DNase (1 U/μL), 2 μL of RNasin® Ribonuclease Inhibitor (40 U/μL), 6 μL of $MgCl_2$ (25 m*M*).
2. Add 20 μL of the digestion mix to every 50 μL of RNA solution.
3. Incubate the RNA/digestion mix at 37°C for 15 min (digestion of DNA).
4. Incubate the RNA/digestion mix at 75°C for 5 min and place on ice (inactivation of DNase).
5. To measure the concentration of total RNA, centrifuge at 10,000*g* for 15 s and return to ice. Dilute total RNA 1 in 100 in nuclease-free water and measure the absorbance as described in **Subheading 3.3.1., step 2**.
6. Dilute RNA to concentrations required to generate calibrators for each curve: 111ng/μL for the *PML-RARα* Calibrator 1 and 100ng/μL for subsequent *PML-RARα* calibrators (*see* **Subheading 3.1.**) and the *BCR* curve (*see* **Subheading 3.2.**). Store single-use aliquots at –80°C.

3.4. Duplex Single-Tube Real-Time Quantitative RT-PCR

QZyme PCR and single-tube RT-PCR can be performed on any real-time thermocycler capable of measuring FAM and CAL Orange. This protocol describes the use of the ABI PRISM 7700, and readers are referred to the manufacturer's user's manual for full details. Two master mixes can be made to target either the S-type or L-type fusion transcript, each duplexed with the endogenous *BCR* control.

1. Keep reagents on ice once thawed (*see* **Note 6**) and ensure fluorescently labeled substrates are protected from exposure to light. Centrifuge briefly and add reagents for each duplex bulk mix as described for S-type and L-type/V-type in **Table 1** and **2** respectively. Centrifuge master mix briefly (*see* **Notes 10** and **11**).
2. Aliquot 20 μL of ice-cold duplex QZyme master mix into the bottom of a MicroAmp optical 96-well plate (*see* **Note 12**). Each RNA sample (calibrator, patient, or control, *see* **Note 13**) should be analyzed in duplicate. The total number of wells is determined by the number of calibrators required for both curves (five points each for each curve), patient samples and controls. Keep the MicroAmp optical 96-well plates on a frozen PCR cooler or an equivalent cooling rack at all times.
3. Add 5 μL of each calibrator (from the calibrator curve series 500,000, 125,000, 31,250, 7813, 1953 copy number or pg total RNA) or control (no-template, positive, or negative control) (*see* **Note 13**) (thawed and centrifuged) to the appropriate wells, rinsing pipet tip in master mix. Total reaction volume 25 μL.
4. Retrieve one aliquot of each patient sample to be tested from –80°C storage (*see* **Subheading 3.3.1.** and **Note 6**), transferring on dry ice until required. Thaw each

Table 1
Mutiplex QZyme™ Master Mix (*S-type PML-RARα* Plus *BCR*)

Solution	Working stock concentration	Final concentration	Volume per 25 µL reaction
DEPC water			To a total of 20 µL
QZyme Mix	2X	1X	12.5 µL
QTaq™	50X	1X	0.5 µL
M-MLV (RNase H minus)	200 U/µL	12.5 U	0.06 µL (**Note 9**)
QZyme *BCR* primer mix	50X	1X	0.50 µL
QZyme *PML* primer mix (S-type)	50X	1X	0.50 µL
QZyme substrate B- FAM	100X	2X	0.50 µL

DEPC, diethylpyrocarbonate; M-MLV, Moloney murine leukemia virus.

Table 2
Mutiplex QZyme™ Master Mix (*L-type/V-type PML-RARα* Plus *BCR*)

Solution	Working stock concentration	Final concentration	Volume per 25 µL reaction
DEPC water			To a total of 20 µL
QZyme Mix	2X	1X	12.5 µL
QTaq	50X	1X	0.5 µL
Additional MgCl$_2$	25 m*M*	0.5 m*M*	0.5 µL
M-MLV (RNase H minus)	200 U/µL	12.5 U	0.06 µL (**Note 9**)
QZyme *BCR* primer mix	50X	1X	0.50 µL
QZyme *PML* primer mix (L-*type* / V-*type*)	50X	1X	0.50 µL
QZyme substrate B-FAM	100X	2X	0.50 µL
QZyme substrate D- CAL Orange	100X	2X	0.50 µL

DEPC, diethylpyrocarbonate; M-MLV, Moloney murine leukemia virus.

sample and briefly centrifuge immediately before addition to the master mix. Add 5 µL patient RNA to wells in duplicate (where patient material permits), rinsing pipet tip in master mix.

5. Repeat for all remaining patient samples and controls.
6. Place MicroAmp optical caps over the wells and seal using the MicroAmp Cap Installing Tool. Keep the plate on ice and covered from light until ready for use on the ABI PRISM 7700.
7. Fill in the setup screen according to the ABI PRISM 7700 user's manual, ensuring that both CAL Orange and FAM fluorophores are selected for all wells.

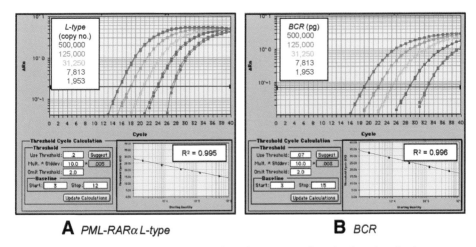

A *PML-RARα L-type*   **B** *BCR*

Fig. 2. Amplification plots and calibration curves for single-tube duplex assay. Examples of duplex assays for (**A**) *PML-RARα* L-type, (**B**) *BCR* control

8. Click on "thermal cycling" and program the following profile (*see* **Note 14**):
   60 min at 55°C, 3 min at 95°C
   10 cycles of 95°C for 15 s and 68°C for 40 s (–1°C/cycle),
   40 cycles of 95°C for 15 s and 55°C for 40 s
9. Load plate, close the lid, and select "run."
10. Save data after completion of run (*see* **Note 15**).
11. Analyze data from the ABI 7700 according to the guidelines from Applied Biosystems (**Note 16**). For both *PML-RARα* assays, set the baseline and thresholds at 3–12 and 0.2, respectively. For the *BCR* assays, set the baseline and threshold at 3–15 and 0.07. Examples of an amplification plot and a standard curve from the L-type duplex assay are given in **Fig. 2** (*see* **Note 17**).

3.5. Relative Quantitation of Transcripts in Patient Samples

To determine the correct primer set to use in QZyme RT-PCR, it is recommended that the *PML-RARα* isoform harbored by each patient be identified by standard qualitative RT-PCR (*see* Chapter 7).

The single-tube QZyme RT-PCR method described in this chapter is not only able to confirm the presence of the *PML-RARα* transcript in each patient, but also estimate its relative abundance. The quantities of *PML-RARα* and *BCR* transcripts, amplified simultaneously in a duplex reaction, are estimated from each calibration curve (*see* **Subheadings 3.1.** and **3.2.**). The relative abundance of transcripts is then calculated by normalization of *PML-RARα* to the control *BCR* transcripts, to account for variation in RNA concentration and quality, according to the equations in **Subheading 3.5., step 2**). The accurate assessment of RNA quality in each specimen, which can vary considerably, is essen-

Table 3
Acceptance and Rejection Criteria of Data and Subsequent Classification of Results*

	PML-RARα (x copies)		
BCR (y pg equivalents)	x < LOD (i.e., PML-RARα not amplified)	LOD < x < LLOQ (i.e., PML-RARα amplified, but not on standard curve)	LLOQ < x < ULOQ (i.e., PML-RARα amplified and on standard curve)
y < LLOQ (i.e., not on BCR standard curve)	No result (1)	Detected but not quantifiable (4)	Detected but not quantifiable (7)
LLOQ < y <5 × 10⁴ (Note 18) (i.e., quantifiable, but poor quality RNA)	No result (2)	Detected but not quantifiable (5)	Quantifiable Quote %RDC (8)
5 × 10⁴ < y < ULOQ (i.e., good quality RNA)	Not detected (3)	Detected but not quantifiable (6)	Quantifiable Quote %RDC (9)

*The final classification of patient results depends on both the *PML/RARα* and *BCR* values obtained. There are nine possible scenarios that result in classification as either "No result," "Not detectable," "Detectable but not quantifiable," or "Quantifiable." For further explanation, see the following footnote.

(1) The *PML-RARα* is less than the limit of detection (LOD) and the *BCR* is less than the lower limit of quantitation (LLOQ). This is classed as a "No result." (2) The *PML-RARα* is less than the LOD, and the *BCR* is less than the cut-off for poor quality RNA; the value of 50,000 pg equivalents (50 ng equivalents) was determined in a previous study. The RNA in this sample is not of sufficient quality to confidently determine that the *PML-RARα* transcript does not exist. This is also classed as a "No result." (3) The *PML-RARα* is less than the LOD, and the *BCR* is greater than the cut-off value for poor quality RNA. The RNA in this sample is of sufficient quality to determine the sample does not contain the transcript and is classed "Not detectable." (4) The *PML-RARα* is amplified and greater than the LOD, but less than the LLOQ. The *BCR* is also less than the LLOQ. This renders the sample "Detectable," but not quantifiable. (5) The *PML-RARα* is as for 4, nonquantifiable. The *BCR* is less than the cut-off for poor quality RNA. The sample is therefore "Detectable," but not quantifiable as no %RDC value can be calculated for it. (6) The *PML-RARα* is as for 4, nonquantifiable. The *BCR* is greater than the cut-off value for poor quality RNA. The sample is therefore "Detectable," but not quantifiable. (7) The *PML-RARα* falls on the standard curve and is quantifiable, but the *BCR* is less than the LLOQ. This renders the sample "Detectable," but not quantifiable as no relative value can be calculated for it. (8) The *PML-RARα* falls on the standard curve and is quantifiable. Although the *BCR* is less than the cut-off for poor quality RNA, a relative %RDC can still be calculated. This sample is "Quantifiable." (9) Both the *PML-RARα* and *BCR* fall on the respective standard curves. A relative %RDC can be calculated and this sample is "Quantifiable."

tial to accurately quantitate *PML-RARα* transcript levels (*see* **Note 18**). This also provides defined acceptance/rejection criteria from which to minimize false-negative results (*see* **Table 3**). This feature of the duplexed quantitative assay provides a distinct advantage over qualitative methods.

1. Quantitative data are expressed as an RDC, which equals the ratio of copies of disease transcripts (expressed as the number of copies of *PML-RARα* in 50 ng of patient RNA) to control transcripts (expressed as pg equivalents of *BCR* in 50 ng of patient RNA). Calculate RDC with the following equation (*see* **Note 8**):

RDC at diagnosis = *PML-RARα*$_{copy\#}$ (per 50 ng of patient RNA)/*BCR*$_{pg\ equivalents}$ (per 50 ng of patient RNA)

2. Samples are rejected (no result) or accepted (and subsequently classified) according to estimates for both the *BCR* and *PML-RARα*. Once analyzed, patient data are classified according to one of four categories: (1) no result, (2) negative (not detectable), (3) detectable, but not quantifiable, or (4) quantifiable (*see* **Table 3**).

3.6. Validation of QZyme Assays

In order to produce data that are quantitative, accurate, specific, and reproducible, it is important for each laboratory to test the critical parameters of the assay on the equipment in their laboratory. This will also permit inter-laboratory standardization of assays for multi-center clinical trials. The critical parameters to test for real-time quantitative PCR are (1) limit of detection, (2) limit of quantitation, and (3) reproducibility (intra- and inter-assay variation). In this subheading, a brief description of how to test these parameters is provided, and a summary of values for the assays used to validate this method is presented in **Table 4**.

3.6.1. Limit of Detection (LOD)

LOD refers to the lowest level of an analyte (e.g., *PML-RARa* transcript) that can be detected above background (*see* **Note 19**). Background signal is determined by analyzing 10 replicates of negative controls, i.e., a sample without the gene transcript of interest. A suitable negative control for *PML-RARα* is RNA from Meg-01 (a cell line that does not express the *PML-RARα* transcript). As *BCR* is constitutively expressed, an RNA-containing negative control does not exist. Water is used as the negative control for *BCR*. The LOD for the duplexed QZyme PCR *PML-RARα-BCR* assay is determined using the following protocol:

1. Set up duplex QZyme PCR *PML-RARα-BCR* reactions as outlined under **Subheading 3.4.**
2. At **Subheading 3.4., step 3**, add 5 µL of 100 ng/µL Meg-01 total RNA to 10 separate reaction tubes, and 5 µL of water to a further 10 reaction tubes.

Table 4
Summary of Values for Each Assay

	QZyme™ assay		
	L-type / V-type	S-type	*BCR*
Limit of detection (threshold cycle [Ct])	40	40	40 (*see* **Subheading 3.6.1., step 6**)
Upper limit of quantitation	5×10^5 (<2% CV) (copies)	5×10^5 (<2% CV) (copies)	5×10^5 (<2% CV) (pg equivalents)
Lower limit of quantitation	1953 (<3% CV) (copies)	1953 (<3% CV) (copies)	1953 (<3% CV) (pg equivalents)
Reproducibility (relative to *BCR*)			
High control (1×10^5 pg)	NSD	<33%	NA
Medium control (2×10^4 pg)	<10%	<29%	NA
Low control (4×10^3 pg)	NSD	<80%	NA

NSD, no significant difference between the ratios of each experiment ($p > 0.05$); <x% refers to the maximum difference in ratio between each experiment.; NA, not applicable.

3. Thermocycle the reactions and export the data (**Subheading 3.4., steps 8–10**).
4. Calculate the threshold cycle (Ct) for the LOD as follows:

$$LOD\ Ct = (Average\ Ct_{(of\ the\ 10\ negatives)}) - (5 \times SD_{(of\ the\ 10\ negatives)})$$

5. Any sample that amplifies with a Ct later than the LOD is deemed undetectable.
6. In our hands, the LOD for the Qzyme *PML-RAR*α L-type and S-type assay was 40 cycles, whereas the *BCR* assays gave a LOD of 50 cycles (no background signal detected before the 50 cycles tested). The LOD was set at 40 cycles for both duplexed assays.

3.6.2. Limit of Quantification (LOQ)—Precision and Accuracy of Calibrators

LOQ refers to the highest and lowest amounts of analyte (*PML-RAR*α or *BCR* transcript) that can be quantitated with reasonable certainty. In the context of quantitative real-time PCR assays, reasonable certainty is determined by the coefficient of variation (CV), a measure of precision. The LOQ is determined by extending calibrator curves above and below the range commonly used, and determining the CV and accuracy for each calibrator. The LOQ for the duplexed QZyme PCR *PML-RAR*α-*BCR* assay can be determined using the following protocol:

1. Set up duplex QZyme PCR *PML-RARα-BCR* reactions as described under **Subheading 3.4.**
2. At **Subheading 3.4., step 3**, the normal calibrator curve (consisting of five calibrators) should be extended above the highest calibrator and below the lowest calibrator, normally assessed, to produce a total of seven calibrators. Five replicates of each of these seven calibrators should be measured to allow precision and accuracy to be calculated.
3. Thermocycle the reactions and export the data (**Subheading 3.4., steps 8–10**). The standard curve should be generated from only the middle five calibrators (those known to produce a linear relationship between Ct and copy number from previous experiments).
4. For each of the seven calibrators, calculate the following values (*see* **Note 20**):

$$CV_{Ct} (\%) = (100 \times SD_{Ct})/average_{Ct}$$

$$CV_{copy\ \#} (\%) = (100 \times SD_{copy\ \#})/average_{copy\ \#}$$

$$Accuracy\ (\%) = 100 \times (average_{measured\ copy\ \#})/(known_{copy\ \#})$$

5. The upper limit of quantitation (ULOQ) is the highest concentration of calibrator that meets the acceptance criteria of $CV_{CT} < 2\%$, $CV_{copy\ \#} < 25\%$, and accuracy within 70% to 130% of the known calibrator value.
6. The lower limit of quantitation (LLOQ) is the lowest concentration that meets the acceptance criteria of $CV_{CT} < 3\%$, $CV_{copy\ \#} < 30\%$, and accuracy within 70% to 130% of the known calibrator value (*see* **Note 20**).

3.6.3. Reproducibility

Reproducibility is a measure of the repeatability of results performed within one run (intra-assay) and between runs (inter-assay). In our experience with the ABI PRISM 7700, the variation between sample wells on the 96-well block is greater than the variation seen for the same well between runs. This variation is also dependent on the amount of signal generated, and thus on the amount of template. Intra- and inter-assay variation are measured by a set of three experiments, as follows:

1. Inter-assay variation is determined by the results of the t-tests performed on a series of controls analyzed over three experiments. Set up Duplex QZyme PCR *PML-RARα-BCR* reactions as described under **Subheading 3.4.**
2. At **Subheading 3.4., step 3,** the calibrator curve should be run in duplicate.
3. Include five replicates of three control samples: "high control" with 100,000 copies of *PML-RARα* plasmid in 500 ng total RNA, "medium control" with 20,000 copies of *PML-RARα* plasmid in 500 ng total RNA, and "low control" with 4000 copies of *PML-RARα* plasmid in 500 ng total RNA. All calibrators and the five replicates of the three controls should be assessed in the same wells for each of the three experiments.

4. Thermocycle the reactions and export the data (**Subheading 3.4., steps 8–10**). Repeat **steps 1–4** twice to total three experiments with exactly the same reactions. Use the same aliquot of calibrators and controls for all three experiments.
5. For the five replicates of each control within each experiment, calculate the following:

$$\text{Average}_{\text{normalized copy \#}}$$

$$\text{SD}_{\text{normalized copy \#}}$$

$$\text{CV}_{\text{normalized copy \#}} (\%) = 100 \times \text{SD}_{\text{normalized copy \#}} / \text{average}_{\text{normalized copy \#}}$$

6. Calculate the following ratios for the high control:

$$\text{Experiment \#1 Average}_{\text{normalized copy \#}}/\text{Experiment \#2 Average}_{\text{normalized copy \#}}$$

$$\text{Experiment \#1 Average}_{\text{normalized copy \#}}/\text{Experiment \#3 Average}_{\text{normalized copy \#}}$$

$$\text{Experiment \#2 Average}_{\text{normalized copy \#}}/\text{Experiment \#3 Average}_{\text{normalized copy \#}}$$

7. Repeat **step 6** for the medium and low controls
8. Perform t-tests between the following values:

$$\text{Replicates of high control}_{\text{normalized copy \#}}: \text{Experiment \#1 vs Experiment \#2}$$

$$\text{Replicates of high control}_{\text{normalized copy\#}}: \text{Experiment \#1 vs Experiment \#3}$$

$$\text{Replicates of High Control}_{\text{normalized copy\#}}: \text{Experiment \#2 vs Experiment \#3}$$

9. Repeat **step 8** for the medium and low controls.
10. If the difference in Average$_{\text{normalized copy \#}}$ for a control from different experiments does not reach statistical significance ($p < 0.05$) then there is no real difference between the Average$_{\text{normalized copy\#}}$ generated by the two experiments, and the ratio is irrelevant. Statistically significant differences may not necessarily be significant in the context of the assay. Real-time quantitative PCR assays have a maximum sensitivity of twofold, and thus any ratio between experiments that falls between 0.5 and 2 is generally acceptable. In our hands, the ratio between experiments for the high and medium controls fall between 0.67 and 1.5 (a variation of 50%). The low control shows greater variability, and we measure ratios of between 0.56 and 1.8 (an 80% variation) (*see* **Note 21**).
11. Intra-assay variation is determined from the CV$_{\text{normalized copy \#}}$ for each control. In our experience, the CV$_{\text{normalized copy \#}}$ for the high and medium controls should fall below 25%, and that for the low control below 35%.

4. Notes

1. Most patients harbor either the L- or S-type, whereas approx 10% of patients harbor the V-type. In V-type patients, the breakpoint usually occurs within exon

6, creating fusion transcripts of varying lengths in individual patients. Approximately one-third to one-half of V-type patients harbor an identical V-type transcript, characterized by the loss of 54 bases from the 3′ end of *PML* exon 6. The 5′ QZyme primer for the L-type/V-type assay has been designed upstream of this common breakpoint, and the transcripts of these V-type patients will be amplifiable. The remaining V-type patients are not amplifiable unless a more 5′ primer with B tag is constructed.

2. QZyme primer sequences (5′ to 3′) are as follows:
   5′ QZyme *BCR* primer: (Tag D—CACTCAGCCACTGGATTTAA)
   3′ *BCR* primer: (GCGTCTTTGCTTTATTCAC)
   5′ QZyme *PML* S-type primer: (Tag B—TCAGCTCTTGCATCACC)
   5′ QZyme *PML* L-type primer (Tag B—AGGAGCCCCGTCATAGGA)
   3′≤ *RAR*α primer: (GGGCACTATCTCTTCAGAAC)

3. The method described in this chapter employs three fluorophores: FAM, ROX, and the less commonly used Cal Orange. The ABI 7700 needs to be calibrated to read each of these.

4. Although plasmids provide stable calibrators of exact copy number, they do not account for the efficiency of the reverse transcriptase. Total RNA remains the only calibrator that accurately controls for reverse transcriptase activity, and its suitability as such has been fully explored in this laboratory. Unfortunately, there are also disadvantages associated with using total RNA from cultured cells as calibrators. The exact transcript copy number remains unknown, and differences in expression can hinder direct comparisons and complicate interpretation of results. Likewise, plasmids diluted in water alone do not account for any differences in amplification efficiency between the calibrator and test sample. In an effort to better mimic the complex milieu of patient samples, the plasmid calibrators containing *PML-RAR*α have been diluted in a background of total RNA that does not contain the *PML-RAR*α transcript.

5. The PCR amplicon from V-type patients will vary in individual patients. The authors acknowledge the potential difference in amplification efficiency between the L-type plasmid calibrator and the V-type patients. To address this, the authors have previously shown there is no significant difference in the amplification efficiency between the L-type template (producing a longer amplicon) and the V-type template (producing a shorter amplicon) when using identical primers. The L-type plasmid is therefore considered suitable for estimating expression in V-type patients.

6. We have found that RNA degrades over time. Some RNA transcripts are particularly labile. To minimize degradation, stocks of RNA that are not for immediate use should be kept in volumes greater then 100 µL at high concentrations (i.e., RNA ≥ 100 ng/µL). Calibrators can be stored as multiple aliquots in smaller volumes but should not be kept for longer than 1 mo.

7. To minimize risk of contamination, we have established several rooms specifically for PCR experiments. All have positive pressure, a dressing room, and contain everything necessary for the designated tasks (ensuring nothing is brought in

or taken out of the rooms). Primer and reagent (**Tables 1** and **2**) handling should be made in a PCR setup room. Calibrator and RNA manipulations (*see* **Subheading 3.1.**) should be made in a designated template room (DNA and RNA extractions also take place here), and thermocyclers (*see* **Subheading 3.3.**) should be kept in a separate room. Extraction or manipulation of concentrated plasmid stock (above the concentration of the top calibrator) or PCR product should be done in an area removed from all others, and preferably in a designated room. Meticulous laboratory protocol should be followed to avoid contamination. Clean benches with 0.05% hypochlorite and 70% ethanol before starting. Clean all pipets with 70% ethanol. Change gloves frequently. Centrifuge all tubes before use to prevent production of aerosols. Minimize sample handling. In the designated PCR rooms, we use disposable laboratory coats, hair nets, shoe covers, and gloves at all times, to ensure no possible carryover between rooms and the lab.

8. As a result of variation in expected abundance of the *PML-RARα* transcript in diagnostic (pretreatment) compared with follow-up (posttreatment) patient samples, the amount of patient RNA amplified per reaction varies accordingly. A total of 50 ng RNA is analyzed for pretreatment specimens, and 500 ng for specimens collected following treatment.

9. All steps using the QIAamp RNA Blood Mini Kit are carried out at room temperature. Working quickly will minimize degradation of RNA.

10. If the volume required for M-MLV is too small to accurately pipet, the M-MLV may be diluted 10-fold in 1X PCR buffer.

11. The QZyme method described in this chapter was individually developed. As a result, the details of the bulk mix and thermocycling conditions are non-standard. Please follow the instructions as described in this chapter and disregard buffers and thermocycling programs recommended in published BD Bioscience protocols.

12. Use a new pipet tip for each addition of master mix and RNA calibrators to the wells. Addition of the master mix can be done with a multi-displacement pipet such as the Eppendorf Research®pro. All reactions should be performed at least in duplicate.

13. To ensure adequate activity of the reverse transcriptase, polymerase, and other reaction components, control reactions should be included in every RT-PCR assay. Appropriate controls include (1) positive controls for the target (calibrators for each target), (2) no amplification controls (NAC) to ensure assay specificity (RNA from a cell line devoid of the target), and (3) no-template controls (NTC) to check for cross-contamination (water instead of target). The reverse transcription of the *PML-RARα* transcript is indirectly controlled for by the RT-PCR of the *BCR* transcript in the same tube. The authors acknowledge that the activity of the reverse transcriptase on the *BCR* transcript from calibrators is indirect evidence for its activity on the *PML-RARα* transcript and is therefore not ideal.

14. Correct procedure for setting up the ABI 7700 for a duplex reaction can be found at the following link:
www.appliedbiosystems.com/support/tutorials/pdf/setting_up_duplex_reactions.pdf
Collection of fluorescent data at the annealing step only can be performed to reduce the size of run files.

15. Be sure to check that the ABI PRISM 7700 has collected data in the SDS file. Otherwise the raw data may need to be imported from the appropriate run file.

16. Applied Biosystems provides an online tutorial for setting the baseline and threshold: www.appliedbiosystems.com/support/tutorials/baseline/

    Also in more detail in the pdf file: www.appliedbiosystems.com/support/tutorials/pdf/data_analysis_7700.pdf

    It is not made clear in the tutorial that the baseline can also be increased past the default value of 15 (*see* **Note 14**). The baseline range and threshold we routinely set for the duplex *PML-RARα* S-type and L-type assays are 3–12 and 0.2, respectively; for *BCR*, 3–15 and 0.07, respectively (*see* **Fig. 2**).

17. Greater precision between standards can be achieved by adjusting the baseline to the maximum number of cycles possible before the most concentrated standard shows an increase above this baseline. Click on "Update Calculations" and view the corresponding standard curve and check the correlation coefficient; also look at the effect this has on precision of the standards (this is best viewed with the *y*-axis on a log scale).

18. Quantification of the endogenous control allows a better estimation of RNA quality than qualitative assessment. The cut-off value of 50 ng for poor quality RNA (**Table 3**) was determined in a retrospective phase II clinical trial (*8*), to accurately indicate RNA of insufficient quality to confidently amplify minimal residual disease. The QZyme is designed to amplify the fusion transcript from 500 ng total RNA where possible. If the *BCR* control indicates the equivalent of <50 ng of total RNA has been amplified (i.e., 10 times less than optimal), this sample is judged as of insufficient quality to accurately assess and is reported as a "no result."

19. The LOD is generally below the limit of quantification. In QZyme PCR, as with other real-time Q-PCR protocols such as SYBR Green 1 analysis, it is possible for background signal to be generated in the absence of the target (nonspecific, or primer-dimer, amplification). The LOD is defined by a Ct, before which false-positive signals are unlikely to be generated. The formula used to define LOD (*see* **Subheading 3.6.1.**) has been used for many QZyme assays in our laboratory and shown not to generate false positives.

20. The CV is the standard deviation as a percentage of the average: $[CV = (100 \times SD)/average]$. The log-linear nature of the relationship between Ct and copy number means that different limits are placed on the CV_{Ct} and $CV_{copy\#}$. A maximum CV_{Ct} of 2% is generally acceptable for calibrators. This corresponds to 10 to 25% for the $CV_{copy\#}$. The lower end of the limit of quantitation may be set to allow less precision. In our experience, a CV_{Ct} of 3% and $CV_{copy\#}$ of 30% is acceptable for the lowest calibrator. Accuracy is used as a measure of quantitation. Accuracy is calculated as the measured copy number for a calibrator expressed as a percentage of the known copy number. The accuracy for each calibrator should be between 70% and 130%. These values serve as a guide. Acceptance criteria for CV and accuracy should be set according to knowledge of individual assays and the degree of accuracy and precision required by the investigator.

21. It is possible to set looser acceptance criteria if the investigator realizes that this limits the discrimination of the assay, for example a ratio between 0.33 and 3 indicates that the assay cannot discriminate differences less than threefold.

References

1. Grimwade, D. and Enver, T. (2004) Acute promyelocytic leukemia: where does it stem from? *Leukemia* **18(3)**, 375–384.
2. Mistry, A. R., Pedersen, E. W., Solomon, E., and Grimwade, D. (2003) The molecular pathogenesis of acute promyelocytic leukaemia: implications for the clinical management of the disease. *Blood Reviews* **17(2)**, 71–91.
3. Degos, L. and Wang, Z. Y. (2001) All trans retinoic acid in acute promyelocytic leukemia. *Oncogene* **20**, 7140–7145.
4. Grimwade, D. and Enver, T. (2002) The significance of minimal residual disease in patients with t(15;17). *Best Pract. Res. Clin. Haematol.* **15(1)**, 137–158.
5. Lo Coco, F., Diverio, D., Avvisati, G., et al. (1999) Therapy of molecular relapse in acute promyelocytic leukemia. *Blood* **94**, 2225–2229.
6. Grimwade, D. and Lo Coco, F. (2002) Acute promyelocytic leukemia: a model for the role of molecular diagnosis and residual disease monitoring in directing treatment approach in acute myeloid leukemia. *Leukemia* **16**, 1959–1973.
7. Applegate, T. L., Iland, H. J., Mokany, E., and Todd, A. V. (2002) Diagnosis and molecular monitoring of acute promyelocytic leukemia using DzyNA reverse transcription-PCR to Quantify PML-RARα fusion transcripts. *Clin. Chem.* **48(8)**, 1338–1343.
8. Applegate, T.L., Iland, H. J., Mokany, E., and Todd, A. V. (2002) Molecular monitoring of acute promyelocytic leukemia by DzyNA reverse transcriptase. *Clinical Chemistry* **48**, 1858–1860.9. Jurcic, J. G. (2003) Monitoring PML-RARalpha in acute promyelocytic leukemia. *Curr. Oncol. Rep.* **5(5)**, 391–398.
9. Jurcic, J. G. (2003) Monitoring PML-RARalpha in acute promyelocytic leukemia. *Curr. Oncol. Rep.* **5**, 391–398.
10. Gu, B. W., Hu, J., and Xu, L. (2001) Feasibility and clinical significance of real-time quantitative RT-PCR assay of PML-RARalpha fusion transcript in patients with acute promyelocytic leukemia. *Hematol. J.* **2(5)**, 330–340.
11. Slack, J. L., Bi, W., and Livak, K. J. (2001) Pre-clinical validation of a novel, highly sensitive assay to detect PML-RARalpha mRNA using real-time reverse-transcription polymerase chain reaction. *J. Mol. Diagn.* **3(4)**, 141–149.
12. Gabert, J. and Beillard, E. (2003) Standardization and quality control studies of 'real-time' quantitative reverse transcriptase polymerase chain reaction of fusion gene transcripts for residual disease detection in leukemia—a Europe Against Cancer program. *Leukemia* **17(12)**, 2318–2357.
13. Larsen, R. (2003) BD QZyme™ Assays for Quantitative PCR. *Clontechniques* **XVIII(4)**, 2–3.
14. Larsen, R., Sheng, D., and Tan, M. (2004) Successful Duplexing of Randomly Selected BD QZyme™ qPCR Assays. *Clontechniques* **XIX**, 10–11.

15. Klein, D. (2002) Quantification using real-time PCR technology: applications and limitations. *TRENDS in Molecular Medicine* **8(6),** 257–260.
16. Kastner, P. and Perez, A. (1992) Structure, localization and transcriptional properties of two classes of retinoic acid receptor alpha fusion proteins in acute promyelocytic leukemia (APL): structural similarities with a new family of oncoproteins. *EMBO J.* **11(2),** 629–642.

9

Diagnosis and Monitoring of *AML1-MTG8* (*ETO*)-Positive Acute Myeloid Leukemia by Qualitative and Real-Time Quantitative RT-PCR

Khalid Tobal and John A. Liu Yin

Summary

Assessing the level of residual disease in leukemia is vital for evaluating patients' response to treatment and for identifying those at high risk of relapse. This should enable early preemptive intervention to prevent the onset of hematological relapse in those patients. One of the most common translocations in acute myeloid leukemia (AML) is the t(8;21). t(8;21) AML is characterized by a relatively good prognosis. This chapter discusses both qualitative and quantitative (real-time quantitative reverse-transcription polymerase chain reaction [RQ-PCR]) protocols for the diagnosis and minimal residual disease (MRD) monitoring in t(8;21) AML. It also discusses the importance of choosing appropriate controls for each assay. The chapter provides a simple equation for assessing the sensitivity/reliability of RQ-PCR assays, which enables scientists to assess the accuracy and reliability of their data.

Key Words: AML; t(8;21); qualitative RT-PCR; real-time RT-PCR (RQ-PCR); minimal residual disease (MRD); control genes; quantification reliability.

1. Introduction

The t(8;21) is one of the most common chromosomal translocations in acute myeloid leukemia (AML), detected in approx 20% of adult and 40% of pediatric AML M2 *(1,2)*. This translocation fuses the *AML1* gene on chromosome 21 and the *MTG8 (ETO)* gene on chromosome 8 *(3)*. Although patients with t(8;21) AML have a relatively good prognosis, relapse remains the most common cause of treatment failure. Therefore, accurately monitoring the level of minimal residual disease may play an important role in the management of this disease, by assessing patients' response to treatment and identifying those at high risk of relapse.

From: *Methods in Molecular Medicine, Vol. 125: Myeloid Leukemia: Methods and Protocols*
Edited by: H. Iland, M. Hertberg, and P. Marlton © Humana Press Inc., Totowa, NJ

2. Materials

1. Ficoll-Hypaque, Amersham Pharmacia.
2. Modified solution D: 6 M guanidinium isothiocyanate, 42.5 M sodium citrate (pH 7.0), 7.5% sarkosyl. Store in a dark container at 4°C.
3. Moloney murine leukemia virus (M-MLV) reverse transcriptase.
4. 5X first-strand buffer (supplied with M-MLV reverse transcriptase).
5. 2 μL dithiothreitol (DTT).
6. 25 mM dNTP mix.
7. Random hexamers, pdN(6).
8. Polymerase chain reaction (PCR) buffer (supplied with Taq polymerase).
9. W1 (Invitrogen, optional).
10. 50 mM MgCl$_2$.
11. Taq DNA polymerase.
12. Real-time qPCR master mix (2X), Eurogentec.
13. Phenol.
14. 70% ethanol.
15. Isopropanol.
16. Sterile water.
17. Primers:
    a. Qualitative reverse-transcription (RT)-PCR (50 pmole/μL)
       11—5' AGC CAT GAA GAA CCA GG 3' (first-round qualitative PCR)
       12—5' AGG CTG TAG GAG AAT GG 3' (first-round qualitative PCR)
       TS—5' CCC CGA GAA CCT CGA AAT CGT 3' (second-round qualitative PCR)
       24—5' GTT GTC GGT GTA AAT GAA 3' (second-round qualitative PCR)
       A2—5' TTC AGC GGC CAG TAG CAT CTG ACT T 3' (ABL qualitative PCR)
       CA3—5' TGT TGA CTG GCG TGA TGT AGT TGC TTG G 3' (ABL qualitative PCR)
    b. Real-time quantitative RT-PCR (RQ-PCR) primers and probes (10 pmole/μL)
       ABL forward: 5' TGTGGCCAGTGGAGATAACACT 3'
       ABL reverse: 5' CATTCCCCATTGTGATTATAGCC 3'
       ABL probe: 5' TAAGCATAACTAAAGGTGAAAAGCTCCGGGTCTT 3'
       AML1-MTG8 forward : 5' CACCTACCACAGAGCCATCAAA 3' (*see* **ref. 4**)
       AML1-MTG8 reverse: 5' ATCCACAGGTGAGTCTGGCATT 3'
       AML1-MTG8 probe: 5' AACCTCGAAATCGTACTGAGAAGCACTCCA 3'

3. Methods

3.1. Sample Preparation and RNA Extraction

Mononuclear cells are obtained from peripheral blood (PB) or bone marrow (BM) samples by Ficoll-Hypaque density gradient centrifugation, and should either be stored at −80°C or used immediately for RNA extraction.

RNA is extracted from mononuclear cells (MNCs) by standard protocols. The following protocol is a minor modification of the one published by Chomczynski and Sacchi *(5)*.

1. 250 µL of MNCs are mixed with 400 µL of modified solution D. This should give a final concentration of approx 4 *M* guanidinium isothiocyanate. Lysates can be stored in solution D for prolonged periods at –80°C.
2. 65 µL of 2 *M* sodium acetate, pH 4.0, are then added to the sample and vortexed well (*see* **Note 1**). Lysates can also be stored after the addition of sodium acetate.
3. Following 2–6 h incubation at room temperature, 650 µL of water-saturated phenol are added and vortexed well.
4. 130 µL of chloroform are then added, the mixture is vortexed well, and incubated on ice for 15 min.
5. Following centrifugation for 20 min at 13,000 rpm in a microfuge, the aqueous layer is removed to a new tube, ensuring that the interface is not disturbed.
6. An equal volume of isopropanol is added to the aqueous layer, vortexed well, and stored at –80°C for at least 2 h.
7. Following centrifugation for 15 min at 13,000 rpm, the supernatant is decanted and the pellets are washed in 70% ethanol.
8. RNA pellets are then dried and re-suspended in sterile water (*see* **Note 2**).
9. RNA should be stored at –80°C or used for the RT reaction immediately.

3.2. Reverse Transcription

RT reactions are performed with random hexamer primers in a 20-µL reaction. RT mixture is prepared by mixing the following on ice (*see* **Note 3**):

1. 4 µL of 5X first-strand buffer, 2 µL DTT, 0.8 µL dNTPs (mixture of all four dNTPs at 25 m*M* concentration), 0.25 µL pdN(6) (at a concentration of 1 µg/µL), 1 µL RNA Guard, 1 µL M-MLV reverse transcriptase, 5.95 µL water (*see* **Note 4**).
2. 2–4 µg of total RNA in a volume of 5 µL is heat denatured for 5 min at 75°C, then snap cooled on ice for 3 min (*see* **Note 5**).
3. RNA is centrifuged, and 15 µL of RT mixture is added.
4. The reaction is performed by incubation at room temperature for 10 min, then at 37°C for 10 min, 42°C for 1 h, and 75°C for 5 min (*see* **Note 6**).

3.3. Qualitative RT-PCR

A number of protocols have been developed for the qualitative detection of *AML1-MTG8 (ETO)*. The sensitivity of these protocols varies from 10^{-4} to 10^{-6}. This varied sensitivity could account for the conflicting data published using these protocols. Using relatively sensitive RT-PCR protocols ($10^{-5}–10^{-6}$), several groups have shown that, following chemotherapy, autologous and allogeneic bone marrow transplantation, *AML1-MTG8 (ETO)* transcripts can be detected in most patients in long-term remission (*6–8*). However, other reports have shown that negative qualitative RT-PCR results correlate with long-term remission and cure (*9*).

For qualitative RT-PCR protocols, suitable controls are necessary. They should include:

1. A negative (no-reaction) control.
2. A negative sample control (a sample or cell line negative for t(8;21)).
3. A positive control (a sample or cell line positive for t(8;21)).
4. A control gene, such as ABL, performed on all samples.

Samples must be tested for a suitable control gene. We have found the *ABL* gene to be suitable for most of the leukemia fusion genes.

3.3.1. ABL PCR Amplification

1. For ABL detection, the PCR reaction is performed in a 25-μL volume containing: 2.5 μL PCR buffer, 1.25 μL W1 (optional), 0.75 μL MgCl₂ (50 m*M*), 0.25 μL dNTPs (25 m*M*), 0.25 μL each primer (A2, CA3), 0.3 μL Taq DNA polymerase, 17.45 μL H₂O (*see* **Note 7**).
2. 2 μL of cDNA is added to the PCR mixture, vortexed, and centrifuged briefly.
3. PCR amplification is then performed according to these parameters:
   a. 95°C for 3 min
   b. 40 cycles of 93°C × 1 min, 55°C × 1 min, 72°C × 1 min.
   c. 72°C for 5 min.
4. 10 μL of PCR products should be electrophoresed on a 2% agarose gel. Expected band size is 276 bp (*see* **Notes 8** and **9**).

3.3.2. AML1-MTG8 (ETO) PCR Amplification

Once ABL amplification is successful, the sample is ready for *AML1-MTG8* (*ETO*) amplification. The protocol described as follows has a sensitivity of 10^{-6}. The protocol takes approx 10 h (two rounds of 4–5 h, depending on the PCR machine used).

1. PCR reaction is performed in a 50-μL volume (*see* **Note 7**).
2. First-round PCR master mix is prepared as follows: 5 μL PCR buffer, 2.5 μL W1 (optional), 1.5 μL MgCl₂ (50 m*M*), 0.5 μL dNTPs (25 m*M*), 0.25 μL each of primer 11 and primer 12, 0.3 μL Taq DNA polymerase, 37.7 μL H₂O.
3. 2 μL of cDNA is added to the PCR mixture, vortexed, and centrifuged briefly.
4. PCR amplification is then performed according to these parameters: 95°C for 3 min, then 40 cycles of 93°C 1 min, 55°C 1 min, 72°C 1 min, followed by 72°C for 5 min.
5. A second round PCR amplification of *AML1-MTG8* (*ETO*) is then performed on 2 μL first-round product, using primers TS and 24. PCR parameters are the same as those used for the first-round PCR.
6. 10 μL of PCR products should be electrophoresed on a 2% agarose gel. Expected band size is 152 bp in a positive sample (*see* **Note 9**).

3.4. Minimal Residual Disease (MRD) Monitoring

The main aim of MRD monitoring is to assess the effectiveness of treatment and to predict relapse at an early stage, thus possibly allowing preemptive or

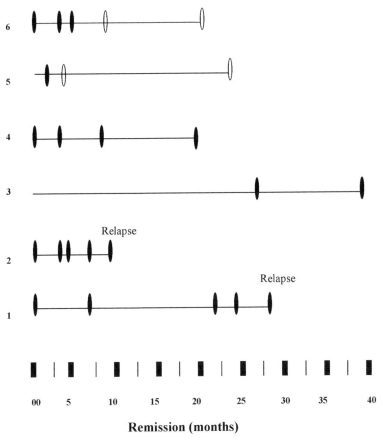

Remission (months)

Fig. 1. Sequential qualitative reverse-transcription (RT)-polymerase chain reaction (PCR) monitoring of *AML1-MTG8 (ETO)* in 6 t(8;21) acute myeloid leukemia (AML) patients. Patients 1 and 2 experienced hematological relapse, whereas patients 3–6 remain in stable remission. Solid circles, RT-PCR positive; open circles, RT-PCR negative.

additional therapy in an attempt to improve clinical outcome. Therefore, the value of any technique will be significantly reduced if it fails to distinguish between patients who are in stable remission and those at high risk of relapse. For this reason, qualitative protocols for the amplification of *AML1-MTG8 (ETO)* with high sensitivity are not suitable for MRD monitoring, as they will detect fusion transcripts even in patients in long-term remission. Moreover, protocols with a low sensitivity will not be able to predict early relapse in a large proportion of patients. Thus, the only credible approach is a sensitive quantification of the *AML1-MTG8 (ETO)* fusion transcripts (**Fig. 1**). There are

two strategies for the quantification of a given transcript: competitive RT-PCR
and RQ-PCR.

3.4.1. Control Gene

Choosing the right control gene is important for both qualitative and quantitative RT-PCR. However, a suitable control gene for qualitative RT-PCR may
not necessarily be suitable for the quantitative protocol. Control genes for quantitative RT-PCR must meet two major requirements: (1) transcript levels of the
control gene must not be affected by the disease in question and (2) degradation rate of the control gene must be equal to that of the gene of interest *(10)*.
Our investigations have shown that ABL is a suitable control gene for qualitative as well as quantitative RT-PCR for most AML fusion genes.

3.4.2. Competitive RT-PCR

Competitive PCR is suitable for the accurate quantification of genes or their
transcripts, especially when real-time equipment is not available *(11)*. In comparison to real-time quantification, competitive PCR could be seen as laborious and time consuming. The principle of the protocol is to simultaneously
amplify two targets in the same reaction using the same set of primers. The two
amplicons are the target gene itself in the test sample, and another DNA fragment, the competitor, which is typically a recombinant variation of the target
gene that is characterized by a deletion or an insertion to produce a different-
sized PCR product (**Fig. 2**). The number of copies in the original stock solution
of the competitor is estimated by spectrophotometry. Dilutions of this competitor are made in a range of 1–10^{10} molecules/2 µL, with a dilution at every
order of magnitude on a logarithmic scale. The lane in which the competitor
and target PCR products are present at equal amounts (the equivalence point)
indicates the number of copies in the test sample.

3.4.3. Real-Time Quantitative RT-PCR

Unlike qualitative PCR, in RQ-PCR a fluorogenic probe is positioned and
hybridized between the forward and reverse primers. The probe is labeled on
the 5′ with a fluorogenic reporter and on the 3′ with a quencher. During the
extension phase of the PCR cycle, the 5′→3′ exonuclease activity of *Taq* polymerase cleaves the hybridized probe, resulting in the release of the fluorogenic
reporter (**Fig. 3**). This causes an increase in the fluorescence emission of the
reporter dye that is proportional to the amount of PCR product accumulated.
Under appropriate conditions, this increase in fluorescence signal is also proportional to the amount of template used. The level of normalized reporter
signal (ΔRn) increases during PCR as the target is amplified, until the reaction
reaches a plateau. At the end of PCR amplification, real-time data analysis is
performed.

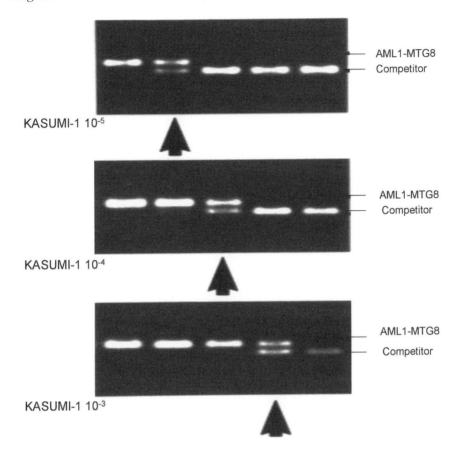

Fig. 2. Linearity study of competitive polymerase chain reaction. Arrows indicate the equivalence points for competitor and fusion transcript.

In RQ-PCR, reactions are characterized by the point during PCR cycling when the fluorescent signal from amplification of the target gene is first detected, rather than the amount of PCR product accumulated after a fixed number of cycles. The larger the starting quantity of the target sequence, the earlier a significant increase in fluorescence is detected. This forms the basis for calculating threshold cycle (Ct), which is defined as the fractional cycle number at which the fluorescence generated passes a fixed threshold above the baseline.

The protocol described as follows for the quantification of *AML1-MTG8* *(ETO)* transcript has a sensitivity of 10^{-5}–10^{-6}. The technique generally takes 3 h for completion (1 h preparation and 2 h running).

1. ABL RQ reaction mix: in a 25-μL reaction volume, add 12.5 μL qPCR master mix, 0.5 μL Abl-forward primer, 0.5 μL Abl-reverse primer, 1 μL Abl-probe, 5.5 μL H_2O (*see* **Note 10**).

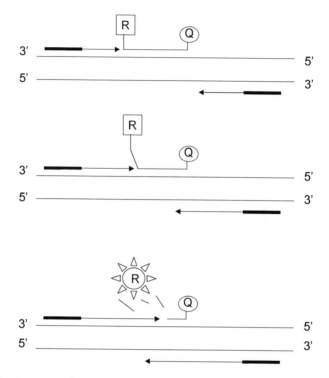

Fig. 3. The TaqMan 5′ nuclease assay.

2. *AML1-ETO* RQ reaction mix: in a 25-μL reaction volume, mix 12.5 μL qPCR master mix, 1 μL t(8;21)-forward primer, 1 μL t(8;21)-reverse primer, 0.5 μL t(8;21)-probe, 5 μL H$_2$O.

3. Reaction mixes for both ABL and *AML1-ETO* RQ should be prepared in sufficient amounts for the number of reactions needed.

4. 20 μL of reaction mix is added in each well.

5. 5 μL of each cDNA (*see* **Note 11**) is added in triplicate wells for each sample. Standard curves should be performed once a month using constructs prepared in the laboratory or commercially available ones (*see* **Note 12**). **Figure 4** shows examples of standard curves for ABL and *AML1-MTG8* (*ETO*) transcripts.

6. Negative controls (reactions without cDNA) should be included in every plate.

7. Wells should be sealed. The plate is then centrifuged at 3000 rpm for 3 min.

8. Real-time amplification is then performed according to the following parameters: 50°C for 2 min, 95°C for 10 min, followed by 40 cycles of 95°C for 15 s and 60°C for 1 min.

9. Analyze the data.

10. Levels should be expressed as a ratio of *AML1-MTG8* (*ETO*)/ABL transcripts.

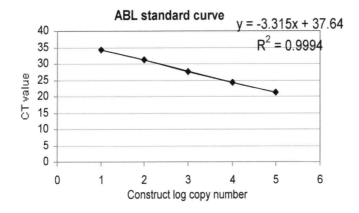

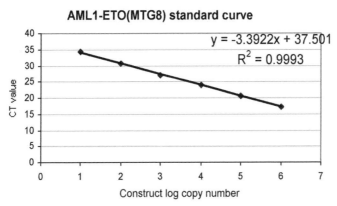

Fig. 4. Standard curves for *ABL* and *AML1-MTG8(ETO)* prepared with serial dilutions of constructs for both transcripts.

3.5. Data Analysis and Assessment of Assay Sensitivity/Reliability

The level of fusion transcripts should be assessed by the ratio of the fusion transcript level to the control transcript level. A number of groups multiply this ratio by 10^5, because it is estimated that 1 μg of RNA contains 10^5 copies of ABL transcript. Recently, and to reduce the confusion of various methods of presenting quantified levels, many researchers have elected to simply divide the fusion transcript level by the control transcript level, i.e., *AML1-MTG8 (ETO)/ABL* ratio (*see* **Fig. 5**).

As can be seen from **Fig. 5**, the relapse risk threshold for BM and PB samples of t(8;21) AML patients are 0.01 ($10^3/10^5$ ABL) and 0.001 ($10^2/10^5$ ABL), respectively. A BM sample with a ratio of 0.01 but an ABL level of $<10^3$ in the RQ-PCR reaction would actually contain $<10^1$ copies of *AML1-MTG8 (ETO)*. Similarly, a PB sample with a ratio of 0.001 but an ABL level of $<10^4$ in the

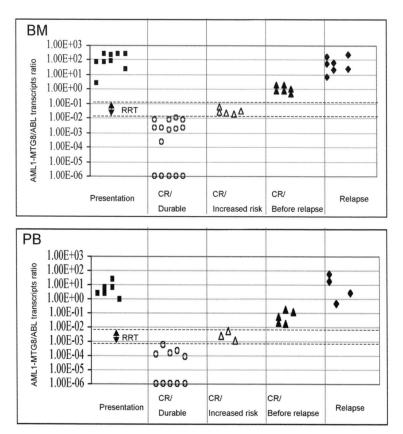

Fig. 5. Levels of *AML1-MTG8 (ETO)* transcript at different phases of t(8;21) acute meloid leukemia (AML). RRT, relapse risk threshold. Levels of 1.00E-06 (i.e., 10^{-6}) represent negative (undetectable) levels.

RQ-PCR reaction would actually contain <10^1 copies. These reactions could show false-negative results, as it is on the borderline of protocol sensitivity. One therefore can estimate the minimum amount of ABL transcript required in a reaction to produce reliable quantification of fusion transcripts. For BM and PB samples, the minimum ABL copy number is 10^3 and 10^4, respectively (*see* **Note 13**).

A number of investigators have started to show this assay sensitivity/reliability levels in their charts using various methods of calculation. A simple and reliable equation is:

$$(10^{-6} \times 10)/(\text{ABL copy number} \times \text{Relapse threshold level}).$$

10^{-6} represents undetectable level of target transcript, whereas 10 represents the lowest reliably quantified *AML1-MTG8 (ETO)* copy number in a reaction.

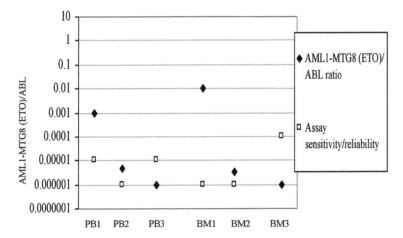

Fig. 6, Analysis of real-time quantitative reverse-transcription polymerase chain reactioin assay sensitivity/reliability. Levels of fusion transcripts in PB3 and BM3 samples are unreliable, as the levels of assay sensitivity/reliability are higher than those for the fusion transcript levels.

Based on the principles discussed above, two criteria for a good assay sensitivity/reliability level must be achieved for the quantification to be considered reliable. Firstly, the assay's sensitivity/reliability level must be <0.0001, and secondly, it must be below the ratio of the target gene/control gene (*AML1-MTG8 [ETO]/ABL*).

For example, a BM sample with a 10^2 ABL level/reaction would show an assay sensitivity/reliability level of $(10^{-6} \times 10)/(100 \times 0.01) = 0.00001$.

If the results of *AML1-MTG8 (ETO)* quantification is negative (0.000001), then the sensitivity/reliability level would be higher than that of the *AML1-MTG8/ABL* ratio. This indicates that the results of this test are unreliable.

Figure 6 shows sensitivity/reliability calculations and fusion transcript levels for three PB and three BM samples, two of which are unreliable.

3.6. Conclusion

The advent of RQ-PCR, which can provide useful information on MRD, will undoubtedly facilitate studies to assess the clinical value of MRD monitoring, which is an integral part of several multi-center trials in AML.

Furthermore, RQ-PCR lends itself to greater standardization and quality controls, which will allow comparison of data between different laboratories and international groups. In the clinical setting, results of accurate MRD quantification may allow risk-directed therapy in t(8;21) AML.

4. Notes

1. Some samples may contain cellular clumps; if this is the case, syringing the cells/solution D mix (after **Subheading 3.1., step 2**) with an approx 21-gauge needle could help to disperse the cells and aid cellular lysis.
2. Genomic DNA contamination may be precipitated with the RNA. High levels of genomic DNA contamination could therefore affect RT-PCR results. A second round of extraction (repeat the protocol previously described) could help in eliminating or significantly reducing the level of genomic DNA contamination.
3. It is necessary to perform all preparation in a sterile cabinet to avoid cross-contamination.
4. M-MLV reverse transcriptase is a thermolabile enzyme and should be kept at all times on ice while in use, then stored at –20°C.
5. The performance of positive and negative control RT reactions is necessary for accurate analysis.
6. Although a shorter RT reaction could be performed, this tends to produce lower levels of cDNA.
7. It is necessary to perform all preparation in a sterile cabinet to avoid cross-contamination.
8. Negative RT-PCR results for the control gene (ABL) indicate a lack of good-quality amplifiable RNA or cDNA. If this is the case, re-extraction of the RNA and the performance of a new RT reaction may help.
9. Positive RT-PCR results in negative control reactions indicate cross-contamination, and the analysis should be repeated.
10. It is necessary to perform all preparation in a sterile cabinet to avoid cross-contamination.
11. Once the cDNA is prepared, the volume is then diluted to 50 µL with water. Using 5 µL of cDNA in the RQ-PCR reaction reduces variation in the level quantified due to sample handling.
12. Performing a standard curve quantification is necessary with all new sets of primers and probes.
13. A low level of ABL indicates a low amount of amplifiable RNA/cDNA. Re-extraction of RNA may help in improving the results.

References

1. Raimondi, S. C., Kalwinsky, D. K., Hayashi, Y., Behm, F. G., Mirro, J. Jr., and Williams, D. L. (1989) Cytogenetics of childhood acute nonlymphocytic leukemia. *Cancer Genet. Cytogenet.* **40,** 13–27.
2. Rowley, J. D. (1990) Recurring chromosome abnormalities in leukemia and lymphoma. *Semin. Hematol.* **27,** 122–136.
3. Erickson, P., Gao, J., Chang, K. S., et al. (1992) Identification of breakpoints in t(8;21) acute myelogenous leukemia and isolation of a fusion transcript, AML1/ETO, with similarity to *Drosophila* segmentation gene, *runt. Blood* **80,** 1825–1831.

4. Gabert, J., Beillard, E., van der Velden, V. H. J., et al. (2003) Standardization and quality control studies of 'real-time' quantitative reverse transcriptase polymerase chain reaction of fusion gene transcripts for residual disease detection in leukemia—A Europe Against Cancer Program. *Leukemia* **17,** 2318–2357.

5. Chomczynski, P. and Sacchi, N. (1987) Single-step method of RNA isolation by acid guanidinium thiocyanate-phenol-chloroform extraction. *Anal. Biochem.* **162,** 156–159.

6. Nucifora, G., Larson, R. A., and Rowley, J. D. (1993) Persistence of the 8;21 translocation in patients with acute myeloid leukemia type M2 in long-term remission. *Blood* **82,** 712–715.

7. Kusec, R., Laczika, K., Knobl, P., et al. (1994) AML1/ETO fusion mRNA can be detected in remission blood samples of all patients with t(8;21) acute myeloid leukemia after chemotherapy or autologous bone marrow transplantation. *Leukemia* **8,** 735–739.

8. Saunders, M. J., Tobal, K., and Liu Yin, J. A. (1994) detection of t(8;21) by reverse transcriptase polymerase chain reaction in patients in remission of acute myeloid leukemia type M2 after chemotherapy or bone marrow transplantation. *Leuk. Res.* **18,** 891–895.

9. Morschhauser, F., Cayuela, J. M., Martini S., et al. (2000) Evaluation of minimal residual disease using reverse transcriptase polymerase chain reaction in t(8 ;21) acute myeloid leukemia : a multicentre study of 51 patients. *J. Clin. Oncol.* **18,** 788–794.

10. Lion, T. and Kidd, V. (chairmen). (1998) Debate round-table: appropriate controls for RT-PCR. *Leukemia* **12,** 1983–1993.

11. Tobal, K., Newton, J., Macheta, M., et al. (2000) Molecular quantitation of minimal residual disease in acute myeloid leukemia with t(8;21) can identify patients in durable remission and predict clinical relapse. *Blood* **95,** 815–819.

10

Diagnosis and Monitoring of *CBFB-MYH11*-Positive Acute Myeloid Leukemia by Qualitative and Quantitative RT-PCR

Bert A. van der Reijden and Joop H. Jansen

Summary

During the last decade, many mutations present in myeloid leukemias have been molecularly characterized. Several of these mutations have clear prognostic impact. The molecular screening of these mutations has now become an essential part in several risk-adapted international clinical trials. Here we describe protocols for the qualitative and quantitative detection of leukemic cells that are characterized by a *CBFB-MYH11* gene fusion.

Key Words: *CBFB-MYH11*; inv(16); t(16;16); M4Eo; qualitative RT-PCR; quantitative RT-PCR; minimal residual disease; control gene.

1. Introduction

The *CBFB-MYH11* gene fusion is frequently found in adult patients with *de novo* acute myeloid leukemia. The incidence is approx 10% (*1*). Approximately one-half of the *CBFB-MYH11*-positive patients exhibit FAB morphology M4Eo, whereas various other FAB morphologies are observed in the remaining 50%. Thus, FAB morphology is not a good predictor for the presence of the *CBFB-MYH11* gene fusion. In most *CBFB-MYH11*-positive cases, the fusion can be cytogenetically observed as an inversion on chromosome 16, inv(16)(p13q22), or, less frequently, as a translocation between the two chromosomes 16—t(16;16)(p13;q22). However, *CBFB-MYH11*-positive cases are known that do not show any cytogenetically visible chromosome 16 abnormalities (*2*). Because patients with the *CBFB-MYH11* fusion have a relatively favorable prognosis and may require adapted treatment, reliable tools are required for its detection. At present, qualitative *CBFB-MYH11* PCR is one of the most powerful methods to identify *CBFB-MYH11*-positive cases. Because the *CBFB-MYH11* gene fusion is tumor cell specific, it is also possible to quan-

From: *Methods in Molecular Medicine, Vol. 125: Myeloid Leukemia: Methods and Protocols*
Edited by: H. Iland, M. Hertzberg, and P. Marlton © Humana Press Inc., Totowa, NJ

tify minimal residual disease during and after treatment with real-time quantitative CBFB-MYH11 reverse-transcription (RT)-polymerase chain reaction (PCR). Because the sensitivity of real-time RT-PCR allows the quantification of at least 1 malignant cell in 10,000 normal cells, this technique allows the early identification of patients who relapse *(3,4)*.

2. Materials

1. cDNA synthesized from RNA isolated from peripheral blood or bone marrow cells.
2. Oligonucleotide primers, final concentration 10 pmol/μL (*see* **Table 1**).
3. Real-time PCR probes, final concentration 10 pmol/μL (*see* **Table 1**).
4. A 25 m*M* dNTP solution. This solution is prepared by mixing equal amounts of 100 m*M* dATP, dCTP, dGTP, and dTTP.
5. 10X PCR buffer.
6. MgCl$_2$.
7. Taq DNA polymerase.
8. Dimethylsulfoxide (DMSO).
9. Mineral oil.
10. TAQ gold DNA polymerase (Applied Biosystems).
11. Agarose gel and DNA sequencing equipment.
12. 6X DNA loading buffer containing 5% sodium dodecyl sufate (SDS).
13. Classical PCR equipment.
14. Real-time PCR equipment (Taqman PCR 7700 or 7900, Applied Biosystems). For storage conditions, *see* **Note 1**.

3. Methods

The methods in this chapter outline (1) the detection of the *CBFB-MYH11* fusion gene at diagnosis by qualitative and quantitative RT-PCR and (2) the quantification of *CBFB-MYH11*-positive cells during and after treatment by quantitative RT-PCR. Because the genomic breakpoints in *CBFB* and *MYH11* are scattered over large areas, it is not feasible to amplify these by regular PCR. However, at the RNA transcript level the breakpoints are found within a limited region. Therefore, reverse transcriptase PCR is used for the detection of the *CBFB-MYH11* fusion. To this end, RNA isolated from peripheral blood or bone marrow cells is first subjected to cDNA synthesis using reverse transcriptase. The synthesized cDNA is subsequently used as the target in *CBFB-MYH11* PCR.

3.1. Diagnosis of CBFB-MYH11-Positive Acute Myeloid Leukemia by Qualitative CBFB-MYH11 RT-PCR

To date, at least 10 different in-frame *CBFB-MYH11* fusion transcripts have been reported, which are caused by variable breakpoints in both *CBFB* and

Table 1
Primers for *CBFB-MYH11* Reverse-Transcription (RT)-Polymerase Chain Reaction (PCR) Detection

Name (*ref.*)	Sequence (5'–3')	Locus and position (5'–3')	Purpose
cd (*9*)	GCAGGCAAGGTATATTTGAAGGC	*CBFB* pos 253–275	First round CBFB-MYH11 PCR
mm (*9*)	CTTCCAAGCTCTTGGCTTTCTTC	*MYH11* pos 2401–2379	First round CBFB-MYH11 PCR
cmdI (*9*)	ATGGTATGGGCTGTCTGGAGT	*CBFB* pos 338–358	Nested CBFB-MYH11 PCR
mmd2 (*9*)	CTGTGGCAAAGATCTCATCTC	*MYH11* pos 2365–2345	Nested CBFB-MYH11 PCR
RAR-in*	CAGCACCAGCTTCCAGTTAG	*RAR* pos 235–254	RAR control PCR
RAR-II*	GGCGCTGACCCCATAGTGGT	*RAR* pos 414–395	RAR control PCR
Mfor (*13*)	AGTAGCCTGTCGGGAAGGAAC	*MYH11* pos 2497–2517	MYH11 qPCR
Mrev (*13*)	GCCTGCTGTGTGGCTTTG	*MYH11* pos 2639–2622	MYH11 qPCR
Mpro (*13*)	CACTCCAGGACGAGAAGCGCCG	*MYH11* pos 2519–2540	MYH11 qPCR probe
Cfor*	GAGAAGGACACGCGAATTTGA	*CBFB* pos 420–440	CBFB-MYH11 qPCR type A
CproMGB*	ATAGAGACAGGTCTCATCG	*CBFB* pos 443–461	CBFB-MYH11 qPCR probe, types A,D,E
MrevA*	GCTTGGACTTCTCCAGCTCAT	*MYH11* pos 1945–1925	CBFB-MYH11 qPCR, type A
ENF803 (*15*)	CATTAGCACAACAGGCCTTTGA	*CBFB* pos 389–410	CBFB-MYH11 qPCR types D, E
ENR863 (*15*)	CCTCGTTAAGCATCCCTGTGA	*MYH11* pos 1237–1217	CBFB-MYH11 qPCR, type D
ENR865 (*15*)	CTCTTTCTCCAGCGTCTGCTTAT	*MYH11* pos 1038–1016	CBFB-MYH11 qPCR, type E
PBGDfor*	GGCAATGCGGCTGCAA	*PBGD* pos 40–55	PBGD control qPCR
PBGDrev*	GGGTACCCACGCGAATCAC	*PBGD* pos 103–85	PBGD control qPCR
PBGDpro*	CTCATCTTTGGGCTGTTTTCTTCCGCC	*PBGD* pos 83–57	PBGD control qPCR probe

*Primers are described here. Please note that the position of the *CBFB* primers and probe are based on the sequence originally published by Liu et al. (*16*). The positions in the concomitant GenBank file (accession number L20298) differ by 21 bases because the first 21 bases (from the start codon) of *CBFB* are not present in the GenBank file. The positions of the MYH11 primers and probe are based on GenBank accession number D10667 (*17*). The cDNA positions of the *RAR* primers are based on GenBank sequence X06614. The positions of the *PBGD* primers and probe are based on GenBank accession number X04808 (*18*).

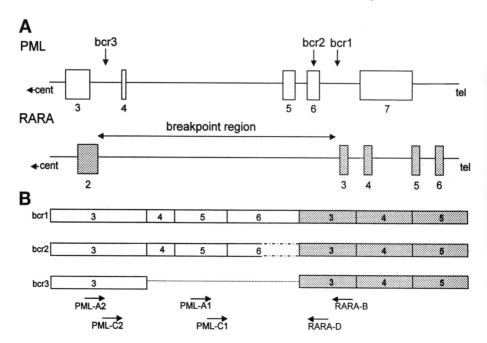

Fig. 1. Schematic representation of exonic junctions in currently known in-frame *CBFB-MYH11* fusion transcripts. Relevant *CBFB* exons (ce) are depicted as gray boxes and numbered. Relevant *MYH11* exons (me) are depicted as open boxes and numbered. In the upper panel, unrearranged *CBFB* and *MYH11* transcripts are shown. In the right column, the type of fusion transcript is indicated. Junctions in *CBFB* occur after exons 4 and 5. Breakpoints in *MYH11* occur before exons 28, 29, 30, 32, 33, and 34. Breakpoints in *CBFB-MYH11* fusion transcript types C and H occur within *MYH11* exons 31 and 28, respectively.

MYH11 (*see* **Fig. 1**) *(1,5–10)*. In addition, alternative splicing in *CBFB* may result in additional bands after PCR *(8)*. For the detection of *CBFB-MYH11* fusion transcripts at diagnosis, qualitative PCR should be applied that detects all known *CBFB-MYH11* fusion transcripts (**Fig. 1**) *(9)*. To increase the sensitivity of the assay, a two-step *CBFB-MYH11* PCR is outlined below (*see* **Subheading 3.1.1.**). For the first-round PCR, cDNA is added to a PCR mix. After PCR, an aliquot of the first-round PCR is used in a second-round PCR. Product amplification is subsequently visualized by agarose gel electrophoresis.

Because acute myeloid leukemia (AML) is defined as the presence of more than 20% of blasts in bone marrow, a sensitivity of at least 1 in 100 should be obtained. The best and most convenient way to show that the desired sensitivity is achieved is to use a dilution series consisting of RNA isolated from a positive control (the cell line ME-1 *[11]*) diluted into RNA from a negative control. Alternatively, *CBFB-MYH11* plasmid constructs may be applied. To exclude false-positive and false-negative results, the dilution series should be included in each analysis. The positive control must be diluted in such a manner that at a certain dilution a conversion from positive to negative signals is observed. If no conversion from PCR positive to negative signals is observed, the dilution series may be contaminated. Consequently, false-negative results may be obtained due to failure to recognize inadequate sensitivity of the assay.

To show that larger transcripts are efficiently amplified in qualitative PCR, we recommend also including a patient sample positive for *CBFB-MYH11* fusion transcript types D or E (*see* **Fig. 1**). To avoid false-positive results, several control samples negative for the *CBFB-MYH11* fusion should be included in each PCR run.

3.1.1. *Qualitative* CBFB-MYH11 *PCR*

1. Prepare the first-round *CBFB-MYH11* PCR mix by pipetting in the following order for one PCR reaction (*see* **Notes 2 and 3**): 11.09 µL H_2O, 1.25 µL 50 m*M* $MgCl_2$, 0.4 µL dNTPs, 2.5 µL DMSO, 2.5 µL 10X PCR buffer, 1.0 µL primer cd (**Table 1**), 1.0 µL primer mm (**Table 1**), and 0.26 µL Taq DNA polymerase (total volume of 20 µL).

2. Mix the first-round *CBFB-MYH11* PCR mix and add per reaction 5 µL of cDNA (50 ng) and a drop of mineral oil (*see* **Note 4**).

3. Perform the first-round *CBFB-MYH11* PCR using an initial denaturing step of 5 min at 94°C, followed by 27 cycles of 1 min at 94°C (denaturation of cDNA-RNA hybrids), 1 min at 62°C (primer annealing), 1 min at 72°C (product extension), followed by a final extension step of 10 min at 72°C (*see* **Note 5**).

4. Prepare the second-round *CBFB-MYH11* PCR mix by pipetting in the following order for one PCR reaction: 11.09 µL H_2O, 1.25 µL 50 m*M* $MgCl_2$, 0.4 µL dNTPs, 2.5 µL DMSO, 2.5 µL 10X PCR buffer, 1.0 µL primer cmdI (**Table 1**), 1.0 µL primer mmd2 (**Table 1**), and 0.26 µL Taq DNA polymerase (total volume 20 µL).

5. Mix the second-round *CBFB-MYH11* PCR mix and add per reaction 5 µL of a five times dilution of the first-round PCR product and a drop of mineral oil.

6. Perform the second-round *CBFB-MYH11* PCR using an initial denaturing step of 5 min at 94°C (denaturation of first-round PCR product), followed by 25 cycles of 1 min 94°C (denaturation), 1 min 62°C (primer annealing), 1 min 72°C (product extension), followed by a final extension step of 10 min at 72°C.

7. Judge *CBFB-MYH11* PCR amplification by agarosose gel electrophoresis using a 1.5% agarose-TBE (0.5X) gel containing 35 ng/mL ethidium bromide. Products can be visualized after ultraviolet (UV) exposure of the agarose gel. Make sure to include DNA size markers that allow for proper size determination in the 250- to 1700-bp range. The PCR product lengths obtained for the various *CBFB-MYH11* fusion transcripts after first- and second-round (nested) PCR, respectively, are indicated in **Table 2**.

Table 2
Currently Known *CBFB-MYH11* Fusion Transcripts and Amplicon Sizes

Transcript type	A	B	C	D	E	F	G	H	I	S
First PCR:										
cb-mm	703	916	1096	1423	1630	607	1327	1430	1318	394
Nested PCR:										
cmdI-mmdII	582	795	975	1302	1509	485	1205	1308	1197	272
Incidence (%)	89	<1	<1	5	5	<1	<1	<1	<1	<1

The indicated amplicon sizes are in base pairs, and are found after applying the primer pairs as indicated under **Subheading 3.1.1.** *(13)*. The incidence indicates the distribution of the various fusion transcripts amongst *CBFB-MYH11*-positive cases. Note that fusion transcript type A occurs in 89% of cases.

3.1.2. Qualitative RAR Control PCR for cDNA Synthesis

All samples used in qualitative *CBFB-MYH11* PCR should be subjected to a single-step (nonnested) qualitative control PCR to show that cDNA was efficiently synthesized in reverse transcription. The control PCR should result in the presence of a defined DNA fragment after agarose gel electrophoresis. Several control PCRs have been developed *(12)*. As an example for qualitative positive control PCR we outline here amplification of part of the *RAR* transcript.

1. Prepare the control *RAR* PCR mix by pipetting in the following order for one PCR reaction (*see* **Notes 2** and **3**): 18.97 µL H₂O, 1.0 µL 50 m*M* MgCl₂, 0.4 µL dNTPs, 2.5 µL 10X PCR buffer, 0.5 µL primer *RAR*-in (**Table 1**), 0.5 µL primer *RAR*-II (**Table 1**), and 0.13 µL Taq DNA polymerase (total volume of 24 µL).
2. Mix the first-round PCR mix and add per reaction 1 µL of cDNA (10 ng) and a drop of mineral oil (*see* **Note 4**).
3. Perform the *RAR* PCR using an initial denaturing step of 5 min at 94°C, followed by 30 cycles of 1 min at 94°C (denaturation of cDNA-RNA hybrids), 1 min at 60°C (primer annealing), 1 min at 72°C (product extension), followed by a final extension step of 10 min at 72°C (*see* **Note 5**).
4. Judge *RAR* PCR amplification by agarose gel electrophoresis using a 1.5% agarose-TBE (0.5X) gel containing 35 ng/mL ethidium bromide. Products can be visualized after UV exposure of the agarose gel. Make sure to include DNA size markers that allow for proper size determination between 100 and 350 bp. The *RAR* PCR product length should be 180 bp.

3.1.3. Validation of Qualitative CBFB-MYH11 PCR Results

A result is considered to be positive when:

1. The quality of the RNA is good as determined by agarose gel electrophoresis (*see* **Note 6**).

2. The control PCR (e.g., *RAR*) of all samples is positive.
3. The sensitivity is more than 1 in 100.
4. All negative controls are negative.
5. Both duplicate analyses are positive; i.e., a clear *CBFB-MYH11* PCR product is visible after UV exposure of the agarose gel.
6. The specificity of the *CBFB-MYH11* PCR product has been confirmed by sequencing.

A sample is considered to be negative when:

1. The quality of the RNA is good as determined by agarose gel electrophoresis (*see* **Note 6**).
2. The control PCR (e.g., *RAR* PCR) of all samples is positive.
3. The sensitivity is more than 1 in 100.
4. All negative controls are negative.
5. Both duplicate analyses are negative.

3.2. Diagnosis of CBFB-MYH11-*Positive AML by Quantitative* MYH11 RT-PCR

Real-time quantitative PCR (qPCR) is currently being used for routine identification and quantification of fusion genes and transcripts associated with hematological malignancies. The value for an individual sample as obtained with real-time PCR is represented by the cycle at which a signal is detected above the background. This value is called the threshold cycle (Ct) value. When applying a calibrator series with known amounts of input (e.g., diluted cells or molecules yielding a calibration curve with Ct values) the amount of a given sample can be calculated. Naturally, individual values should be corrected for variations in PCR efficiency, cDNA input, and so on, using a reference gene.

3.2.1 Quantitative MYH11 *PCR to Identify* CBFB-MYH11-*Positive Cases Among Newly Diagnosed AML*

The amplicon size used in qPCR should be less than 300 bp to guarantee efficient amplification. Because the distance between the smallest and longest *CBFB-MYH11* fusion transcript is over 1200 bp, the efficient detection of all fusion transcripts requires at least four different qPCRs. The *MYH11* gene is very weakly expressed in normal bone marrow cells and *CBFB-MYH11*-negative leukemia cells. However, as a result of the fusion to *CBFB*, the involved *MYH11* moiety is strongly expressed (approx 100- to 1000-fold higher) *(13)*. A single *MYH11* real-time PCR can be applied to function as an initial screen to identify *CBFB-MYH11*-positive cases based upon the relatively high *MYH11* expression at diagnosis. To completely rule out false-positive results, the presence of *CBFB-MYH11* should subsequently be confirmed with qualitative PCR as described under **Subheading 3.1.1.** The *MYH11* qPCR is not suitable to determine the type of *CBFB-MYH11* fusion transcript. The type of *CBFB-MYH11* transcript can be determined with qualitative *CBFB-MYH11* PCR followed by sequence analysis of the amplified PCR product.

Because cryopreservation can negatively affect the percentage of *CBFB-MYH11*-positive cells, quantitative *MYH11* PCR is suitable only as an indicator of the presence of *CBFB-MYH11* in freshly isolated samples.

To enable quantification of *MYH11* expression in patient samples, a calibration series with known amounts of input covering the desired range of quantification must be included in each PCR. The best and most convenient way to show that the desired sensitivity is achieved is to use a complete dilution series, consisting of cDNA generated from a positive control (e.g., the cell line ME-1 *[11]*) diluted into H_2O. Such a dilution series should be included in each analysis.

1. Prepare the *MYH11* qPCR mix by pipetting in the following order for one PCR reaction (*see* **Notes 2** and **3**): 24.25 µL H_2O, 10.0 µL 25 m*M* $MgCl_2$, 0.5 µL dNTPs, 5.0 µL 10X PCR buffer A, 1.5 µL primer Mfor (**Table 1**), 1.5 µL primer Mrev (**Table 1**), 2.0 µL probe Mpro, and 0.25 µL Taq gold DNA polymerase (total volume of 45.0 µL).
2. Mix the *MYH11* qPCR mix and add per reaction 5.0 µL of cDNA (50 ng).
3. Perform the *MYH11* qPCR using an initial denaturing step of 10 min at 94°C to activate the Taq gold DNA polymerase, followed by 45 cycles of 15 s at 94°C (denaturation) and 1 min at 60°C (primer and probe annealing and extension).
4. Collect the quantities of the unknown samples generated by the real-time PCR equipment that are based upon the obtained given quantities and generated Ct values of the calibration series.

3.2.2. Quantitative PBGD PCR for Normalization

The quantification of a control gene should be performed on each patient sample analyzed in real-time PCR to correct for variations in PCR and cDNA synthesis efficiency, cDNA input variations, and so on. However, if values are normalized over large ranges (>10-fold differences based upon the reference gene), quantitative results may be quite imprecise. To avoid correction over large ranges, we strongly recommend applying the same amount of cDNA in each PCR. Another advantage of this approach is that a calibration curve for quantification of the reference gene is not needed, because normalization occurs only over a limited range. By following this strategy, the amplification (quantification) of the control gene also shows that cDNA was efficiently synthesized. Several control genes for real-time RT-PCR normalization have been evaluated *(14)*. We discuss here amplification of the *PBGD* (porphobilinogen deaminase) gene, because the variation in expression in bone marrow and blood samples is minimal (*see* **Table 1** for *PBGD* primer-probe combination, and **Note 7**).

1. Prepare the *PBGD* qPCR mix by pipetting in the following order for one PCR reaction (*see* **Notes 2** and **3**): 25.25 μL H_2O, 10.0 μL 25 m*M* $MgCl_2$, 0.50 μL dNTPs, 5.0 μL 10X PCR buffer A, 1.5 μL primer *PBGD*for (**Table 1**), 1.5 μL primer *PBGD*rev (**Table 1**), 1.0 μL probe PBGDpro, and 0.25 μL Taq gold DNA polymerase (total volume of 45.0 μL).
2. Mix the *PBGD* qPCR mix and add per reaction 5.0 μL of cDNA (50 ng).
3. Perform the *PBGD* qPCR using an initial denaturing step of 10 min at 94°C to activate the Taq gold DNA polymerase, followed by 45 cycles of 15 s at 94°C (denaturation) and 1 min at 60°C (primer and probe annealing and extension).
4. Collect the Ct values of the unknown samples generated by the real-time PCR equipment.

3.2.3. Validation of Results, Normalization of Quantities, and Identification of Positive Samples

Check whether the required sensitivity is observed (*see* **Note 8**) and check the quality of the *MYH11* and *PBGD* PCRs according to **Note 9**. Check the cDNA quality according to **Note 10**.

Normalize the *MYH11* expression quantity of unknown samples (as generated by TaqMan software) for PCR and cDNA input variations by multiplying the quantity with the correction factor $2^{\Delta cycle\ threshold(Ct)}$, in which ΔCt = Ct *PBGD* of a sample minus the average *PBGD* Ct (*see also* **Note 10** for details). After normalization, a maximal variation of fourfold in the quantity between duplicate samples is allowed.

Samples with normalized *MYH11* quantities within a 25-fold range of a standard positive control (either higher or lower) are considered to be *CBFB-MYH11* positive (*see* **Note 11** for more details). For these samples, the presence of the *CBFB-MYH11* fusion and transcript type should be confirmed with qualitative *CBFB-MYH11* PCR. Negative samples have normalized *MYH11* quantities that are at least 1000-fold lower than that of the standard control. So far we have observed occasional samples with normalized *MYH11* quantities between 25- and 1000-fold lower compared to the standard control. All of these samples appeared negative in qualitative *CBFB-MYH11* PCR. Nevertheless, we recommend screening these samples for the presence of *CBFB-MYH11* by qualitative PCR.

3.3. Monitoring of CBFB-MYH11-Positive AML by Quantitative RT-PCR

With the development of real-time PCR, it is possible to monitor *CBFB-MYH11*-positive disease with a sensitivity of at least 1 malignant cell among 10,000 normal cells (*3,4*). Recent studies have shown that the *CBFB-MYH11* expression at diagnosis is similar among patients, and *CBFB-MYH11* expression levels can be used as an indicator of the percentage of *CBFB-MYH11*-positive cells (*3,4,15*). As mentioned previously, at least 10 different

CBFB-MYH11 fusion transcripts have been reported to date. We discuss here three *CBFB-MYH11* qPCRs that allow for the detection of the most frequently occurring fusion transcript types—A, D, and E. Together, these transcripts occur in about 98% of all *CBFB-MYH11*–positive cases (*see* **Table 2**). The only difference between these PCRs is the application of different primers located in *CBFB* and *MYH11* (*see* **Subheading 3.3.1.**). The *CBFB-MYH11* real-time probe described here intercalates with the minor groove of DNA (minor groove binding [MGB] probe). Because these MGB probes bind DNA more efficiently than standard real-time PCR probes, shorter sequences that exhibit similar melting temperatures as compared to longer, non-MGB real-time PCR probes can be used. In addition, these probes harbor a non-fluorescent quencher. As a result, these probes exhibit lower background fluorescence than do probes containing fluorescent quenchers.

3.3.1. Quantification of CBFB-MYH11 Positive Disease by qPCR

1. Prepare the *CBFB-MYH11* qPCR mix by pipetting in the following order for one PCR reaction (*see* **Notes 2** and **3**): 28.50 µL H$_2$O, 6.0 µL 25 mM MgCl$_2$, 0.25 µL dNTPs, 5.0 µL 10X PCR buffer A, 1.5 µL primer Cfor (**Table 1**), 1.5 µL primer MrevA, 2.0 µL probe CproMGB (use 5 pmol/µL instead of 10 pmol/µL), and 0.25 µL Taq gold DNA polymerase (total volume of 45.0 µL). To detect fusion transcript types D and E, use as forward primer ENF803 instead of Cfor and use reverse primers ENR863 or ENR865 instead of MrevA to detect respectively fusion transcript types D and E (**Table 1, Fig. 1**).
2. Mix the *CBFB-MYH11* qPCR mix and add per reaction 5.0 µL of cDNA (50 ng).
3. Perform the *CBFB-MYH11* qPCR using an initial denaturing step of 10 min at 94°C to activate the Taq gold DNA polymerase, followed by 45 cycles of 15 s at 94°C (denaturation) and 1 min at 60°C (primer and probe annealing and extension).
4. Collect the quantities of the unknown samples generated by the real-time PCR equipment that are based upon the obtained Ct values and given quantities of the calibration series.

3.3.2. Validation of Results and Quantification of Minimal Residual Disease

Check whether the required sensitivity is observed (*see* **Note 8**) and check the quality of the *CBFB-MYH11* and *PBGD* PCRs according to **Note 9**. Check the cDNA quality according to **Note 10**.

Normalize the *CBFB-MYH11* expression of unknown samples (as generated by TaqMan software) for PCR and cDNA input variations by multiplying the quantity with the correction factor $2^{\Delta cycle\ threshold(Ct)}$, in which $\Delta Ct = Ct$ PBGD of a sample minus the average *PBGD* Ct (*see* **Note 10** for details). After normalization, a maximal variation of fourfold in the quantity between duplicate samples is allowed.

4. Notes

1. All solutions and buffers (except for mineral oil and DMSO) used in PCR must be stored at –20°C to avoid loss of quality that may result in inefficient PCR. Mineral oil and DMSO should be stored at room temperature. Before use of frozen material, thaw the required ingredients on ice. Materials used for agarose gel electrophoresis can be stored at room temperature.

2. All steps should be carried out on ice to avoid loss of quality of PCR ingredients, which may cause inefficient amplification.

3. The amount of PCR mix should be multiplied according the number of samples that need to be analyzed (include mix for two additional samples because of loss of mix during pipetting). Perform all analyses in duplicate.

4. Add mineral oil to avoid evaporation of the PCR mix during cycling when a PCR machine without heated lid is used.

5. The described PCR cycling conditions were optimized using a DNA Thermal Cycler 480 from Perkin Elmer. Because a large variation in PCR machines with different performances exists, it may be necessary to adjust the annealing temperature if the required sensitivity is not obtained or when nonspecific amplification is observed. If adequate sensitivity is not obtained, the annealing temperature is probably too high and should be lowered stepwise by 2°C until the desired sensitivity is obtained. Conversely, if background or nonspecific amplification is observed in controls negative for *CBFB-MYH11*, the annealing temperature should be increased stepwise by 2°C.

6. The quality of RNA can be checked by regular agarose gel electrophoresis. Take 1 μg RNA in 10μL H_2O and add 2 μL of 6X DNA loading buffer containing 5% SDS. Run the samples in a fresh 1.5% agarose gel (0.5X TBE), which may also be used for PCR product electrophoresis. Check for the presence of 18S and 28S ribosomal RNA bands that, compared to DNA fragments, run at sizes of respectively 1.8 and 4.8 Kb. The presence of SDS in the DNA loading buffer will prevent RNA degradation.

7. We have observed an average Ct value of 26.4 for *PBGD* when analyzing 50 ng of cDNA of over 100 different patient samples (using a fixed threshold at 0.05). Because degraded RNA can yield *PBGD* Ct values of 29, we advise setting the maximal *PBGD* Ct value for individual patient samples at 28.4 (ΔCt of 2 relative to the average, equaling a fourfold less efficient amplification compared to the average value).

8. The quantitative range of a real-time PCR assay is determined by the lowest dilution in the standard curve that shows a positive result in duplicate (ΔCt < 2). Below this dilution, quantification is unreliable. Positive samples below this dilution may be reported as weakly positive. For both the *MYH11* and *CBFB-MYH11* qPCR, a sensitivity of 1 in 10,000 should be obtained.

9. The quality of real-time PCRs is determined using the calibration curve. The slope of the calibration curve should lie between –2.8 and –3.8, a predefined maximum Ct should be obtained for the undiluted sample of the calibration curve at a fixed threshold, and negative controls should be negative.

10. The cDNA quality is determined as follows: the ΔCt of the reference gene between a sample and the laboratory standard value should be less than 2. The laboratory standard value is obtained by using the mean Ct of over 100 samples with fixed input (50 ng cDNA).

11. As a standard, we have used the *CBFB-MYH11*-positive cell line ME-1 *(13)*. Alternatively, a *CBFB-MYH11*-positive patient sample can be used. The smallest difference in *MYH11* expression between the *CBFB-MYH11*-positive patient with the lowest *MYH11* expression and the *CBFB-MYH11*-negative patient with the highest *MYH11* expression was 25-fold *(13)*.

References

1. Liu, P. P., Hajra, A., Wijmenga, C., and Collins, F. S. (1995) Molecular pathogenesis of the chromosome 16 inversion in the M4Eo subtype of acute myeloid leukemia. *Blood* **85,** 2289–2302.

2. Langabeer, S. E., Walker, H., Gale, R. E., et al. (1997) Frequency of CBF beta/ MYH11 fusion transcripts in patients entered into the U.K. MRC AML trials. The MRC Adult Leukaemia Working Party. *Br. J. Haematol.* **96,** 736–739.

3. van der Reijden, B. A., Simons, A., Luiten, E., et al. (2002) Minimal residual disease quantification in patients with acute myeloid leukaemia and inv(16)/ CBFB-MYH11 gene fusion. *Br. J. Haematol.* **118,** 411–418.

4. Guerrasio, A., Pilatrino, C., De Micheli, D., et al. (2002) Assessment of minimal residual disease (MRD) in CBFbeta/MYH11-positive acute myeloid leukemias by qualitative and quantitative RT-PCR amplification of fusion transcripts. *Leukemia* **16,** 1176–1181.

5. Claxton, D. F., Liu, P., Hsu, H. B., et al. (1994) Detection of fusion transcripts generated by the inversion 16 chromosome in acute myelogenous leukemia. *Blood* **83,** 1750–1756.

6. Poirel, H., Radford-Weiss, I., Rack, K., et al. (1995) Detection of the chromosome 16 CBF beta-MYH11 fusion transcript in myelomonocytic leukemias. *Blood* **85,** 1313–1322.

7. Hebert, J., Cayuela, J. M., Daniel, M. T., Berger, R., and Sigaux, F. (1994) Detection of minimal residual disease in acute myelomonocytic leukemia with abnormal marrow eosinophils by nested polymerase chain reaction with allele specific amplification. *Blood* **84,** 2291–2296.

8. van der Reijden, B. A., Lombardo, M., Dauwerse, H. G., et al. (1995) RT-PCR diagnosis of patients with acute nonlymphocytic leukemia and inv(16)(p13q22) and identification of new alternative splicing in CBFB-MYH11 transcripts. *Blood* **86,** 277–282.

9. van der Reijden, B. A., de Wit, L., van Der Poel, S., et al. (2001) Identification of a novel CBFB-MYH11 transcript: implications for RT- PCR diagnosis. *Hematol. J.* **2,** 206–209.

10. Springall, F. H., Lukeis, R. L., Tyrrell, V., Joshua, D. E., and Iland, H. J. (1998) Identification of a novel CBFB-MYH11 fusion transcript in a patient with AML and inversion of chromosome 16. *Leukemia* **12,** 2034–2035.

11. Yanagisawa, K., Horiuchi, T., and Fujita, S. (1991) Establishment and characterization of a new human leukemia cell line derived from M4E0. *Blood* **78,** 451–457.
12. Kidd, V. and Lion, T. (1997) Debate round-table. Appropriate controls for RT-PCR. *Leukemia* **11,** 871–881.
13. van der Reijden, B. A., Massop, M., Tönnissen, E., et al. (2003) Rapid identification of CBFB-MYH11-positive acute myeloid leukemia (AML) cases by one single MYH11 real-time RT-PCR. *Blood* **101,** 5085–5086.
14. Beillard, E., Pallisgaard, N., van der Velden, V., et al. (2003) Evaluation of candidate control genes for diagnosis and residual disease detection in leukemic patients using 'real-time' quantitative reverse-transcriptase polymerase chain reaction (RQ-PCR)—a Europe Against Cancer program. *Leukemia* **17,** 2474–2486.
15. Gabert, J., Beillard, E., van der Velden, V., et al. (2003) Standardization and quality control studies of 'real-time' quantitative reverse transcriptase polymerase chain reaction of fusion gene transcripts for residual disease detection in leukemia—a Europe Against Cancer program. *Leukemia* **17,** 2318–2357.
16. Liu, P., Tarle, S. A., Hajra, A., et al. (1993) Fusion between transcription factor CBF beta/PEBP2 beta and a myosin heavy chain in acute myeloid leukemia. *Science* **261,** 1041–1044.
17. Matsuoka, R., Yoshida, M. C., Furutani, Y., et al. (1993) Human smooth muscle myosin heavy chain gene mapped to chromosomal region 16q12. *Am. J. Med. Genet.* **46,** 61–67.
18. Grandchamp, B., De Verneuil, H., Beaumont, C., et al. (1987) Tissue-specific expression of porphobilinogen deaminase. Two isoenzymes from a single gene. *Eur. J. Biochem.* **162,** 105–110.

11

Detection of the *FIP1L1-PDGFRA* Fusion in Idiopathic Hypereosinophilic Syndrome and Chronic Eosinophilic Leukemia

Jan Cools, Elizabeth H. Stover, and D. Gary Gilliland

Summary

Idiopathic hypereosinophilic syndrome (HES) and chronic eosinophilic leukemia (CEL) are related hematological malignancies characterized by sustained, unexplained hypereosinophilia (>1,500 eosinophils/µL) *(1–4)*. The term *CEL* is used when there is evidence that the disease is of clonal origin. We recently identified the *FIP1L1-PDGFRA* fusion gene in approx 50% of HES/CEL cases *(5)*. Fusion of *FIP1L1* to *PDGFRA* is the consequence of a deletion on chromosome 4, del(4)(q12q12), with the centromeric breakpoint in *FIP1L1* and the telomeric breakpoint in *PDGFRA*. The breakpoints in *FIP1L1* are diverse (introns 7 to 10), but the breakpoints in *PDGFRA* are always in exon 12 (encoding the juxtamembrane region). because the chromosomal deletion is only 800 kb in size, it remains undetected with standard cytogenetics. In agreement with this, most patients with HES/CEL present with a normal karyotype. Here we describe three different techniques to detect the presence of the *FIP1L1-PDGFRA* fusion gene in peripheral blood or bone marrow cells.

Key Words: Eosinophilia; fusion gene; kinase; imatinib; detection.

1. Introduction

The presence of the *FIP1L1-PDGFRA* fusion gene can be detected in blood or bone marrow from patients with hypereosinophilia at three different levels: the chromosome level, the DNA level, and the RNA level (**Fig. 1**) *(5,6)*. The *FIP1L1-PDGFRA* fusion transcript can be detected by reverse transcriptase polymerase chain reaction (RT-PCR), which is by far the easiest and most sensitive detection method. Alternatively, the *FIP1L1-PDGFRA* fusion gene can be detected and cloned at the DNA level by long-distance inverse PCR (LDI-PCR), which also allows sequencing of the exact breakpoints within *FIP1L1* and *PDGFRA*. The chromosomal deletion del(4)(q12q12), associated with the

From: *Methods in Molecular Medicine, Vol. 125: Myeloid Leukemia: Methods and Protocols*
Edited by: H. Iland, M. Hertzberg, and P. Marlton © Humana Press Inc., Totowa, NJ

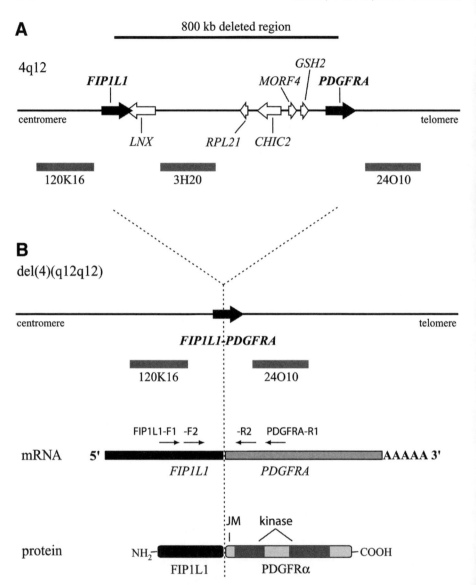

Fig. 1. Overview of the del(4)(q12q12) and the associated *FIP1L1-PDGFRA* fusion gene. Schematic representation of the genomic region at 4q12 involved in the deletion. The genes in this region are shown, as well as the three BAC probes that can be used for fluorescence *in situ* hybridization analysis. The deletion (approx 800 kb) creates the *FIP1L1-PDGFRA* fusion gene. The presence of the *FIP1L1-PDGFRA* fusion transcript can be detected by reverse-transcription polymerase chain reaction with the primers FIP1L1-F1 and PDGFRA-R1, and the nested primers FIP1L1-F2 and PDGFRA-R2.

generation of the *FIP1L1-PDGFRA* fusion, can be detected by three-color fluorescence *in situ* hybridization (FISH).

2. Materials

1. Anti-coagulated (preferably with EDTA) peripheral blood or bone marrow cells.
2. Red blood cell lysis buffer: 150 mM NH$_4$Cl, 0.1 mM ethylenediamine tetraacetic acid (EDTA), 10 mM KHCO$_3$, adjust to pH 7.4
3. Phosphate-buffered saline (PBS): 0.144 g/L KH$_2$PO$_4$, 0.795 g/L Na$_2$HPO$_4$, 9 g/L NaCl.
4. Freezing medium: 90% fetal bovine serum, 10% dimethylsulfoxide (DMSO).
5. Trizol (Invitrogen).
6. 70% ethanol: 7 vol 100% ethanol in 3 vol nuclease or RNase-free water.
7. Chloroform.
8. Isopropanol.
9. 8 mM NaOH.
10. DNA wash solution: 0.1 M sodium citrate, 10% ethanol (use autoclaved water).
11. cDNA synthesis kit.
12. Restriction endonuclease *Ase*I.
13. One-phor-all buffer Plus (OPA+, AP Biotech).
14. T4 ligase.
15. ATP.
16. Oligonucleotides (primers): FIP1L1-F1 (exon 7, 5′-acctggtgctgatctttctgat), FIP1L1-F2 (exon 7, 5′-aaagaggatacgaatgggacttg), PDGFRA-R1 (exon 14, 5′-tgagagcttgtttttcactgga), PDGFRA-R2 (exon 13, 5′-gggaccggcttaatccatag), Ase-Fa (5′-cagctgacatttgtggagtcct), Ase-Fb (5′-ttccgctagtctttcccatctt), PDGFRA-Ra (5′-agcaaatttccattgcctagttct), PDGFRA-Rb (5′-ggaggttaccccatggaactta), ZNF384-F (5′-cccatttcggctcccatgatt) and ZNF384-R (5′-ggtctcggtgtgtgacttgga)
17. Bacterial artificial chromosomes (BACs): RPCI11–120K16, RPCI11–3H20, RPCI11–24010 (available from http://bacpac.chori.org).
18. The EOL-1 cell line (available from http://www.dsmz.de).
19. RPMI-1640 medium, supplemented with 10% fetal bovine serum.

3. Methods

3.1. Extraction of RNA, DNA, and Proteins From Blood or Bone Marrow

3.1.1. Isolation of White Blood Cells From Blood or Bone Marrow

1. Add 5 vol of red blood cell lysis buffer to the anti-coagulated blood or bone marrow (*see* **Notes 1 and 2**).
2. Incubate the mixture on ice for 10 min.
3. Centrifuge at 450g for 10 min at 4°C.
4. After centrifugation, the cell pellet should be white, with only a small amount of red cells present. If this is the case, proceed with **step 5**. If the cell pellet is still red and no white blood cells are visible, resuspend the pellet again in red blood

cell lysis buffer and repeat the procedure from **step 2**. Keep the cells on ice all the time.

5. Aspirate the supernatant and resuspend the white blood cells in cold PBS.
6. Remove an aliquot to count the cells.
7. Pellet 5×10^6 to 10^7 cells by centrifugation (450g for 10 min at 4°C) (*see* **Note 3**).
8. Keep the cells on ice. Remove the supernatant, and vortex the cell pellet for 5 s. Proceed with RNA/DNA or protein extraction.

3.1.2. Simultaneous RNA and DNA Extraction From White Blood Cells

1. Add 1 mL Trizol (Invitrogen) to the cells and pipet up and down several times (*see* **Note 4**).
2. Incubate the lysate at room temperature for 5 min.
3. Add 200 µL of chloroform.
4. Shake the mixture vigorously for 15 s.
5. Incubate at room temperature for 10 min.
6. Centrifuge at 12,000g for 15 min at 4°C.
7. After centrifugation, the mixture is separated in a colorless upper phase, a white interphase, and a red lower phase. The RNA is present in the aqueous upper phase. Transfer the colorless upper phase (600 to 650 µL) to a clean 1.5-mL tube. Avoid touching the interphase in order not to risk contamination of the RNA with DNA. Save the interphase and the lower phase for DNA extraction.
8. Add 500 µL of isopropanol to the colorless phase. Invert the tube three times and incubate at room temperature for 10 min. While incubating the RNA/isopropanol mixture, use the following method for DNA extraction:
   a. Add 300 µL of 100% ethanol to the interphase and red lower phase (these phases contain the genomic DNA and proteins). Invert the tube three times. A precipitate should form directly. Incubate 3 min at room temperature.
   b. Centrifuge at 2000g for 5 min at 4°C.
   c. Discard the supernatant, and wash the pellet three times with DNA wash solution. Incubate for 20 min in this solution. Invert the tube several times during this wash step.
   d. Collect the DNA pellet by centrifugation at 2000g for 5 min at 4°C.
   e. Repeat **steps c** and **d** two more times.
   f. After these three wash steps, perform a final wash step with 70% ethanol.
   g. Remove all ethanol and air-dry the DNA pellet for 5 min.
   h. Resuspend the DNA in 8 mM NaOH. Do not pipet up and down too much, because this will break the DNA.
   i. Let the DNA dissolve at 4°C overnight.
   j. Add HEPES to adjust the pH (*see* **Note 5**), and measure the concentration and A_{260}/A_{280} ratio.
9. Centrifuge at 12,000g for 20 min at 4°C.
10. After centrifugation, a small, white RNA pellet is visible. Carefully discard the supernatant and add 1 mL 70% ethanol (make sure RNase-free water is used to dilute the ethanol). Invert the tube five times.

11. Centrifuge at 12,000*g* for 5 min at 4°C.
12. Remove the ethanol and spin briefly. Remove the rest of the ethanol and air-dry the pellet for 5 min. Do not dry the pellet for much longer than 5 min, as this may cause problems with dissolving the RNA.
13. Resuspend the RNA pellet in 10–20 µL RNase-free water, and measure the concentration (absorption at 260 nm, A_{260}) and the A_{260}/A_{280} ratio *(7)*.

3.2. Detection of the FIP1L1-PDGFRA *Fusion at the RNA Level*

The *FIP1L1-PDGFRA* fusion transcript is a tumor-specific transcript that is not expressed in normal cells *(5)*. One of the best techniques to detect the presence of this fusion gene in hypereosinophilic syndrome (HES)/ chronic eosinophilic leukemia (CEL) patients is the use of reverse-transcription (RT)-polymerase chain reaction (PCR) with *FIP1L1-* and *PDGFRA*-specific primers (**Figs. 1** and **2**). This analysis requires the availability of RNA (total RNA or mRNA) from peripheral blood or bone marrow (*see* **Note 6**).

RT-PCR consists of two separate steps: a cDNA synthesis step, followed by two consecutive PCR steps. In many cases, the *FIP1L1-PDGFRA* transcript can be detected after the first PCR reaction, but to increase sensitivity and specificity, a second (nested) PCR is recommended (*see* **Note 7**).

3.2.1. cDNA Synthesis

During random cDNA synthesis, RNA is reverse transcribed to single-strand cDNA (first-strand cDNA). Use 1–5 µg of total RNA. If you are not experienced with cDNA synthesis, use a commercial kit that provides all components: reverse transcriptase, buffer, dNTPs, random hexamer oligonucleotides (e.g., Superscript First-strand Synthesis System, Invitrogen). During cDNA synthesis, the RNA and the primers are denatured at 70°C, rapidly cooled down on ice to keep them denatured, and finally the primers are annealed to the RNA at 37°C to 42°C. The reverse transcription is usually performed at 37°C to 42°C for 1 h. Follow the recommendations specific for the cDNA synthesis kit.

After cDNA synthesis, the reverse transcriptase enzyme can be inactivated by a 10-min incubation step at 70°C, but no further purification is required.

3.2.2. First-Round PCR Reaction

For optimal PCR results, it is important to use the correct controls. You will need a positive control (cDNA in which the *FIP1L1-PDGFRA* fusion is present), a negative control (cDNA in which the fusion is not present), and a water control. A good positive control to use is cDNA obtained from RNA isolated from the EOL-1 cell line. This cell line expresses the *FIP1L1-PDGFRA* fusion gene *(8)*. The negative control can be cDNA generated from RNA from blood of a healthy individual or from a human cell line that does not express *FIP1L1-PDGFRA*.

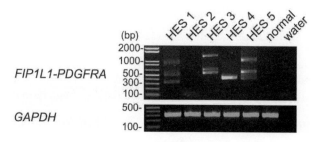

Fig. 2. Reverse-transcription polymerase chain reaction (RT-PCR) results. Example of the RT-PCR results for five hypereosinophilic syndrome cases. Cases 1, 3, 4, and 5 are positive, whereas case 2 is negative. Note that the positive cases show multiple bands because of alternative splicing and thus the presence of different fusion transcripts.

The *FIP1L1-PDGFRA* fusion is amplified using the oligonucleotides FIP1L1-F1 and PDGFRA-R1. At the same time, also set up a PCR reaction for a control gene (e.g., *ZNF384*) using primers ZNF384-F and ZNF384-R as a control for RNA quality and cDNA synthesis. Set up four reactions for each primer pair, according to **Table 1**, and perform the PCR according to the program in **Table 2**.

3.2.3. Second-Round PCR Reaction

Set up four reactions with the primers FIP1L1-F2 and PDGFRA-R2, according to **Table 1**, using 1 µL of the first-round PCR products instead of 1 µL of cDNA/water. Perform the PCR according to the program in **Table 2**.

3.2.4. Gel Electrophoresis and Interpretation of the Results

Analyze the PCR products, by loading 5 µL on a 1.5% agarose gel (*see* **Fig. 2**).

Expected results are shown in **Table 3**. Amplification of *ZNF384* serves as a control for RNA quality and cDNA synthesis. If no product is generated after first-round PCR, then either the RNA of that sample was of bad quality or the cDNA synthesis failed. The *FIP1L1-PDGFRA* transcript should be detected after the first-round PCR in the positive control (EOL-1 cells), as well as after second-round PCR, and should remain negative after second round of PCR in the negative and water controls. Only then can the result for the HES/CEL patient be completely trusted. In most patients, multiple bands are visible on the gel, due to the presence of splice variants of the *FIP1L1-PDGFRA* fusion (as shown in **Fig. 2**) *(5)*.

3.3. Detection of the FIP1L1-PDGFRA *Fusion Gene at the DNA Level*

In contrast with the detection of the *FIP1L1-PDGFRA* fusion transcript at the RNA level, which can be performed by PCR amplification using primers

Table 1
Polymerase Chain Reaction Setup

Component	Amount needed			
	Positive control	Negative control	Water control	HES patient
Forward primer	10 pmol	10 pmol	10 pmol	10 pmol
Reverse primer	10 pmol	10 pmol	10 pmol	10 pmol
10X buffer	5 μL	5 μL	5 μL	5 μL
dNTPs (10 mM)	1 μL	1 μL	1 μL	1 μL
Taq enzyme	2.5 U	2.5 U	2.5 U	2.5 U
cDNA from EOL-1	1 μL*	—	—	—
cDNA from healthy individual	—	1 μL*	—	—
Water	—	—	1 μL	—
cDNA from HES patient	—	—	—	1 μL*
Water	to 50 μL	to 50 μL	to 50 μL	to 50 μL

* This is approximately a one-twentieth fraction of the cDNA obtained from 1–5 μg. dNTPs, deoxynucleotidetriphosphates.

Note: When setting up four reactions with the same primer pair, prepare a fivefold master mix containing each component (except cDNA).

HES, hypereosinophilic syndrome.

Table 2
Polymerase Chain Reaction (PCR) Program

Step	Temperature	Time
1	94°C	3 min (denaturing of the cDNA)
2	94°C	30 s (denaturing of the cDNA/PCR products)
3	58°C	30 s (primer annealing)
4	72°C	90 s (primer extension by Taq DNA polymerase)
→ repeat steps 2–4 34 times (35 cycles in total)		
5	72°C	3 min (final extension step)
6	4°C	indefinite (cooling)

This is a basic PCR program. Based on the type of PCR machine, variations on specific times may be needed.

for *FIP1L1* and *PDGFRA*, the fusion gene cannot be detected so easily at the DNA level. This is due to the presence of large introns in *FIP1L1* and the variation of the breakpoints over a region of 50 kb (*see* **Note 8**). Based on the fact that the breakpoints in *PDGFRA* are always located within exon 12

Table 3
Expected Results After First and Second Polymerase Chain Reaction (PCR)

	Positive control	Negative control	Water	HES patient
First PCR				
ZNF384	+	+	—	+
FIP1L1—PDGFRA	+	—	—	±
Second PCR				
FIP1L1—PDGFRA	+	—	—	±

A second-round PCR reaction is not necessary for the control gene. HES, hypereosinophilic syndrome.

(4,5), long-distance inverse PCR (LDI-PCR) *(9)* can be used efficiently to amplify and clone the genomic breakpoint region. The method was designed to amplify a DNA fragment using specific primers in cases where the sequence of one end of the DNA fragment is unknown. In HES cases, the breakpoint in *PDGFRA* is always located in exon 12, which represents the known end of the DNA fragment. The breakpoint in *FIP1L1* is unknown (intron 7 to intron 10). **Fig. 3** shows the steps in LDI-PCR.

1. To 500 ng of genomic DNA, add 30 U of restriction endonuclease *Ase*I in its appropriate buffer in a total volume of 40 μL.
2. Incubate at 37°C for 3 h (to achieve complete digestion).
3. Purify the digested DNA using a PCR purification system (Qiagen).
4. Elute the DNA from the column with 100 μL water.
5. Add 5 U T4 DNA ligase, 50 μL of 10X OPA+ buffer (AP Biotech), 5 μL of 100 m*M* ATP, add water to 500 μL.
6. Incubate overnight at 15°C.
7. Purify the ligated DNA using a PCR purification system (Qiagen). Make sure to add 5 vol of PB buffer (included in the Qiagen PCR purification system). Load the DNA/PB buffer mixture all onto the same purification column in consecutive steps (load, spin, load again, spin, and so on).
8. Elute the DNA in 80 μL water.
9. Set up the PCR reactions using a PCR system to amplify long (more than 5 kb) PCR products (e.g., the Long Range PCR system, Roche). Use 20 μL (1/4) of the eluate as template in these PCR reactions with the primers AseF1 and PDGFRA-Ra. Follow the recommendations of the long-range PCR kit you are using for setting up the PCR reactions and the PCR program.
10. Transfer 1 μL of the first reaction to a new PCR reaction, using the same PCR kit, but now using the primer AseF2 in combination with PDGFRA-Rb.
11. Load 5 μL of the PCR reaction on a 1% agarose gel for analysis (*see* **Note 9**).
12. Isolate the PCR products from the gel and purify.

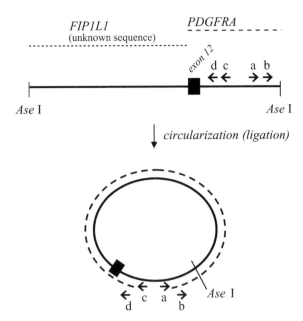

Fig. 3. Overview of the long-distance inverse polymerase chain reaction (PCR) (LDI-PCR) technique. Genomic DNA is cut with *Ase*I, the digested DNA is purified and diluted, and subjected to a ligation reaction under conditions that favor self ligation (circularization). Subsequent PCR reaction using the primers a (Ase-Fa) and c (PDGFRA-Ra) in a first-round PCR, and the primers b (Ase-Fb) and d (PDGFRA-Rb) in the second (nested) PCR reaction, yields a PCR product containing the region at the fusion of *FIP1L1* and *PDGFRA*.

13. Load a fraction of the isolated PCR product again on a 1% agarose gel to check its concentration and purity.
14. Sequence the PCR product using primer PDGFRA-Rb (*see* **Note 9**).

3.4. Detection of the del(4)(q12q12) at the Chromosome Level

3.4.1. Fluorescence In Situ Hybridization (FISH)

The FISH technique is described in detail in a previous chapter in this volume. The deletion is present in most peripheral blood cells, particularly eosinophils (up to 70% of white blood cells in the blood of HES/CEL patients), and neutrophils. FISH can be performed on peripheral blood or on bone marrow. The probes described here have been successfully used for both interphase and metaphase FISH (*6*) (*see* **Note 10**).

3.4.2. FISH Probes for Detection of the del(4)(q12q12)

Three probes have been selected for three-color FISH analysis of the deletion (RPCI11–120K16, RPCI11–3H20, RPCI11–24010) (**Fig. 1**). The selective absence of probe RPCI11–3H20 identifies the deletion associated with the
FIP1L1-PDGFRA fusion.

4. Notes

1. Be sure to wear gloves at all times. Blood and bone marrow should be treated as
   hazardous material. RNA and proteins are unstable in blood and bone marrow
   cells. Isolation of good quality RNA and proteins requires that the blood or bone
   marrow samples be processed as quickly as possible (best within hours after the
   sample was obtained). DNA is much more stable and can be isolated even after a
   few days.
2. Five to ten milliliters of blood is sufficient.
3. The rest of the cells can be stored as cell pellets at –80°C in aliquots of 5×10^6 to
   10^7 cells. Alternatively, the cells can be resuspended in freezing medium, and
   frozen slowly (at a rate of –1°C per minute) down to –80°C and then stored in
   liquid nitrogen. Cells frozen like this remain viable and can be used later for
   molecular analysis, or can even be used for short-term in vitro cultures.
4. Be sure to wear gloves during RNA extraction and while handling RNA. Use
   RNase-free tubes and tips. RNases are very stable and cannot be inactivated by
   autoclaving.
5. Add 2.3 μL HEPES (1 *M*) to 100 μL DNA in 8 m*M* NaOH.
6. As RNA is unstable and rapidly degraded, best results are obtained on fresh blood
   or bone marrow cells, or with white blood cells that were isolated and stored
   frozen at –80°C within hours of the time the blood/bone marrow sample was
   obtained. We have, however, obtained good results from blood that was stored
   for 48 h at room temperature.
7. A second (nested) PCR reaction, using an aliquot of the first PCR reaction as
   template, will increase the sensitivity of the detection method. This is highly
   recommended for detection of *FIP1L1-PDGFRA* fusion transcripts when starting with low-quality RNA and during hematological remission.
8. Detection of the *FIP1L1-PDGFRA* fusion transcript by RT-PCR and subsequent
   sequence analysis of the PCR product may provide a good indication of the position of the breakpoint in *FIP1L1*. First, some introns of *FIP1L1* are relatively
   short (intron 9 [2 kb] and intron 11 [1.3 kb]), making it possible to amplify the
   fusion directly from genomic DNA. This can be achieved by using a primer in the
   FIP1L1 exon upstream of the breakpoint and a primer at the exon-intron boundary of exon/intron 12 of *PDGFRA* (located completely downstream of the
   breakpoint). Second, in some *FIP1L1-PDGFRA* fusions, a few nucleotides
   derived from an intron of *FIP1L1* are incorporated in the fusion transcript. These
   nucleotides are located between the cryptic splice site (GT) that is used to splice
   FIP1L1 to *PDGFRA* and the actual breakpoint in the intron of *FIP1L1*. Thus,

comparison of the sequence of the *FIP1L1* gene (available at http://www.ensembl.org) with these intronic nucleotides in the *FIP1L1-PDGFRA* transcript may reveal the exact location of the breakpoint in *FIP1L1*. If this can be determined, a direct PCR can be designed to amplify the *FIP1L1-PDGFRA* fusion from the genomic DNA of that particular patient.

9. The LDI-PCR procedure can generate false-positive bands. False-positive bands are usually weaker than true positives. Only after sequencing of the bands and confirming a breakpoint in exon 12 of *PDGFRA* can a definitive conclusion be made.

10. Eosinophils may show autofluorescence, which may cause background fluorescence during FISH analysis.

References

1. Chusid, M. J., Dale, D. C., West, B. C., and Wolff, S. M. (1975) The hypereosinophilic syndrome: analysis of fourteen cases with review of the literature. *Medicine (Baltimore)* **54**, 1–27.
2. Weller, P. F. and Bubley, G. J. (1994) The idiopathic hypereosinophilic syndrome. *Blood* **83**, 2759–2779.
3. Gotlib, J., Cools, J., Malone, J. M., III, Schrier, S. L., Gilliland, D. G., and Coutre, S. E. (2004) The FIP1L1-PDGFRalpha fusion tyrosine kinase in hypereosinophilic syndrome and chronic eosinophilic leukemia: implications for diagnosis, classification, and management. *Blood* **103**, 2879–2891.
4. Cools, J., Stover, E. H., Wlodarska, I., Marynen, P., and Gilliland, D. G. (2004) The FIP1L1-PDGFRalpha kinase in hypereosinophilic syndrome and chronic eosinophilic leukemia. *Curr. Opin. Hematol.* **11**, 51–57.
5. Cools, J., DeAngelo, D. J., Gotlib, J., et al. (2003) A tyrosine kinase created by fusion of the PDGFRA and FIP1L1 genes as a therapeutic target of imatinib in idiopathic hypereosinophilic syndrome. *N. Engl. J. Med.* **348**, 1201–1214.
6. Vandenberghe, P., Wlodarska, I., Michaux, L., et al. (2004) Clinical and molecular features of FIP1L1-PDFGRA (+) chronic eosinophilic leukemias. *Leukemia* **18**, 734–742.
7. Sambrook, J., Fritsch, E. F., and Maniatis, T. (1989) *Molecular Cloning, A Laboratory Manual.* 2nd edition. Cold Spring Harbor, NY: Cold Spring Harbor Laboratory Press.
8. Cools, J., Quentmeier, H., Huntly, B. J., et al. (2004) The EOL-1 cell line as an in vitro model for the study of FIP1L1-PDGFRA-positive chronic eosinophilic leukemia. *Blood* **103**, 2802–2805.
9. Willis, T. G., Jadayel, D. M., Coignet, L. J., et al. (1997) Rapid molecular cloning of rearrangements of the IGHJ locus using long-distance inverse polymerase chain reaction. *Blood* **90**, 2456–2464.

12

FLT3 Mutations in Acute Myeloid Leukemia

Hitoshi Kiyoi and Tomoki Naoe

Summary

The prevalence of an internal tandem duplication (ITD) of the juxtamembrane domain-coding sequence and a missense mutation of D835 within the kinase domain of the *FLT3* gene is 15–35% and 5–10% of adults with acute myeloid leukemia (AML), respectively. In addition, point mutations, deletions, and insertions have been found in the juxtamembrane domain and in the other codons within the kinase domain, though these are less common. Several large-scale studies in well-documented patients published to date have demonstrated that *FLT3* mutations are strongly associated with a poor prognosis and a high leukemia cell count in patients with AML, suggesting that *FLT3* mutations are involved in disease progression. Because the detection of *FLT3* mutations is fast, easy, and inexpensive, mutation analysis should be performed as a routine test. This chapter describes methods for detecting ITD and D835 mutations in the *FLT3* gene.

Key Words: *FLT3*; internal tandem duplication; point mutation; deletion mutation; tyrosine kinase; leukemia; molecular target.

1. Introduction

FLT3, a member of the receptor tyrosine kinase class III family, is preferentially expressed on the surface of a high proportion of acute myeloid leukemia (AML) and B-lineage acute lymphoblastic leukemia (ALL) cells as well as hematopoietic stem cells *(1–3)*. An interaction of *FLT3* and its ligand has been shown to play an important role in the survival, proliferation, and differentiation of not only normal hematopoietic cells but also leukemia cells. Mutations of the *FLT3* gene were first reported as an internal tandem duplication (ITD) of the juxtamembrane domain-coding sequence, and subsequently as a missense mutation of D835 within the activation loop *(4,5)*. In addition, point mutations, deletions, and insertions have been found in the juxtamembrane domain and in the other codons of the kinase domain, although these are less common *(5–9)* (*see* **Note 1**). The prevalence of ITD and D835 mutations is 15–35% and 5–10% of adults with AML, respectively. Thus, *FLT3* mutation is currently the

From: *Methods in Molecular Medicine, Vol. 125: Myeloid Leukemia: Methods and Protocols*
Edited by: H. Iland, M. Hertzberg, and P. Marlton © Humana Press Inc., Totowa, NJ

most frequent genetic alteration identified in AML. Several large-scale studies in well-documented patients published to date have demonstrated that *FLT3* mutations are strongly associated with a poor prognosis and a high leukemia cell count in patients with AML, suggesting that *FLT3* mutations are involved in disease progression *(6,10,11)*. Both ITD and D835 mutations are detected by means of a conventional genomic PCR-mediated technique *(2)*. Because the detection of *FLT3* mutations is fast, easy, and inexpensive, mutation analysis can be performed as a routine test to facilitate assessment of individual patient prognosis.

2. Materials

1. DNA extraction reagent or kit (e.g., DNA_{ZOL}™ Reagent, Gibco BRL, Gaithersburg, ND; and QIAamp® DNA Mini Kit, Qiagen, Chatsworth, CA).
2. Ethanol.
3. Oligonucleotide primers.
4. Thermostable DNA polymerase (e.g., AmpliTaq Gold™, Perkin Elmer, Foster City, CA).
5. Polymerase chain reaction (PCR) reaction buffer (usually supplied with polymerase).
6. dNTP solution (usually supplied with polymerase).
7. $MgCl_2$ solution (usually supplied with polymerase).
8. Water (autoclaved deionized, ultrafiltered, or glass-distilled water is recommended).
9. PCR equipment (thermal cycler).
10. *Eco* RV endonuclease.
11. Reaction buffers for *Eco*RV (usually supplied with *Eco* RV endonuclease).
12. Agarose (e.g., NuSieve® GTG agarose and SeaKem® GTG agarose).
13. Sample loading buffer.
14. TBE buffer: 89 m*M* Tris-borate, 2 m*M* ethylenediamine tetraacetic acid (EDTA), pH 8.0.
15. DNA molecular-weight marker (e.g., 100-bp ladder markers for the detection of ITD, 10-bp ladder markers for the detection of D835 mutations).
16. Ethidium bromide.
17. Electrophoresis equipment.
18. DNA sequencing kit and equipment.

3. Methods

3.1. DNA Extraction

Genomic DNA for the detection of *FLT3* mutations is extracted from bone marrow and/or peripheral blood cells by any one of a number of standard methods. Many reagents and/or kits for DNA extraction are commercially available. We usually use DNA_{ZOL} Reagent (Gibco BRL, Gaithersburg, ND) or QIAamp DNA Mini Kit (Qiagen, Chatsworth, CA).

3.1.1. DNA$_{ZOL}$ Reagent

This reagent can be stored at 15°C to 30°C for at least 1 yr. It contains guanidine isothiocyanate, and may be harmful if contact with skin or eyes occurs. It is highly recommended that the manufacturer's instructions be read carefully before use. Ethanol is also required for the procedure. The extraction procedure can be performed quickly and easily according to the manufacturer's instructions. In brief, cell pellets are lysed in this reagent by gently pipetting. The genomic DNA is precipitated from the lysate with ethanol.

3.1.2. QIAamp DNA Mini Kit

This kit provides fast and easy methods for purification of genomic DNA from whole blood and buffy coat. Columns and all reagents, except for ethanol and phosphate-buffered saline, are included in the kit. Some reagents are harmful and irritant. It is highly recommended that the manufacturer's instructions be read carefully before use. DNA extraction can be performed by the simple QIAamp spin and vacuum procedures within 20 min according to the manufacturer's instructions.

3.2. PCR

3.2.1. Primers

To date, several primer pairs for the detection of *FLT3* mutations have been described. The following primer sequences have been reported by us *(5,12)*:

For the detection of ITD mutations in the juxtamembrane domain:
    Forward primer: 5′-CAATTTAGGTATGAAAGCCAGC-3′
    Reverse primer: 5′-CTTTCAGCATTTTGACGGCAACC-3′
For the detection of D835 mutations in the kinase domain:
    Forward primer: 5′-CCGCCAGGAACGTGCTTG-3′
    Reverse primer: 5′-GCAGCCTCACATTGCCCC-3′

3.2.2. Reaction Mixture and PCR Condition

Many thermostable DNA polymerases and their reaction buffers are available. Neither special polymerase nor buffer conditions are required for the amplification of the *FLT3* gene. We usually use AmpliTaq Gold and the accompanying reagents (Perkin Elmer, Foster City, CA). AmpliTaq Gold and reagents must be stored at –20°C in a constant-temperature freezer.

1. Thaw and gently mix each of the reagents.
2. Spin the polymerase solution down in a microcentrifuge before use.
3. Prepare reaction mixture according to **Table 1**.
4. It is recommended that a master mix of sufficient volume for the number of samples being analyzed be prepared. This should contain all the reagents except

Table 1
Reaction Mixture for Polymerase Chain Reaction (PCR)

Reaction mixture (for 1 reaction)	
Sample DNA	100–200 ng
10X PCR Gold Buffer	5 μL
25 mM MgCl$_2$ solution	3 μL
2.5 mM dNTP solution	4 μL
Forward primer	50 pmol
Reverse primer	50 pmol
AmpliTaq Gold™	2.5 Units (0.5 μL)
Distilled water	add up to the total volume 50 μL

for the sample DNA. Importantly, both positive and negative control samples should be included at every analysis (*see* **Note 2**). To avoid cross-contamination, sample DNA should be added last to the reaction mixture, which has been aliquotted from the master mix.

3.3. PCR Conditions

The thermal profile for obtaining optimal PCR amplification is dependent in part upon the characteristics of individual PCR machines and reaction tubes. The following profiles have been confirmed to be optimal when using MicroAmp reaction tubes and GeneAmp PCR system 2400, 2700, 9600, or 9700 (Applied Biosystems). For other combinations, the optimal amplification conditions should first be determined by each investigator.

The thermal profile for ITD-mutations: pre-PCR step, 95°C—9 min; thermal cycle, 94°C—30 s, 56°C—1 min, 72°C—2 min; 35 cycles; post-PCR step, 72°C—10 min.

The thermal profile for D835-mutations: pre-PCR step, 95°C—9 min; thermal cycle, 94°C—30 s, 60°C—1 min, 72°C—2 min; 35 cycles; post-PCR step, 72°C—10 min.

Because AmpliTaq Gold is provided in an inactive state, the pre-PCR heat step is essential. It is recommended by the manufacturer that optimal results are obtained with a 9- to 12-min heat step at 92–95°C before the PCR cycles. Amplified products can be stored at –20°C until post-PCR analysis.

3.4. Digestion With Eco RV

To detect D835 mutations, a restriction fragment length polymorphism-mediated PCR assay is used, because D835 and I836 codons are encoded by the nucleotide sequence GATATC, which represents an *Eco* RV restriction site. Amplified products are digested with *Eco* RV, and subjected to electrophoresis in an agarose gel.

Table 2
Reaction Mixture for *Eco* RV Digestion

Reaction Mixture (for one reaction)	
Polymerase chain reaction products	10 µL
10X digestion buffer	3 µL
100X bovine serum albumin	0.3 µL
Eco RV	1 µL (20 U)
Distilled water	15.7 µL
Total	30 µL

1. Prepare the reaction mixture according to **Table 2**.
2. Incubate at 37°C for 2 h.
3. Heat-inactivate the enzyme at 65°C for 10 min.
4. PCR products can be directly used for the digestion procedure without any purification. However, it is recommended that optimal PCR amplification be confirmed by gel electrophoresis before the digestion procedure.

3.5. Electrophoresis

In most instances, ITD mutations can be detected by agarose gel electrophoresis of the amplified products (*see* **Note 3**). This procedure usually demonstrates a wild-type band (329 bp) and a larger-size band that is the ITD mutation (**Fig. 1**). In some cases harboring an ITD mutation, loss of the wild-type allele has been observed (*see* **Note 4**). In those cases, only the ITD band is present (**Fig. 1B**, lane 5).

D835 mutations are detected by electrophoresis of the amplified products following digestion with *Eco* RV. The amplified products of wild-type alleles are digested to two bands (68 bp and 46 bp) by *Eco* RV. When amplified products contain D835 mutations, undigested bands (114 bp) are visualized on agarose gel electrophoresis (**Fig. 2**). Inclusion of a negative control is essential to ensure complete digestion by *Eco* RV, thereby eliminating the possibility of false-positive results in patient samples.

3.6. DNA Sequencing

When identifying *FLT3* mutations, DNA sequencing is not necessarily required. However, we recommend the sequencing of mutated *FLT3* genes to confirm the mutation types and to exclude false positives. Mutated bands are cut out from the agarose gel and purified with gel extraction kits, such as QIAquick Gel Extraction Kit (Qiagen). Purified samples can usually be sequenced directly. We use BigDye® Terminator Cycle Sequencing Kit

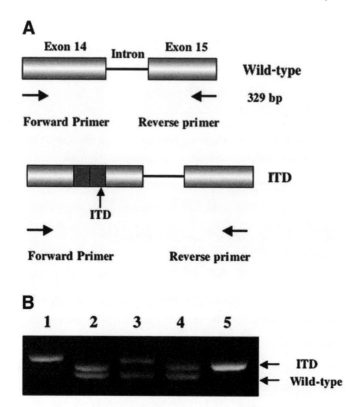

Fig. 1. Detection of internal tandem duplication (ITD) mutations. **(A)** Although ITD mutations vary in size and location, they always occur in the region around exons 14 and 15. **(B)** When leukemia cells have ITD mutations, polymerase chain reaction (PCR) products usually contain a wild-type band (329 bp) and a larger ITD band (lanes 1 to 4). When leukemia cells lose the wild-type allele, PCR products show only an ITD band (lane 5).

(Applied Biosystems) for this purpose. When direct sequencing is unsuccessful, it is necessary to clone the purified products into an appropriate vector. The TA-cloning system is suitable for this procedure.

4. Notes
1. Point mutations, deletions, and insertions have been found in other codons surrounding D835 as well as in the juxtamembrane domain. Although these mutations are less common, it is important to identify all kinds of mutations, because activating *FLT3* mutations could serve as a target for potent FLT3 kinase inhibitors. For screening all mutations in the juxtamembrane domain and the activation loop, amplified products must be separated in single-strand conformational poly-

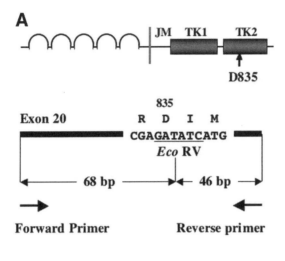

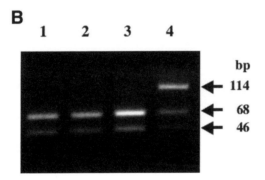

Fig. 2. Detection of D835 mutations. **(A)** The D835 codon is located in the TK2 domain of *FLT3*, and D835 and I836 codons are encoded by the nucleotide sequence GATATC which forms the *Eco* RV restriction site. **(B)** The amplified products of wild-type *FLT3* are digested to two bands (68 bp and 46 bp) by *Eco* RV (lanes 1 to 3). When amplified products contain D835 or I836 mutations, undigested bands (114 bp) are visualized on agarose gel electrophoresis (lane 4).

morphism gels under denaturing conditions *(3)*. Alternatively, amplified products can be sequenced directly. However, if deletion and/or insertion mutations are present, it may be necessary to clone the PCR products prior to sequencing to ensure accuracy. Finally, it has been reported that denaturing high-performance liquid chromatography (HPLC)-based procedures are potentially useful for screening for *FLT3* mutations *(13)*.

2. Both positive and negative controls should always be included in the experiments. To date, some human leukemia cell-lines are reported to have ITD or D835 mutations. MOLM13, MOLM14, and MV4;11 have ITD mutations. The former two

cell-lines have both wild-type and ITD alleles, but the latter lacks the wild-type allele (*see* **Note 4**). KOCL-33 and KOCL-48 have D835 mutations *(14)*.

3. It has been reported that ITD mutations consist of 3–400 bp of additional sequence. Generally, agarose gel electrophoresis is sufficient for separating the ITD band from the wild-type band. However, electrophoresis using polyacrylamide gels will give rise to better results than agarose gels in some samples, especially those with short duplications *(15)*.

4. The importance of the genotype in which ITD mutations occurred on one allele and the other wild-type allele was deleted, was demonstrated by the Cancer and Leukemia Group B (CALGB) *(16)*. In that report, it was shown that the hemizygous $FLT3^{ITD/-}$ genotype was an adverse prognostic factor in AML. A subsequent study has also demonstrated that the ratio of ITD to wild-type alleles is an independent prognostic factor in AML *(6)*. The allelic ratio can be semi-quantitatively assessed by using densitometry, while more sensitive and quantitative methods using fluorescent-labeled PCR have also been developed *(6)*. For this method, fluorescent-labeled primers are required. Amplified products, which are generated from the fluorescent-labeled primers, are subjected to gene scanning procedures, and the intensities of ITD and wild-type products are determined by laser excitation.

References

1. Gilliland, D. G. and Griffin, J. D. (2002) The roles of FLT3 in hematopoiesis and leukemia. *Blood* 100, 1532–1542.
2. Kiyoi, H. and Naoe, T. (2002) FLT3 in human hematologic malignancies. *Leuk. Lymphoma* **43,** 1541–1547.
3. Stirewalt, D. L. and Radich, J. P. (2003) The role of FLT3 in haematopoietic malignancies. *Nat. Rev. Cancer* **3,** 650–665.
4. Nakao, M., Yokota, S., Iwai, T., et al. (1996) Internal tandem duplication of the flt3 gene found in acute myeloid leukemia. *Leukemia* **10,** 1911–1918.
5. Yamamoto, Y., Kiyoi, H., Nakano, Y., et al. (2001) Activating mutation of D835 within the activation loop of FLT3 in human hematologic malignancies. *Blood* **97,** 2434–2439.
6. Thiede, C., Steudel, C., Mohr, B., et al. (2002) Analysis of FLT3-activating mutations in 979 patients with acute myelogenous leukemia: association with FAB subtypes and identification of subgroups with poor prognosis. *Blood* **99,** 4326–4335.
7. Spiekermann, K., Bagrintseva, K., Schoch, C., Haferlach, T., Hiddemann, W., and Schnittger, S. (2002) A new and recurrent activating length mutation in exon 20 of the FLT3 gene in acute myeloid leukemia. *Blood* **100,** 3423–3425.
8. Piccaluga, P. P., Bianchini, M., and Martinelli, G. (2003) Novel FLT3 point mutation in acute myeloid leukaemia. *Lancet Oncol.* **4,** 604.
9. Stirewalt, D. L., Meshinchi, S., Kussick, S. J., et al. (2004) Novel FLT3 point mutations within exon 14 found in patients with acute myeloid leukaemia. *Br. J. Haematol.* **124,** 481–484.

10. Kiyoi, H., Naoe, T., Nakano, Y., et al. (1999) Prognostic implication of FLT3 and N-RAS gene mutations in acute myeloid leukemia. *Blood* **93**, 3074–3080.
11. Kottaridis, P. D., Gale, R. E., Frew, M. E., et al. (2001) The presence of a FLT3 internal tandem duplication in patients with acute myeloid leukemia (AML) adds important prognostic information to cytogenetic risk group and response to the first cycle of chemotherapy: analysis of 854 patients from the United Kingdom Medical Research Council AML 10 and 12 trials. *Blood* **98**, 1752–1759.
12. Kiyoi, H., Towatari, M., Yokota, S., et al. (1998) Internal tandem duplication of the FLT3 gene is a novel modality of elongation mutation which causes constitutive activation of the product. *Leukemia* **12**, 1333–1337.
13. Bianchini, M., Ottaviani, E., Grafone, T., et al. (2003) Rapid detection of Flt3 mutations in acute myeloid leukemia patients by denaturing HPLC. *Clin. Chem.* **49**, 1642–1650.
14. Taketani, T., Taki, T., Sugita, K., et al. (2004) FLT3 mutations in the activation loop of tyrosine kinase domain are frequently found in infant ALL with MLL rearrangements and pediatric ALL with hyperdiploidy. *Blood* **103**, 1085–1088.
15. Stirewalt, D. L., Kopecky, K. J., Meshinchi, S., et al. (2001) FLT3, RAS, and TP53 mutations in elderly patients with acute myeloid leukemia. *Blood* **97**, 3589–3595.
16. Whitman, S. P., Archer, K. J., Feng, L., et al. (2001) Absence of the wild-type allele predicts poor prognosis in adult de novo acute myeloid leukemia with normal cytogenetics and the internal tandem duplication of FLT3: a cancer and leukemia group B study. *Cancer Res.* **61**, 7233–7239.

13

WT1 Overexpression in Acute Myeloid Leukemia and Myelodysplastic Syndromes

Daniela Cilloni, Enrico Gottardi, and Giuseppe Saglio

Summary

The Wilms tumor gene was identified as a tumor suppressor gene responsible for a particular type of kidney tumor. Several years ago, it was demonstrated that it is also overexpressed in acute and chronic leukemias. Although the exact role of this gene in the hematopoietic system is still quite completely obscure, it represents a reliable marker for the detection of the presence of leukemic cells. *WT1* quantitative assessment may therefore represent a useful tool for the diagnosis and follow up of leukemia patients. In this chapter, we describe the method for the quantification of *WT1* transcript by real-time polymerase chain reaction.

Key Words: *WT1*; myelodysplastic syndrome; acute leukemia; minimal residual disease; real-time PCR.

1. Introduction

The applicability of molecular techniques for the diagnosis and monitoring of minimal residual disease (MRD) in acute leukemia has been limited to those patients whose leukemia is characterized by genetic markers amenable to sensitive detection by polymerase chain reaction (PCR). Genetic markers such as fusion genes derived from chromosome translocations *(1,2)* are ideally suited to such an approach. At present, more than 50% of acute leukemia patients, and in particular most cases of acute myeloid leukemia (AML), lack known genetic lesions or markers of clonality that are suitable for MRD monitoring. Moreover, several hematological malignancies present particular difficulties in terms of differential diagnosis. This is the situation for many patients affected by myelodysplastic syndromes (MDS), which are rarely characterized by the presence of cytogenetic abnormalities *(3)*. In this setting, the Wilms tumor gene (*WT1*) has gained a central role as a universal molecular marker of leukemia *(4–6)*.

From: *Methods in Molecular Medicine, Vol. 125: Myeloid Leukemia: Methods and Protocols*
Edited by: H. Iland, M. Hertzberg, and P. Marlton © Humana Press Inc., Totowa, NJ

1.1. The Wilms Tumor Gene

The Wilms tumor gene (*WT1*) was first cloned in 1990 at band 11p13 *(7)*. *WT1* codes for a protein with the characteristics of a transcription factor: four carboxy-terminal zinc fingers with high homology to the zinc finger of the Egr-1 transcription factor, a DNA binding domain, and a proline-glutamine-rich region that is capable of regulating transcription *(8)*. *WT1* expression is restricted to a small number of normal tissues *(9)*, such as kidney, testis, ovaries, myometrium, stromal cells of the uterus, mesothelial cells lining body cavities and visceral organs such as the heart, lung, intestine, and liver, and in the supportive stroma and capsule of the spleen *(10)*. Although the role of the *WT1* gene in the development of malignancies in the kidney appears quite well defined, currently its potential function in human hematopoiesis still needs to be clarified. *WT1* may contribute to blood cell development, as suggested by its expression in early hematopoietic precursors and its rapid down-regulation following differentiation in primary blood cells and leukemia-derived cell lines *(11–12)*. *WT1* overexpression in leukemic hematopoiesis suggests that *WT1* possesses a paradoxical oncogenic activity in this particular setting, and recent studies are in line with this hypothesis.

1.2. WT1 *Expression in Leukemias*

The introduction of real-time PCR has enabled widespread agreement on the significance of *WT1* overexpression, which had been contentious for many years. This happened mainly because the reported data had been obtained with reverse-transcription (RT)-PCR techniques that proved to be inadequate for the majority of settings in which *WT1* expression is currently applicable.

At present, although minor differences in the data reported by different laboratories still persist, mainly due to the different methods used, all the studies support low *WT1* expression in normal bone marrow (BM) cells. In our hands, using the method described here, the mean value of WT1 transcripts in normal BM is 35 *WT1* copies/10^4 *ABL* copies (range 0–90). The majority (60%) of normal peripheral blood (PB) samples do not express *WT1*, and the remainder express very low levels, with a mean value of 5 WT1 copies/10^4 ABL copies (range 0–20) *(4)*.

By contrast, as shown in **Table 1**, a large number of clonal hematopoietic disorders overexpress *WT1* at diagnosis, although considerable heterogeneity exists *(13)*. *WT1* has achieved recognition as a molecular marker that is particularly useful in those conditions that present particular difficulties in terms of differential diagnosis. In this regard, patients affected by MDS, especially those characterized by a low proportion of blast cells in the bone marrow, may profit from the presence of a sensitive molecular marker. In MDS patients, WT1 overexpression is also a valuable prognostic indicator, because it corre-

Table 1
The Wilms Tumor Gene (*WT1*) Expression in Clonal Hematopoietic Disorders

	Mean Value (*WT1* copies per 10,000 *ABL* copies)	Range
Normal bone marrow	35	0–90
Normal peripheral blood	5	0–20

Conditions associated with *WT1* overexpression

	Mean Value (*WT1* copies per 10,000 *ABL* copies)	Range	Percentage of cases with *WT1* overexpression
Acute myeloid leukemia	27,669	1081–121,806	100%
(AML)			
Acute lymphoblastic leukemia (ALL)	13,807	318–94,682	100%
CML chronic phase and blastic phase	3262	191–54,171	100%
Chronic myelomonocytic leukemia (CMML)	4667	1070–23,674	100%
Ph negative CML like diseases	9731	890–70,980	100%
Primitive hyper-eosinophilic syndromes	280	102–7800	95%
Refractory anemias	366	100–1289	65%
RAEB	2262	227–11,006	100%
RAEB-T	14,033	3757–51,700	100%

Conditions associated with normal *WT1* expression

Regenerating bone marrow (immature but normal cells)
 Granulocyte/colony-stimulating factor stimulated cells
Polyclonal anemias
Inflammatory diseases
Reactive thrombocytosis
 Secondary leukocytosis
Secondary hypereosinophilia

lates with the percentage of blast cells and the number and types of cytogenetic abnormalities, which are the key components of the International Prognostic Scoring System (IPSS) score, the most widely accepted index of the risk of progression towards acute leukemia *(5)*.

Many polyclonal conditions that may be considered in the differential diagnosis have been analyzed in order to establish the specificity of *WT1* overexpression. As shown in **Table 1**, patients affected by hemolytic anemias or cytopenias secondary to polyclonal conditions express normal values of *WT1* *(4–5)*.

Because all AML patients and the majority of ALL patients express very high values of *WT1* at diagnosis, the periodic assessment of *WT1* expression provides a sensitive method for monitoring the persistence of disease after chemotherapy or bone marrow transplantation, or the reappearance of leukemic cells during follow-up *(4–14)*. The presence of immature but normal cells, as occurs in regenerating BM samples after chemotherapy-induced aplasia, does not alter *WT1* values, which persist within the normal range *(4)*. Moreover, neither the stimulus induced by granulocyte colony-stimulating factor (G-CSF) treatment, nor the presence of inflammatory leukocytosis, is associated with increased *WT1* values. We are therefore entitled to regard abnormal *WT1* expression values as always being associated with the presence of leukemic or myelodysplastic cells. Finally, the sensitivity of this marker may sometimes allow detection of altered *WT1* values in BM or PB samples in the absence of blast cells by morphological and immunophenotypic criteria. In these cases, the abnormal *WT1* values precede the clinical appearance or reappearance of disease. A rise of *WT1* values above the normal range during the follow-up of AML patients is always indicative of relapse.

2. Materials

1. Semi-automatic pipets.
2. ART self-sealing barrier tips.
3. NaCl 0.9% solution.
4. Phosphate-buffered saline (PBS).
5. Lympholyte-H (Cedarlane, Ontario, Canada).
6. RNAwiz (Ambion) (*see* **Note 1**).
7. Chloroform.
8. Isopropanol.
9. 75% ethanol.
10. RNase-free water.
11. RT buffer: 100 mM Tris-HCl, 500 mM KCl (pH 8.3).
12. MgCl$_2$: 25 mM.
13. 0.1 M Dithiothreitol (DTT) solution.
14. Random hexamers: 50 μM.
15. RNAse inhibitor: 20 U/μL.
16. MuLV reverse transcriptase enzyme.
17. dNTPs.
18. 96-well optical reaction plate with optical caps.

19. TaqMan Universal PCR Master Mix (Applied Biosystems, Foster City, CA).
20. ABI prism 7700 Sequence Detection System (Applied Biosystems, Foster City, CA) (*see* **Note 2**).
21. PCR II TOPO vector (Invitrogen, Groningen, The Netherlands).
22. QIAFILTER Plasmid MIDI kit (Qiagen, Courtaboeuf, France).
23. *Bam*HI and *Hin*dIII restriction enzymes.
24. Solution for dilution of standard curve plasmids: Tris 10 m*M*, ethylenediamine tetraacetic acid (EDTA) 1 m*M* (pH 8).
25. *Escherichia coli* 16S and 23S rRNA (Roche).
26. *ABL*-containing plasmid for generation of the control gene standard curve is available from Ipsogen (Marseilles, France).

3. Methods
3.1. Cell Separation and RNA Extraction

1. Collect 3–4 mL of BM in sodium citrate or 10–20 mL of PB in EDTA (*see* **Note 3**).
2. Dilute the sample with NaCl 0.9% solution or PBS. For PB, the dilution volume/ volume is 1:1; for BM, the dilution is 1 vol of BM to 2 vol of NaCl (or PBS).
3. Using a 10- to 15-mL centrifuge tube, layer 6 mL of the diluted blood or marrow over 3 mL Lympholyte-H.
4. Centrifuge the tubes for 30 min at 800g at room temperature.
5. Using a pipet, carefully remove the mononuclear cells from the interface and transfer to a 2-mL of Eppendorf tube.
6. Add 1.5 mL of NaCl 0.9% solution and centrifuge for 1 min at 800g.
7. Discard the supernatant and add 1 mL of RNAwiz (*see* **Note 4**) and homogenize using a 2.5-mL syringe with a 22-gauge needle (*see* **Note 5**).
8. Incubate the homogenate at room temperature for 5 min.
9. Add 250 μL of chloroform and shake vigorously for 5 min (*see* **Note 6**).
10. Centrifuge the mixture at 12,000g for 15 min at 4°C.
11. Without disturbing the interphase, carefully transfer the aqueous phase into a 2-mL Eppendorf tube.
12. Add a half volume of sterile water and an equal volume of isopropanol and mix well.
13. Store the tube at –20°C for at least 2 h (or overnight).
14. Centrifuge the tube for 15 min at 12,000g at 4°C.
15. Decant the supernatant and wash the pellet with 1 mL of cold 75% ethanol.
16. Centrifuge at 7500g for 5 min at 4°C.
17. Discard the supernatant and dry the pellet using a vacuum pump.
18. Resuspend the RNA in an appropriate amount of RNase-free water.
19. Assess the RNA concentration and purity by spectrophotometric analysis (at 260 nm and 280 nm).

3.2. RT Reaction

1. Use 1 μg of total RNA and incubate at 70°C for 10 min.
2. Cool on ice and add the following reagents plus H$_2$O to a final theoretical volume of 20 μL. Depending on the commercial availability of a stock solution of random hexamers at sufficiently high concentration, the exact final volume of the reagent mix may be as much as 21.8 μL:
   a. RT buffer 1X: 10 m*M* Tris-HCl, 50 m*M* KCl (pH 8.3).
   b. MgCl$_2$: 5 m*M* (final concentration).
   c. DTT: 10 m*M* (final concentration).
   d. dNTP: 1 m*M* each (final concentration).
   e. Random hexamers: 25 μ*M* (final concentration).
   f. RNAse inhibitor: 20 U.
   g. Reverse transcriptase enzyme 100 U.
3. Use the following thermal cycler temperatures and time conditions:
   a. 20°C for 10 min.
   b. 42°C for 45 min.
   c. 99°C for 3 min.
   d. 4°C at the end of the RT step.
4. After the RT reaction, add RNase-free water to a final volume of 50 μL (*see* **Note 7**).

3.3. Real-Time Quantitative RT-PCR Step

1. All the real-time quantitative RT-PCR (RQ-PCR) reactions are performed on a 7700 ABI platform (*see* **Note 2**).
2. Perform each run using a specific set of primers and probe for *WT1* and *ABL* (*see* **Note 8**).
3. Perform the PCR reaction for *WT1* and *ABL* as follows:
   a. Use 5 μL of diluted cDNA (corresponding to approx 100 ng of starting RNA).
   b. 12.5 μL of TaqMan Universal PCR Master Mix (Applera).
   c. 300 n*M* of each primer.
   d. 200 n*M* of the probe.
   e. Add sterilized water to reach a final volume of 25 μL.
4. The RQ-PCR primers and probe for *WT1* are (*see* **Note 9**):
   forward primer (located on exon 7):
   5′- CAGGCTGCAATAAGAGATATTTTAAGCT-3′
   reverse primer (located on exon 8):
   5′-GAAGTCACACTGGTATGGTTTCTCA-3′
   TaqMan probe (located on exon 7):
   5′-CTTACAGATGCACAGCAGGAAGCACACTG-3′.
5. The RQ-PCR primers and probe for *ABL* (*see* **Note 10**) are:
   forward primer 5′-TGGAGATAACACTCTAAGCATAACTAAAGGT-3′
   reverse primer 5′-GATGTAGTTGCTTGGGACCCA-3′
   TaqMan probe 5′-CCATTTTTGGTTTGGGCTTCACACCATT-3′

The fluorescent Taqman probes are labeled with 6-carboxy-fluorescein phosphoramide (FAM) as reporter dye at the 5'-end, and the quencher dye is 6-carboxytetramethylrhodamine (TAMRA) at the 3'-terminus.

The PCR procedure starts with:

a. 2 min at 50°C to activate the UNG enzyme, then
b. 10 min at 95°C to inactivate the UNG enzyme and to provide a "hot start" for activating the AmpliTaq polymerase.
c. Subsequently, 50 cycles of denaturation at 95°C for 15 s followed by annealing/extension at 60°C for 60 s.

6. Perform all sample analysis in triplicate; where the results show a discrepancy of more than 1 threshold cycle (Ct) in one of the wells, that replicate must be excluded (*see* **Note 11**).

3.4. Generation of Plasmid Standard Curves

1. To construct a *WT1* plasmid for the standard curve in the RQ-PCR assay, add the following primers and reagents in a final volume of 50 µL to amplify a *WT1* RT-PCR product:

   forward primer: exon 7 -5'-GGCATCTGAGACCAGTGAGAA-3'
   reverse primer: exon 10 5'-GGACTAATTCATCGACCGGG-3'

   a. PCR buffer 1X:10 m*M* Tris-HCl, 50 m*M* KCl (pH 8.3)
   b. MgCl$_2$: 2.5 m*M* (final concentration)
   c. dNTP: 200 µ*M* (final concentration)
   d. 400 n*M* of each primer (final concentration)
   e. Taq enzyme: 1 U
   f. 3 µL of cDNA product

   Use the following thermal cycler temperatures and time conditions:

   a. Initial melting 95°C for 30 s
   b. 35 PCR cycles at the following conditions: 94°C for 30 s, 65°C for 1 min, 72°C for 1 min.

2. Clone the PCR products into the PCR II TOPO vector (Invitrogen, Groningen, The Netherlands) according to the manufacturer's instructions.

3. Sequence the selected plasmid for confirmation of the insert, and extract the plasmid DNA using the Qiafilter Plasmid MIDI kit (Qiagen, Courtaboeuf, France) and quantify spectrophotometrically. The copy number for 1 µg is estimated according to the molecular weight of the vector plus the insert.

4. Linearize 20 µg of plasmid with *Bam*HI or *Hin*dIII restriction enzymes for 1 h at 37°C under agitation.

5. Dilute the digested plasmid in a solution of Tris 10 m*M*, EDTA 1 m*M* (pH 8), containing 20 ng/mL of *E. coli* 16S and 23S rRNA (Roche).

6. Prepare five successive serial dilutions (20,000, 2000, 200, 20, and 2 copies/µL). The corresponding standard curve generates a mean slope of –4.04 and an intercept of 46.75 Ct. A mean Ct value of 26.4 should be obtained for 100,000 copies of the plasmid dilution (*see* **Fig. 1**). The actual values achieved (as in **Fig.**

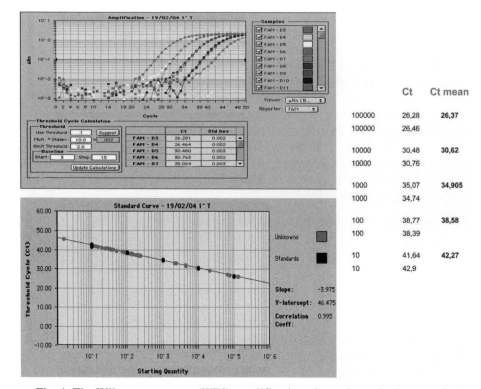

	Ct	Ct mean
100000	26,28	26,37
100000	26,46	
10000	30,48	30,62
10000	30,76	
1000	35,07	34,905
1000	34,74	
100	38,77	38,58
100	38,39	
10	41,64	42,27
10	42,9	

Fig. 1. The Wilms tumor gene (*WT1*) amplification plot and standard curve with 6-carboxytetramethylrhodamine (TAMRA) probe. In the amplification plot, the threshold was set to a value of 0.1 and the baseline to between cycles 3 and 15. The standard curve generates a slope of –3.975 and an intercept of 46.475. The mean threshold cycle (Ct) values for each of the plasmid copy numbers obtained by serial dilutions of the plasmid are indicated to the right of the figure.

1) may vary slightly from these theoretical values for several reasons, including variability in the efficiency of the reaction and individual operator manual variability. This should not cause inaccuracies in the final quantitation of copy numbers, because the latter are normalized using the *ABL* gene.

7. To prepare the *ABL* control gene standard curve, use commercial *ABL* plasmid (Ipsogen, Marseille, France).

8. Use three different serial dilutions (20,000, 2000, and 200 copies/µL). The corresponding standard curve generates a mean slope of –3.64 and an intercept of 40 Ct. A mean Ct value of 21.78 should be obtained for the 100,000 copies of the plasmid dilution (*see* **Fig. 2**). The actual values achieved may vary slightly from these theoretical values, as discussed above.

9. Store the plasmid dilutions at –20°C. Aliquot the serial dilutions in order to avoid

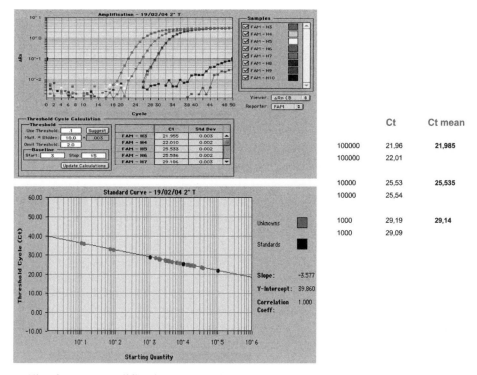

Fig. 2. *ABL* amplification plot and standard curve with 6-carboxytetramethyl-rhodamine (TAMRA) probe. In the amplification plot, the threshold was set to a value of 0.1 and the baseline to between cycles 3 and 15. The standard curve generates a slope of −3.577 and an intercept of 39.86. The mean threshold cycle values for each of the plasmid copy numbers obtained by serial dilutions of the plasmid are indicated to the right of the figure.

excessive repetitive freezing and thawing. Each aliquot should be thawed no more than 10–15 times.

3.5. Setup and Preparation of the Plate for the RQ-PCR Reaction

1. Use a 96-well plate with optical caps. Divide the plate (theoretically) into two parts. The upper part is used for performing the *WT1* reaction on samples, on *WT1* plasmid dilutions, and on "no-template" controls (NTC) (*see* **Note 12**). The test samples are assayed in triplicate (loaded into 3 wells), whereas the plasmid dilutions and the NTC are tested in duplicate (*see* **Note 13**).
2. The lower part is used for performing the *ABL* reaction on the same samples, on *ABL* plasmid dilutions, and on NTC.
3. The amount of plasmid to be loaded in the appropriate wells in the plate is 5 μL,

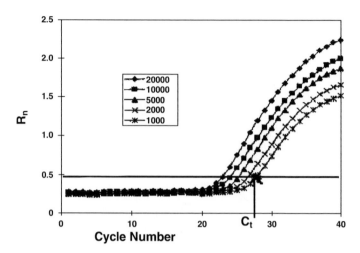

Fig. 3. Relative quantification using the threshold cycle (Ct) value. The threshold cycle represents the first cycle of the polymerase chain reaction able to generate a detectable level of fluorescence. The higher the transcript amount, the smaller the Ct.

corresponding to a logarithmic scale of *WT1* and *ABL* copies. For *WT1*, we generate a curve with 100,000, 10,000, 1000, 100, and 10 copies, and for *ABL* we use 100,000, 10,000 and 1000 copies.

At the end of the run, an Excel final report is provided by the software. The Ct values and the "quantity" values of standard curve and tested samples are provided. Ct refers to "threshold cycle," and it indicates the first cycle of the PCR reaction in which a detectable level of fluorescence develops and it can be measured by the instrument (*see* **Fig. 3**).

4. Set the threshold to 0.1 and the baseline from cycles 3 to 15 for both *WT1* and *ABL* genes (*see* **Note 14**).
5. Using Excel software, calculate the mean of the Ct and sample quantity from triplicate wells (*see* **Note 15**).
6. Calculate the ratio of *WT1* copies/*ABL* copies and multiply by 10,000 (*see* **Note 16**).
7. Samples with an *ABL* Ct value above 29 must be discarded (*see* **Note 17**). The RQ-PCR assay for *WT1* was consistently able to detect 10 plasmid molecules, and its sensitivity was further established by diluting the K562 cell line into normal lymphocytes obtained from the peripheral blood of a normal subject that scored repeatedly negative (Ct $\geq$ 50) for *WT1* expression. Under these experimental conditions, RQ-PCR was able to detect a positive *WT1* signal at a dilution of one K562 cell in 10^5 normal lymphocytes.

4. Notes

1. Other RNA isolation reagents can also be used (Trizol, Ultraspec, and so on) with comparable results.

2. The reactions can be carried out on alternative real-time detection systems, and will yield comparable results that maintain the relationships between samples but with different absolute values.

3. The collection of samples should be optimized in order to minimize the time between sample acquisition and processing, as it has been demonstrated that the stability of transcripts (including *WT1*) may be altered over time and with exposure to different temperatures. Sodium citrate and EDTA are the optimal anticoagulants for PB and BM, respectively, in order to avoid any interference with the RQ-PCR procedure.

4. Use 1 mL of RNAwiz for a maximum of 10^7 cells.

5. Samples homogenized in RNAwiz can be stored at $-20°C$ or $-80°C$ for up to 1 mo.

6. The chloroform should not contain isoamylalchohol (IAA).

7. cDNA products can be stored at $-20°C$ or $-80°C$ for up to 1 yr.

8. It is mandatory to amplify a control gene so that impaired amplification of *WT1* can be recognized by a corresponding reduction in the quantity of the control gene that is detected. Variation in amplification could reflect variations in RNA quality, quantity, and/or cDNA synthesis efficiency. Thus, quantification of *ABL* expression is used to identify poor-quality samples, based on reference values observed in a large number of fresh samples. The choice of ABL was decided by a European network, because *ABL* expression is stable and constant in normal and leukemic cells and in different cell types.

9. Alternative primer sets for *WT1* assessment are present in the published literature. This specific set possesses the advantage that it does not amplify genomic DNA. It has been designed to avoid the two splicing regions present in exon 5 and 9, and the exon regions that are most frequently mutated in *AML* patients.

10. For *WT1* quantitation in *BCR-ABL*-positive leukemias, it is more appropriate to use GUS as the control gene instead of *ABL*, because the *ABL* primers will also amplify the *BRC-ABL* fusion transcripts derived from the rearranged *ABL* allele. That would result in an increased value for *ABL*, thereby altering the *WT1/ABL* ratio, and consequently the *WT1* value would be underestimated.

11. If one out of three amplified replicate samples shows a difference of more than 1 Ct with respect to the other two, we regard this as due to operator error, and the discrepant replicate should be discarded. This rule applies for samples with a *WT1* Ct value below 40. For Ct values above 40, the amount of transcript is so low that small differences in copy number may produce a large difference in Ct. Accordingly, for samples with Ct values >40, we use the mean value of the three replicates even when the Ct values for a specific sample differ by 2 or 3. In these cases, discard only the replicates with a Ct value >50. For very low *WT1* levels (such as those present in normal PB samples), only one well out of three may give a positive result; the final value is then represented by the single value obtained.

12. The no-template control is a well that contains the reaction mixture without cDNA.

13. Although test samples are assayed in triplicate, each plasmid dilution is loaded in duplicate because they are very stable and the Ct values obtained are very reproducible.

14. The threshold and baseline values have been established by the European network in order to provide comparable results between different laboratories.
15. The software automatically generates standard curves for *WT1* and *ABL* using the mean Ct values of the different plasmid serial dilutions that have been included in the plate. The mean Ct for both *WT1* and *ABL* in each of the samples is then automatically compared with the respective plasmid standard curves to obtain the corresponding quantity (copy number) of transcripts in each sample tested.
16. The final result expresses the *WT1* copy number normalized per 10,000 ABL copies.
17. The samples with an *ABL* Ct value >29 should be discarded, because the quality of the sample is unacceptable.

References

1. Van Dongen, J. J., Seriu, T., Panzer-Grumayer, E. R., et al. (1998) Prognostic value of minimal residual disease in acute lymphoblastic leukaemia in childhood. *Lancet* **28,** 1731–1738.
2. Cavé, H., van der Werfften, Bosch, J., et al. (1998) Clinical significance of minimal residual disease in childhood acute lymphoblastic leukemia. European Organization for Research and Treatment of Cancer-Childhood Leukemia Cooperative Group. *N. Engl. J. Med.* **27,** 591–598.
3. Nowell, P. C. (1992) Chromosome abnormalities in myelodysplastic syndrome and acute myelogenous leukemia. *Semin. Oncol.* **19,** 25–33.
4. Cilloni, D., Gottardi, E., De Micheli, D., et al. (2002) Quantitative assessment of *WT1* expression by real time quantitative PCR may be a useful tool for monitoring minimal residual disease in acute leukemia patients. *Leukemia* **16,** 2115–2121.
5. Cilloni, D., Messa, F., Gottardi, E., et al. (2003) Very significant correlation between WT1 expression level and the IPSS score in patients with myelodysplastic syndromes. *J. Clin. Oncol.* **21,** 1988–1995.
6. Inoue, K., Ogawa, H., Sonoda, Y., et al. (1997) Aberrant overexpression of the Wilms tumor gene (WT1) in human leukemia. *Blood* **89,** 1405–1412.
7. Call, K. M., Glaser, T., Ito, C. Y., et al. (1990) Isolation and characterization of a zinc finger polypeptide gene at the human chromosome 11 Wilms' tumor locus. *Cell* **60,** 509–520.
8. Madden, S. L., Cook, D. M., Morris, J. F., Gashler, A., Sukhatme, V. P., and Rauscher, F. J. III. (1991) Transcriptional repression mediated by the WT1 Wilms' tumor gene product. *Science* **253,** 1550–1553.
9. Park, S., Schalling, M., Bernard, A., et al. (1993) The Wilms tumor gene WT1 is expressed in murine mesoderm-derived tissues and mutated in a human mesothelioma. *Nat. Genet.* **4,** 415–420.
10. Pritchard-Jones, K. and Fleming, S. (1991) Cell types expressing the Wilms' tumor gene (WT1) in Wilms' tumor: implications for tumor histogenesis. *Oncogene* **6,** 2211–2220.

11. Sekiya, M., Adachi, M., Hinoda, Y., Imai, K., and Yachi, A. (1994) Downregulation of the Wilms' tumor gene (wt1) during myelomonocytic differentiation in HL60 cells. *Blood* **83,** 1876–1882.
12. Maurer, U., Brieger, J., Weidmann, E., Mitrou, P. S., Hoelzer, D., and Bergmann, L. (1997) The Wilms' tumor gene is expressed in a subset of CD34+ progenitors and downregulated early in the course of differentiation in vitro. *Exp. Hematol.* **25,** 945–950.
13. Cilloni, D. and Saglio, G. (2003) Usefulness of quantitative assessment of Wilms Tumor gene expression in chronic myeloid leukemia patients undergoing imatinib therapy. *Semin. Hematol.* **40,** 37–41.
14. Cilloni, D., Gottardi, E., Fava, M., et al. (2003) Usefulness of quantitative assessment of WT1 gene transcript as a marker for minimal residual disease detection. *Blood* **15,** 773–774.

14

Classification of AML by DNA-Oligonucleotide Microarrays

Alexander Kohlmann, Wolfgang Kern, Wolfgang Hiddemann, and Torsten Haferlach

Summary

Accurate diagnosis and classification of leukemias are the bases for the appropriate management of patients. The diagnostic accuracy and efficiency of present methods may be improved by the use of microarrays. The followin g chapter gives an overview of the method of gene expression profiling of leukemia samples, its laboratory procedure, and how to approach the analysis of the data.

Key Words: AML; gene expression; microarray; classification

1. Introduction

The standard methods for establishing the diagnosis of acute leukemias are cytomorphology and cytochemistry in combination with multiparameter immunophenotyping. Furthermore, cytogenetics, fluorescence *in situ* hybridization, and polymerase chain reaction (PCR)-based assays add important information regarding biologically defined and prognostically relevant subgroups and allow a comprehensive diagnosis of well-defined subentities today. In the clinical setting, a better understanding of the clinical course of distinct biologically defined disease subtypes is the basis for a selection of disease-specific therapeutic approaches. Microarray technology, which quantifies gene expression intensities of thousands of genes in a single analysis, holds the potential to become an essential tool for the molecular classification of leukemias. It may therefore be used as a routine method for diagnostic purposes in the near future. This chapter outlines the major steps of the procedure for gene expression profiling analyses using the Affymetrix microarray platform.

From: *Methods in Molecular Medicine, Vol. 125: Myeloid Leukemia: Methods and Protocols*
Edited by: H. Iland, M. Hertzberg, and P. Marlton © Humana Press Inc., Totowa, NJ

2. Materials

A detailed description of reagents and required buffers is also available in the Affymetrix technical manual on gene expression profiling analyses (www.affymetrix.com).

1. Safe-Lock tubes (Eppendorf).
2. Acetylated bovine serum albumin (BSA), 50 mg/mL (Sigma).
3. Ammonium acetate, 7.5 M (Sigma).
4. cDNA Synthesis System Kit (Roche Applied Science).
5. Control oligonucleotide B2, 3 nM (Affymetrix).
6. Ethylenediamine tetraacetic acid (EDTA), 0.5 M (Sigma).
7. Enzo BioArray HighYield RNA Transcript Labeling Kit (Affymetrix).
8. Ethanol (Roth).
9. Eukaryotic Hybridization Control Kit, 20X stock solution (Affymetrix).
10. Ficoll Isotonic Solution (density: 1077 g/mL) Biochrom (Berlin).
11. Fragmentation buffer, 5X concentrated (Affymetrix).
12. Glycogen, 20 mg/mL (Roche Applied Science).
13. Guanidine isothiocyanate buffer (RLT-Buffer, Qiagen).
14. Herring sperm DNA, 10 mg/mL (Sigma).
15. Hybridization buffer, 2X concentrated.
16. Nuclease-free water (Ambion).
17. Phosphate-buffered saline (PBS) with Ca^{2+} and Mg^{2+}.
18. Phase Lock Gel light (Eppendorf).
19. Phenol/chloroform/isoamylalcohol, 25:24:1 (Ambion).
20. QIAshredder columns (Qiagen).
21. RNeasy Mini Kit (Qiagen).
22. Streptavidin-phycoerythrin (SAPE) staining solution.

3. Methods

3.1. Patient Samples

All leukemia patient samples should be sent to the laboratory via express mail. At the time point of diagnosis, the patients should provide bone marrow (BM) aspirates or peripheral blood samples. All relevant clinical parameters, as well as detailed diagnostic reports, can be entered in a specific leukemia database *(1)*.

3.2. Isolation of Mononucleated Cells by Ficoll Gradient Centrifugation

1. Mix 1–20 mL of BM or blood with the same volume of PBS.
2. Place the same volume as this total mixture (or at most 20 mL) of Ficoll into an extra tube. Carefully overlay the Ficoll with the BM/PBS mixture and centrifuge for 20 min at 1088g. Don't use the brake; it will last around another 20 min until the run stops.

3. Carefully remove the cell circlet with a 10-mL pipet and transfer it into a new tube.
4. Add 10 mL of PBS.
5. Centrifuge 10 min at 370g (with brake).
6. Count the cells.
7. Place 5×10^6 cells into a 1.5-mL reaction tube and centrifuge 5 min at 2000 rpm in a standard centrifuge and remove supernatant.
8. Lyse with 300 µL guanidine isothiocyanate buffer (RLT buffer, Qiagen) by pipetting five times up and down. Subsequently, the stabilized lysates can be stored at –80°C until preparation for microarray analyses.

3.3. Microarray Target Preparation

Figure 1 outlines the major steps of the procedure for gene expression profiling analyses (as recommended by Affymetrix, Inc., Santa Clara, CA).

3.3.1. Isolation of Total RNA

Isolation of total RNA from frozen lysates of mononuclear cells can be performed according to the RNeasy Mini Kit protocol (Qiagen, Hilden, Germany), including an initial homogenization step. In this protocol, a specialized high-salt buffer system allows up to 100 µg of RNA longer than 200 bases to bind to the RNeasy silica-gel membrane. The biological samples are first lysed and homogenized in the presence of a highly denaturing guanidine isothiocyanate (GITC)-containing buffer, which immediately inactivates RNases to ensure isolation of intact RNA. Then ethanol is added to provide appropriate binding conditions and the sample is applied to an RNeasy mini column, where the total RNA binds to the membrane and contaminants are efficiently washed away. High-quality RNA is subsequently eluted in 40 µL of nuclease-free water. Up to eight individual samples can be processed in parallel. All steps of the protocol should be performed quickly at room temperature. All centrifugation steps are performed in a standard microcentrifuge (Eppendorf, Hamburg, Germany). RPE wash buffer is supplied as a concentrate. Before using it for the first time, 4 vol of absolute ethanol have to be added to obtain a working solution. A 70% ethanol solution is prepared in 2.0-mL reaction tubes using absolute ethanol and nuclease-free water.

1. Thaw frozen cell lysates of individual patient samples (stored at –80°C) on ice. Then incubate samples for 4 min at 45°C.
2. To homogenize the sample, pipet the lysate directly onto a QIAshredder spin column, placed in a 2-mL collection tube, and centrifuge for 2 min at maximum speed (*see* **Note 2**).
3. Add one volume (usually 300 µL) of 70% ethanol to the homogenized lysate in the collection tube and mix well by pipetting. Do not centrifuge. Apply the

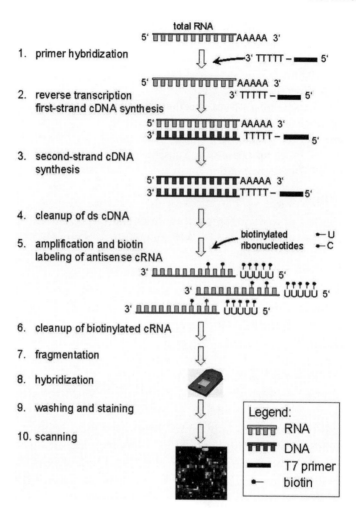

Fig. 1. Gene expression analysis overview. The gene expression profiling analysis starts with sample target preparation (*see* **Note 1**). The target is the labeled nucleic acid that is being interrogated. It is hybridized to the probes on the array. For each respective sample, double-stranded (ds) cDNA is synthesized from total RNA isolated from mononuclear cells. An in vitro transcription (IVT) reaction is then performed to produce biotin-labeled cRNA from the cDNA. After fragmentation, a hybridization cocktail is prepared, including the fragmented target, probe array controls, bovine serum albumin, and herring sperm DNA. The cocktail is hybridized to the probe array during a 16-h incubation. Immediately following hybridization, the probe array undergoes an automated washing and staining protocol on the fluidics station. After the array is scanned, the raw data are analyzed for probe signal intensities and all results are reported in tabular and graphical formats. Then the data set is prepared for detailed statistical analyses.

sample, including any precipitate that may have formed, to an RNeasy mini column placed in a 2-mL collection tube. Close the tube gently and centrifuge for 15 s at 8000g. Discard the flow-through. Transfer the column into a new 2-mL collection tube.

4. Add 700 µL washing buffer RW1 to the column. Close the tube gently, and centrifuge for 15 s at 8000g. Discard the flow-through and collection tube. Transfer the column into a new 2-mL collection tube.

5. Pipet 500 µL RPE washing buffer onto the column. Close the tube gently, and centrifuge for 15 s at ≥8000g. Discard the flow-through. Transfer the column into a new 2-mL collection tube.

6. Add another 500 µL RPE washing buffer to the column. Close the tube gently, and centrifuge for 2 min at ≥8000g to dry the membrane. Subsequently, to eliminate any chance of possible RPE washing buffer carryover, place the column in a new 2-mL collection tube, and discard the old collection tube with the flow-through. Centrifuge in a microcentrifuge at full speed for 1 min.

7. Remove the column from the collection tube carefully so the column does not contact the flow-through, as this will result in carryover of ethanol (*see* **Note 3**). Transfer the column to a new 1.5-mL collection tube and proceed with elution of total RNA.

8. Pipet 40 µL nuclease-free water directly onto the membrane. Close the tube gently, incubate for 1 min and centrifuge for 1 min at 8000g to elute.

Store the isolated total RNA on ice while aliquots are pipetted for quantification and during the subsequent cDNA synthesis step. The concentration of RNA is determined by measuring the absorbance at 260 nm (A_{260}) in a spectrophotometer. In general, to ensure significance, readings should be between 0.10 and 1.0. An absorbance of 1 unit at 260 nm corresponds to 40 µg of RNA per mL. The isolated total RNA is diluted 1:50 for the measurement in nuclease-free water (2 µL total RNA, 98 µL water).

3.3.2. Synthesis of ds cDNA

For the synthesis of ds cDNA, the one-tube double-stranded cDNA Synthesis System (Roche Applied Science, Mannheim, Germany) can be used. This system has been designed according to the method of Gubler and Hoffmann (*2*) and is optimized to reduce manipulation steps, allowing the rapid and reliable synthesis of full-length cDNAs, especially from total RNA. During the first-strand reaction, avian myeloblastosis virus (AMV) reverse transcriptase is used. The initiation of the first-strand synthesis depends upon hybridization of an oligo [(dT)24 T7promoter]65 primer to the mRNA, usually at the poly(A) tail. This primer also contains a promoter for the T7 RNA polymerase, which enables a subsequent in vitro transcription (IVT) reaction. The first- and second-strand syntheses are performed in the same tube, which speeds the synthesis procedure and maximizes recovery of cDNA. Synthesis for the second strand takes place using the DNA/RNA hybrid as substrate. Mild treatment with RNase H inserts nicks into the RNA, providing 3′ OH-primers for DNA polymerase I present in the second-strand enzyme cocktail. The 5′-3′ exonuclease activity of DNA polymerase I removes the primer stretches in the direction of synthesis, which are then replaced with new nucleotides by the polymerase activity. *Escherichia Coli* ligase links the gaps to a complete ds cDNA strand. The last step in the cDNA synthesis is to ensure that the termini of the cDNA are blunt. This is done by adding T4 DNA polymerase, which removes any remaining overhanging 3′ ends on the ds cDNAs.

1. Thaw all necessary components and place them on ice. Pipet the following components in a sterile 1.5-mL reaction tube (40 µL total reverse-transcription reaction volume) (*see* **Table 1**).
2. Incubate 10 min at 70°C (Eppendorf Thermostat Plus; can also be used for all following downstream incubations), then place the tube immediately on ice. Add the components from **Table 2**, mix gently, and incubate for 60 min at 42°C. In the meantime, thaw all required components for the second-strand synthesis reaction, mix them, and place on ice.
3. After 60 min, place the tube on ice for 5 min to terminate the reaction. Continue immediately with the second-strand reaction (*see* **Table 3**). Pipet directly into the first-strand reaction tube the following components, mix gently, and incubate for 2 h at 16°C.
4. After 2 h incubation, add 20 µL (20 U) T4 DNA polymerase and incubate for 5 min at 16°C. Then stop the reaction by adding 6.8 µL EDTA (0.5 M, pH 8.0).
5. Subsequently, digest residual total RNA. Add 1.5 µL (15 U) RNase I and incubate for 30 min at 37°C. Add 5 µL (3 U) proteinase K to the reaction and incubate for another 30 min at 37°C.
6. Add 153.5 µL water to the cDNA. The final volume now is 336.8 µL and the cDNA is ready for the subsequent cleanup step.

3.3.3. Cleanup of ds cDNA

The cDNA cleanup step is performed using 1.5-mL Phase Lock Gel (PLG) technology caps (Eppendorf). PLG is a product that eliminates interface-protein contamination during the phenol extraction. Upon centrifugation, the gel migrates to form a tight seal between the phases of an aqueous/organic extraction. The organic phase and the interface material are effectively trapped in or below the barrier. This allows the complete and easy transfer of the entire aqueous phase containing the cDNA species by simply pipetting. The risk of contaminating the sample with interface material is eliminated.

1. Add 330 µL phenol/chloroform/isoamylalcohol (25:24:1) to the cDNA solution, vortex for 10 s, and transfer the supernatant to a 1.5-mL PLG tube. Centrifuge for

Table 1
First-Strand cDNA Synthesis Initiation

Component	Volume	Final concentration (or amount)
Total RNA	Variable	1–10 µg
Oligo[(dT)24 T7 promoter]65 primer	2 µL	200 pmol
Water	Add to 21 µL	
Final volume	21 µL	

Table 2
First-Strand cDNA Synthesis Reaction

Component	Volume	Final concentration (or amount)
Reverse-transcription buffer, 5X concentrated	8 µL	1X
Dithiothreitol, 0.1 M	4 µL	10 mM
Avian myeloblastosis virus (AMV), 25 U/µL	2 µL	50 U
RNase inhibitor, 25 U/µL	1 µL	25 U
dNTP-mix, 10 mM each	4 µL	1 mM each
Total final volume	40 µL	

Table 3
Second-Strand cDNA Synthesis Reaction

Component	Volume
2nd strand buffer, 5X concentrated	30 µL (1X final concentration)
dNTP-mix, 10 mM each	1.5 µL
2nd strand enzyme blend	6.5 µL
Water	72 µL
Total final volume	150 µL

2 min at maximum speed. Transfer the supernatant to a new tube.

2. Repeat cleanup but now add 310 µL phenol/chloroform/isoamylalcohol (25:24:1), vortex for 10 s, and transfer the supernatant to a 1.5-mL PLG tube. Centrifuge for 2 min at maximum speed. Transfer the supernatant to a new tube.

3. Repeat cleanup, but now add 290 µL phenol/chloroform/isoamylalcohol (25:24:1), vortex for 10 s, and transfer the supernatant to a 1.5-mL PLG tube. Centrifuge for 2 min at maximum speed. Transfer the supernatant to a new tube.

4. In this new tube, now containing the purified cDNA, precipitate the ds cDNA by

adding 175 µL ammonium acetate (7.5 *M*), 0.5 µL glycogen (20 mg/mL), and 1000 µL of absolute ethanol (*see* **Note 4**). Store overnight or longer at –20°C.

5. Pellet the ds cDNA by centrifugation at maximum speed for 30 min, discard the supernatant carefully. Wash the pellet by overlaying with 500 µL 80% ethanol. Centrifuge at maximum speed for 15 min. Then discard the supernatant carefully.

6. Wash the ds cDNA pellet by overlaying with 500 µL 80% ethanol. Centrifuge at maximum speed for 15 min. Then discard the supernatant carefully.

7. Wash the ds cDNA pellet by overlaying with 500 µL 100% ethanol. Centrifuge at maximum speed for 15 min. Then discard the supernatant carefully.

8. Air dry the pellet by evaporating residual ethanol. This takes approx 5–10 min.

9. Dissolve the cDNA pellet in 22 µL nuclease-free water and vortex for 10 s. Continue immediately with the IVT procedure.

3.3.4. Synthesis of Biotin-Labeled cRNA

After the ds cDNA has been purified, it is transcribed in vitro to generate more than 400 biotinylated cRNA molecules for each ds cDNA molecule. Adequately intact input RNA should result in an expected yield of biotinylated cRNA of between 4- and 10-fold greater than the total RNA input *(3)*.

1. Pipet the template cDNA and reaction components from the RNA transcript labeling kit into RNase-free microcentrifuge tubes (*see* **Table 4** and **Note 5**). Perform all steps at room temperature to avoid precipitation of DTT.

2. Carefully mix the reagents and collect the mixture in the bottom of the tube by brief centrifugation (5 s). Then place the reaction tube in a 37°C incubator and incubate for 5 h. After the IVT, immediately proceed with the purification of the biotin-labeled cRNA.

3.3.5. Cleanup of Biotin-Labeled cRNA

After the IVT reaction, cleanup of biotinylated cRNA is performed according to the RNeasy Mini Kit protocol (Qiagen). GITC-containing lysis buffer and ethanol are added to the sample to create conditions that promote selective binding of the cRNA to the silica-gel membrane in the RNeasy mini column. The cRNA binds to the membrane, contaminants are efficiently washed away, and high-quality cRNA is eluted in water. Eight individual samples can be processed in parallel. All steps of the RNeasy protocol should be performed quickly at room temperature. All centrifugation steps can be performed in a standard microcentrifuge. RPE wash buffer is supplied as a concentrate. Before using it for the first time, 4 vol of absolute ethanol are added to obtain a working solution. According to the manufacturer's recommendation, RLT buffer is prepared freshly for each cleanup procedure (10 µL 2-mercaptoethanol per 1 mL RLT buffer; mixed in a 15-mL Falcon tube).

1. Adjust the sample to a volume of 100 µL with water. Therefore, add 60 µL water to the 40-µL cRNA reaction volume.

Table 4
In Vitro Transcription Reaction

Component	Volume
Reaction buffer, 10X concentrated	4 µL
Dithiothreitol, 10X concentrated	4 µL
RNase inhibitor mix, 10X concentrated	4 µL
Biotin-labeled ribonucleotides, 10X concentrated	4 µL
T7 RNA polymerase, 20X concentrated	2 µL
Template ds cDNA	Variable
Water	Variable (to give a final volume of 40 µL)
Final volume	40 µL

2. Add 350 µL RLT buffer and mix thoroughly. The total volume now is 450 µL.
3. Add 250 µL absolute ethanol to the diluted cRNA, and mix thoroughly by pipetting. Do not centrifuge. The total volume now is 700 µL.
4. Continue immediately to apply the sample to an RNeasy mini column placed in a 2-mL collection tube. Close the tube gently, and centrifuge for 15 s at 8000*g*.
5. Apply the flow-through again to the same column placed in a new 2-mL collection tube. Close the tube gently, and centrifuge for 15 s at 8000*g*. Now discard the flow-through. Transfer the RNeasy column into a new 2-mL collection tube.
6. Pipet 500 µL RPE buffer onto the column. Close the tube gently, and centrifuge for 15 s at 8000*g* to wash the column. Discard the flow-through. Transfer the column into a new 2-mL collection tube.
7. Add another 500 µL RPE buffer to the column. Close the tube gently, and centrifuge for 2 min at ≥8000*g* to dry the membrane. Place the column in a new 2-mL collection tube, and discard the old collection tube with the flow-through. Centrifuge in a microcentrifuge at full speed for 1 min.
8. To elute, transfer the column to a new 1.5-mL collection tube (Eppendorf). Pipet 40 µL nuclease-free water directly onto the membrane and incubate for 1 min. Close the tube gently, and centrifuge for 1 min at 8000*g* to elute.

Store the isolated cRNA on ice while aliquots are pipetted for downstream applications. The concentration of cRNA is determined by measuring the absorbance at 260 nm (A_{260}) in a spectrophotometer. In general, to ensure significance, readings should be between 0.10 and 1.0. An absorbance of 1 U at 260 nm corresponds to 40 µg of cRNA per mL. The isolated cRNA is diluted 1:50 for the measurement in nuclease-free water (2 µL total RNA, 98 µL water). The A_{260}/A_{280} ratio should be close to 2.0 (ratios between 1.9 and 2.1 are acceptable).

Table 5
Fragmentation Reaction

Component	Volume
15 μg cRNA	Up to 24 μL
5X fragmentation buffer	6 μL
Water	To 30 μL
Final volume	30 μL (0.5 μg/μL cRNA)

3.3.6. Fragmenting the cRNA

After elution and quantification of the biotinylated cRNA, an aliquot of 15 μg is fragmented. The full-length cRNA is broken down to 35–200 base fragments by metal-induced hydrolysis. The final cRNA concentration in the fragmentation mix is usually adjusted to 0.5 μg/μL. The following procedure gives an example of a fragmentation reaction for 15 μg cRNA at a final concentration of 0.5 μg/μL.

1. Add 2 μL of 5X fragmentation buffer for every 8 μL of cRNA plus water. The cRNA is fragmented in the same tube that is later used for preparation and storage of the hybridization cocktail (*see* **Table 5** and **Note 6**).
2. Incubate at 94°C for 35 min.
3. Cool the fragmented cRNA on ice. Immediately proceed with the completion of the hybridization cocktail.

3.3.7. Target Hybridization

After fragmenting the cRNA, a hybridization cocktail is prepared, including the fragmented target, probe array controls, acetylated bovine serum albumin (BSA), and herring sperm DNA. It is then hybridized to the probe array during a 16-h incubation. A GeneChip probe array chip comes mounted in a plastic package to form a cartridge. The chip contains a collection of oligonucleotide probes that have been arrayed on the inner glass surface *(4,5)*. A chamber in the plastic package directly under the chip acts as a reservoir where hybridization and subsequent washing and staining steps occur.

1. Mix the following components for each target cRNA as given in **Table 6**. Standard-format microarrays require a 300-μL volume cocktail preparation. Hybridization cocktails can be stored at −20°C for later use or subsequently be hybridized.
2. Equilibrate the microarray to room temperature.
3. Heat the hybridization cocktail for 5 min to 99°C. Then incubate it for 5 min at 45°C. Subsequently, spin the hybridization cocktail for 5 min at maximum speed in

Table 6
Components for the Hybridization Cocktail

Component	Volume	Final concentration
Fragmented cRNA	15 µg	0.05 µg/µL
Control oligonucleotide B2 (3 nM)	5 µL	50 pM
Eukaryotic hybridization controls, 20X	15 µL	1.5, 5, 25, 100 pM, respectively
Herring sperm DNA (10 mg/mL)	3 µL	0.1 mg/mL
Acetylated bovien serum albumin (50 mg/mL)	3 µL	0.5 mg/mL
Hybridization buffer, 2X concentrated	150 µL	1X
Water	Add to 300 µL	
Final volume	300 µL	

a microcentrifuge to pellet any insoluble material from the hybridization mixture.

4. Meanwhile, wet the microarray by filling it through one of the septa with 200 µL 1X hybridization buffer using a micropipettor and appropriate tips (Rainin). Incubate the filled microarray in the hybridization oven for 15 min at 45°C with constant rotation (60 rpm).
5. After 15 min, remove the buffer solution from the microarray cartridge and fill with 200 µL of the clarified hybridization cocktail, avoiding any pelleted, insoluble matter at the bottom of the tube.
6. Place the microarray into the hybridization oven and incubate for 16 h at 45°C with constant rotation (60 rpm).

3.3.8. Microarrays

The U133 set (HG-U133A and HG-U133B) is a widely used design of gene expression microarrays. A detailed description regarding sequences and probe selection rules is available as a technical note from the manufacturer (www.affymetrix.com).

Affymetrix HG-U133A and HG-U133B Microarrays

The U133 two-array set provides comprehensive coverage of well-substantiated genes in the human genome. It can be used to analyze the expression level of 39,000 transcripts and variants, including greater than 33,000 human genes. The two arrays comprise more than 45,000 probe sets and 1 million distinct oligonucleotide features. The sequences from which these probe sets were derived were selected from GenBank, dbEST, and RefSeq. The sequence clusters were created from the UniGene database (Build 133, April 20, 2001) and then refined by analysis and comparison with a number of other publicly available databases, including the Washington University EST trace repository and the University of California–Santa Cruz Golden-Path human genome database (April 2001 release). In addition, an advanced understanding of probe uniqueness and hybridization characteristics allowed an improved selection of probes based on predicted behavior. The U133 chip design uses a multiple linear regression model that was derived from a thermodynamic model of nucleic acid duplex formation *(6)*. This model predicts probe binding affinity and linearity of signal changes in response to varying target concentrations. The two arrays are manufactured as standard format arrays with a feature size of 18 µm and use 11 probe pairs per sequence. The oligonucleotide length is 25-mer.

3.3.9. Microarray Washing and Staining

After hybridizing for 16 h at 45°C, the microarray is ready for washing and staining. GeneChip probe arrays are processed by the Fluidics Station instrument, which contains four modules, with each module processing one microarray cartridge.

1. Use the Microarray Suite software and define an experiment for each array to be processed (.exp extension). Perform a priming protocol to ensure that the wash lines are full of the appropriate buffer and that the fluidics station is ready to process a cartridge.
2. In the meantime, after 16 h of hybridization, remove the hybridization cocktail from the probe array and fill the probe array completely with nonstringent wash buffer (*see* **Note 7**).
3. Insert the probe array into the designated module of the fluidics station, select the correct experiment name in the drop-down experiment list, and start the protocol for washing and staining of expression microarrays. Standard-format microarrays were processed using the EukGE-WS2v4 signal-amplification protocol (*see* **Table 7**).
4. When the liquid crystal display (LCD) window indicates, place the microcentrifuge vial containing 600 µL of the respective staining solution into the sample holder. Verify that metal sampling needle is in the vial with its tip near the bottom.
5. At the end of the run, remove the probe arrays from the fluidics station modules and check the probe array window for large bubbles or air pockets. If the probe array has no large bubbles, it is ready to scan on the scanner. Otherwise, fill the array manually with non-stringent wash buffer.

3.3.10. Microarray Scanning and Image Analysis

After the wash and staining protocols are complete, the probe array is scanned using the GeneArray scanner. The laser excitation enters through the back of the glass support and focuses at the interface of the array surface and

Table 7
Fluidics Protocol for Antibody Amplification for Eukaryotic Targets

Step	Details
Posthybridiation wash no. 1	10 cycles of 2 mixes/cycle with non-stringent wash buffer A at 25°C
Posthybridization wash no. 2	4 cycles of 15 mixes/cycle with wash buffer B
First stain	Stain the probe array for 10 min in streptavidin-phycoerythrin (SAPE) solution at 25°C
Post-stain wash	10 cycles of 4 mixes/cycle with wash buffer A at 25°C
Second stain	Stain the probe array for 10 mins in antibody solution at 25°C
Third stain	Stain the probe array for 10 min in SAPE solution at 25°C
Final wash	15 cycles of 4 mixes/cycle with wash buffer A at 30°C.
Protocol	EukGE-WS2v4

the target solution. Then, fluorescence emission is collected by a lens and passes through a series of optical filters to a sensitive detector. This results in a quantitative two-dimensional fluorescence image of hybridization intensity. Each completed probe array image is stored in a separate image data file identified by the experiment name (.dat extension). Then the software defines the probe cells by grid alignment and computes an intensity for each probe cell (.cel extension). After the raw image is obtained, the algorithms in the Microarray Suite software are applied to process the raw probe set data to generate expression values (signal intensities), detection calls (absent, marginal, present), and associated *p*-values for every transcript represented on the arrays (.chp extension). These files are used to generate detailed reports on the sample quality and technical parameters (.rpt extension).

1. In the Microarray Suite software, select the experiment name that corresponds to the probe array to be scanned. A dialog box appears, prompting you to load an array into the scanner. Use default settings for pixel values and wavelength of the laser beam (pixel value = 3 μm, and laser wavelength = 570 nm).
2. The scanner begins scanning the probe array and acquiring data. After the scan has been completed, an image file containing the raw expression data is stored in an uncompressed format, i.e., individual pixels per probe cells.

3.3.11. Quality Assessment

Quality assessment is critical in obtaining reproducible microarray results. A series of quality control (QC) procedures can be performed at various key checkpoints during the gene expression profile analysis and include both monitoring of sample-related parameters and technical features.

- Gel electrophoresis according to standard protocols *(7)* can be performed to detect any degradation of input total RNA.
- After the IVT and cleanup of the cRNA, the ratio of 260/280 absorbance values is assessed by spectrophotometer measurements. Good-quality cRNA should demonstrate ratios of 1.9 to 2.1. Low cRNA yield can be a sensitive indicator of problematic labeling procedures and/or starting material.
- Basic microarray image analyses include visual array inspections (.dat file) and check for a correct grid alignment at each of the four corners and the center of the array.
- Basic raw data analyses include parameters to monitor the overall background intensity, scaling factor, percentage of present called genes (%P), and 3'/5' ratio for the GAPD gene (*see* **Note 8**).

A technically acceptable gene expression profile can be defined according to the following characteristics: $\geq 1.0 \,\mu g$ of input total RNA results in sufficient cRNA yield ($\geq 20.0 \,\mu g$), concentration ($\geq 0.6 \,\mu g/\mu L$), and ratio of absorbance at 260 nm/280 nm (approx 2.0). The scanned array image should not show largely visible artifacts and should have a correct grid aligned for feature extraction. After adjusting the scanned image to common target intensity, the scaling factor within a project should lie within two standard deviations of the mean. When analyzing Affymetrix A-series microarrays, the %P called probe sets should be $\geq 30.0\%$, and the 3'/5' ratio for GAPD should be ≤ 3.0. If the 3'/5' ratio is > 3.0, but still $> 30.0\%$ of the genes were called present, the profile may be rated as acceptable. However, in most cases with 3'/5' ratio > 3.0, the %P is also $< 30.0\%$. Then, the data must also be normalized with higher scaling factors, which may be outside an acceptable range within a given data set. As a consequence, a sample fails if, in combination, a low 3'/5' ratio, high percentage of %P probe sets, and comparable range of scaling factors are missed. Accordingly, these gene expression profiles should not be used for gene selection or training of a classification engine. Most of these metrics directly follow the recommendations of the Tumor Analysis Best Practices Working Group for Affymetrix MAS 5.0 probe set algorithms and data analyses. This working group has recently been established to develop recommendations for experimental design, data analysis algorithms, signal-to-noise assessments, and biostatistical methods *(3)*.

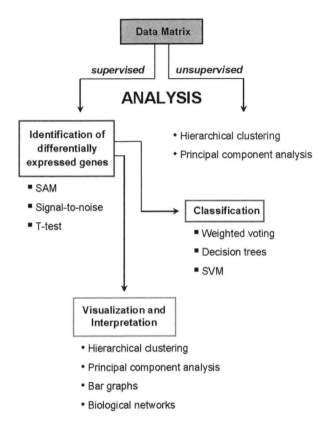

Fig. 2. Overview of the data analysis workflow. After preparation of corresponding data sets from the main master table, the data are analyzed, either unsupervised or supervised. Unsupervised analyses are performed by hierarchical clustering or principal component analysis. In the supervised analyses, differentially expressed genes can be identified by various methods and selected for further interpretations, e.g., visualization by hierarchical clustering, principal component analysis, plotting as bar graphs, or generation of biological networks. In addition, differentially expressed genes can be selected for classification tasks where several different machine-learning approaches can be applied.

3.4. Microarray Data Analysis

A wide range of approaches are available for gleaning insights from the data obtained from transcriptional profiling *(8)*. Data analyses are performed by two different approaches—supervised and unsupervised (**Fig. 2**). Unsupervised analyses are used to test the hypothesis that specific characteristics, e.g., genetic aberrations, are also reflected at the level of gene expression signatures. Supervised analyses identify a minimal set of genes that could be used to stratify those patients after a training of classification engines *(9,10)*. The gene lists from supervised analyses can also further be interpreted in terms of biology. For all gene expression profiles, master data tables have to be maintained. In these tables, rows represent all genes for which data has been collected, and columns represent microarray experiments from individual patients. Each cell represents the measured fluorescence intensity from the corresponding target probe set on the microarray. Before analyzing the data, it is a routine procedure to normalize the data *(11)*. This is a mandatory step in the data-mining process in order to appropriately compare the measured gene expression levels. U133 set microarray signal intensity values can be normalized by scaling the raw data intensities to a common target intensity using a recommended mask file (U133A/B mask file; e.g., selected global target intensity value: 5000) (*see* **Note 9**).

3.4.1. Identification of Differentially Expressed Genes

In microarray experiments, a common goal is to detect genes that show differential expression across two or more biological conditions. Therefore, multiple hypothesis testing algorithms are performed on all genes simultaneously to determine whether each one is differentially expressed. The null hypothesis is that there is no change in expression levels between various leukemia subclasses. The alternative hypothesis is that there is significant differential gene expression. The analyses can be performed either between two distinct classes (pairwise comparisons; subtype A vs subtype B) or between one distinct class and all other remaining classes in a one-vs-all (OVA) approach.

3.4.1.1. SIGNIFICANCE ANALYSIS OF MICROARRAYS

Supervised data analyses can be performed using the significance analysis of microarrays (SAM) software. SAM is a statistical technique for finding significant genes in large-scale microarray-based gene expression profiles, and correlates gene expression data with an external variable, e.g., the leukemia subclass or karyotype information. The SAM software is an add-in package for Microsoft Excel and analyzes statistical significance of the changes in gene expression from repeated permutations. It was proposed by Tusher and colleagues *(12)*. SAM identifies genes with statistically significant changes in expression by assimilating a set of gene-specific t-tests. Each gene is assigned a score on the basis of its change in gene expression relative to the standard deviation of repeated measurements for that gene. Genes with scores greater than an adjustable threshold are deemed potentially significant. The cutoff for significance is determined by the tuning parameter delta, chosen by the user based on the false discovery rate (FDR). The FDR, i.e., the percentage of genes identified by chance, is estimated by analyzing repeated permutations of the data.

3.4.1.2. STATISTICAL SIGNIFICANCE

Microarrays can measure the expression of thousands of genes to identify expression changes between different biological states. Methods based on conventional *t*-tests provide the probability (P) that a difference in gene expression occurred by chance. Although $p < 0.01$ is significant in the context of experiments designed to evaluate small numbers, a microarray experiment for more 10,000 genes would identify 100 genes by chance. Thus, methods are needed to determine the significance of these changes while accounting for the enormous number of genes. Commonly, to address the multiple testing problem, false-discovery rates (FDR) of genes are calculated according to a statistical method adapted specifically for microarrays *(13)*. As it automatically takes into account the fact that thousands of genes are simultaneously being tested, the FDR is a widely accepted method to measure statistical significance in genome-wide studies. A measure of statistical significance called the *q*-value is associated with each tested feature. Similarly to the *p*-value, the *q*-value gives each measured gene its own individual measure of significance. Whereas the *p*-value is a measure of significance in terms of the false-positive rate, the *q*-value is a measure in terms of the false-discovery rate (FDR). In a microarray data set, the *q*-value of a particular feature is the expected proportion of false positives incurred when calling that feature significant. The *q*-values can be used as an exploratory guide for which features to investigate further, e.g., through the use of pathway applications or classification engines.

3.4.2. Estimation of Prediction Performance

The generalization performance of the different algorithms can be estimated by performing cross-validation methods (CV). These methods are based on the idea that the most unbiased test of the predictive error is by applying it to data that were not used in the building of the initial predictive model. A common application is to partition a dataset into two parts—to fit the model on the first part, and to assess the predictive capability of that model on the second part. Depending on the CV method, the complete data set is split into different proportions of a training set and a test set. Each approach is performed to determine the accuracy, i.e., the probability of correct classification of a previously unknown sample.

3.4.2.1. LEAVE-ONE-OUT CROSS-VALIDATION

The leave-one-out cross-validation (LOOCV) method is one of several approaches to estimating how well a model that was trained on training data is going to perform on future as-yet-unseen data. LOOCV implies that one sample is excluded from the complete data set n and the remaining samples are used for training. This training and prediction process is repeated n times to include predictions for each sample (so that each sample is classified once in the *n* iterations).

3.4.2.2. 10-Fold CV

Ten-fold CV is another method used to estimating the apparent accuracy, i.e., the overall rate of correct predictions of the complete data set. This classification task means that the data set is divided into 10 equally sized subsets, balanced for the respective subclasses of the data. Then, differentially expressed genes are identified in the training set (9 subsets), and a model is trained based on the top genes that demonstrate differential expression between each of the respective subclasses in the training set. This model is used to generate predictions for the remaining subset. This training and prediction process has to be repeated 10 times to include predictions for each subset (so that each sample is classified once in the 10 iterations).

3.4.2.3. Resampling Analysis

A resampling approach can be used to assess the robustness of class predictions. Here again, the data set is randomly (but balanced for the respective subtypes) split into a training set, consisting of two-thirds of samples, and an independent test set with the remaining third. Differentially expressed genes are identified in the training set, a support vector machine (SVM) model is built from the training set, and predictions are made in the test set. This complete process is repeated 100 times. By this means, 95% confidence intervals for accuracy, sensitivity, and specificity can also be estimated. Sensitivity and specificity are calculated as follows:

Sensitivity = (number of positive samples predicted)/(number of true-positives)

Specificity = (number of negative samples predicted)/(number of true-negatives)

3.4.3. Hierarchical Clustering

Two-dimensional hierarchical cluster analysis is a popular method of organizing expression data, i.e., arranging genes and patients according to similarity in their patterns of gene expression (**Fig. 3**). This method helps to organize but not to alter tables containing the primary expression data. The output format is a graphic display that allows the clustering and the underlying expression data to be conveyed in an intuitive form to biologists *(14)*. By adopting a mathematical description of similarity, the object of this algorithm is to compute a dendrogram that assembles all elements into a single tree. For any set of n genes, an upper-diagonal similarity matrix is computed by the Euclidean distance metric, which contains similarity scores for all pairs of genes. The matrix

Data Matrix

Visualization

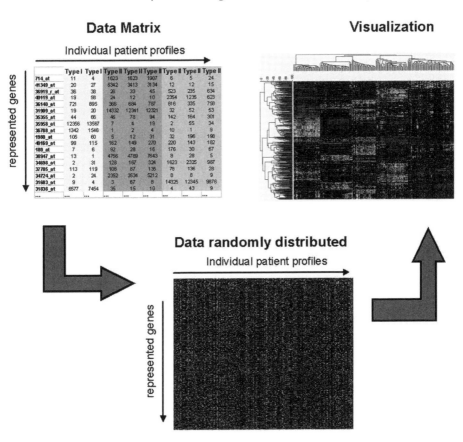

Individual patient profiles

represented genes

Data randomly distributed

Individual patient profiles

represented genes

Fig. 3. Hierarchical cluster analysis workflow. The primary expression data are graphically represented. Each data point is represented with a color that quantitatively and qualitatively reflects the original measured fluorescence intensity. One can look at such images, identify patterns or branches of the dendrogram of interest, and readily zoom in on the detailed expression patterns and identities of the genes contributing to these patterns.

is scanned to identify the highest value that represents the most similar pair of genes. Then a node is created joining these two genes, and a gene expression profile is computed for the node by averaging observations for the joined elements. The similarity matrix is updated with this new node replacing the two joined elements, and the process is repeated $n - 1$ times until only a single elcment remains.

Any unsupervised gene expression analysis begins with a definition of similarity between expression patterns, but with no prior knowledge of the true functional classes of the genes, or patients, respectively. For visualization of unsupervised data analyses, a variation filter can be applied. This filter aims at removing probe sets that demonstrate minimal variation across the complete data set. Practically, for each gene the standard variance is calculated across all samples. Then the data matrix is sorted according to the standard variances, and probes demonstrating a low variance are excluded from the subsequent analysis. Hierarchical clustering is the method of choice when one has little or no a priori knowledge of the complete repertoire of expected gene expression patterns. However, no information about the statistical significance is provided. In contrast, using hierarchical clustering in a supervised approach helps to visualize differential gene expression of an already preselected set of genes.

3.4.4. Principal Component Analysis

The need to visualize large amounts of data in many dimensions occurs frequently in bioinformatics. Commonly, principal component analysis (PCA) is used in statistics to extract the main relationships in data of high dimensionality *(15)*. It is a useful tool for categorization of multidimensional data such as gene expression studies, because it separates the dominating features in the data set. The background mathematical technique used in PCA is called *eigen analysis*. PCA reduces the dimensionality of the data set while retaining most of the information contained therein via the construction of a linear transformation matrix. This transformation matrix is composed of the most significant eigenvectors of the covariance matrix of the input matrix of feature vectors. The principal components (PC) are the projections of the data on the eigenvectors. These vectors give the directions in which the data cloud is stretched most. The significance of an eigenvector is defined by its variance, which is equivalent to its corresponding eigenvalue. Eigenvalues give an indication of the amount of information the respective PC represent. PCs corresponding to large eigenvalues represent much information in the data set, and thus can tell much about the relations between the data points. Because the original data's variation can be retained and explained by a smaller number of transformed variables, a PCA projects the data into a new two- or three-dimensional space and may provide valuable insight into the data (**Fig. 4**).

Fig. 4. *(opposite page)* Principal component analysis workflow. The multi-dimensional data are reduced by transformation to a new set of variables, the principle components (PCs). The traditional approach is to use the first few PCs, because they capture most of the variation in the original data. In the final graph, data points with similar characteristics will cluster together. Each patient's expression pattern is represented by a color-coded sphere.

Data Matrix

patient profiles →

represented genes ↓

	Type I	Type I	Type II	Type II	Type II	Type II	Type II	Type II
714_at	11	4	1623	1623	1907	6	5	24
41349_at	20	27	6342	3413	3134	12	12	15
36919_r_at	36	38	26	33	45	523	235	634
40119_at	19	58	24	12	10	2354	1235	823
36140_at	721	895	366	694	787	616	335	758
31909_at	19	20	14332	12341	12321	32	52	53
35355_at	44	66	46	78	94	142	164	301
35958_at	12356	13567	7	4	19	2	55	34
36766_at	1342	1546	1	2	4	10	1	9
1988_at	105	60	5	12	31	32	196	198
40169_at	99	115	162	149	270	220	143	182
180_at	7	8	92	28	18	176	30	67
38947_at	13	1	4756	4789	7643	8	28	5
34698_at	2	31	128	167	324	1623	2325	987
37705_at	113	119	108	87	135	78	136	28
34724_at	2	24	2352	3534	5212	8	12345	9
31663_at	9	4	3	67	8	14325	43	9
31638_at	6577	7454	35	15	10	4		9876

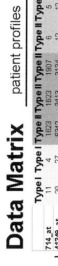

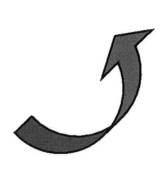

Visualization

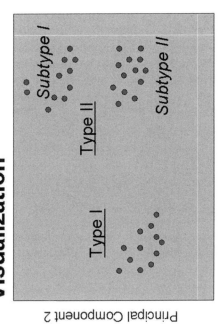

Type I

Type II

Subtype I

Subtype II

Principal Component 2

Principal Component 1

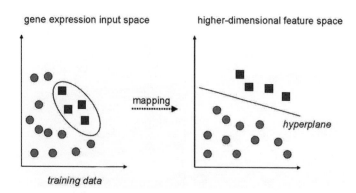

Fig. 5. Concept of support vector machine (SVM)-based classification. The SVM operates by mapping the given training set into a possibly high-dimensional feature space and attempting to locate in that space a plane that separates positive from negative samples. The hyperplane, i.e., a plane in a space with more than three dimensions, corresponds to a nonlinear decision boundary in the input space.

3.4.5. Classification of Samples Based on Gene Expression Patterns: SVM-Based Classification

For classification of microarray data, the support vector machine (SVM) algorithm can be used. SVMs are learning machines that can perform binary classification tasks *(16–18)*. A classification task involves training and testing gene expression profiles, which consist of some data instances. Each instance in the training set contains "target values" (class labels, i.e., leukemia classes) and several "attributes" (features, i.e., genes). The goal of this approach is to produce a model that predicts target values of data instances in the testing set that are given only the attributes. Applied to gene expression data, an SVM would begin with a set of genes that have a common function—e.g., genes that demonstrate differential expression between distinct leukemia subtypes. After nonlinearly mapping the n-dimensional input space into a high-dimensional feature space, a linear classifier is constructed in this high-dimensional feature space (**Fig. 5**).

Using this training set, a SVM would learn to discriminate between the types and subtypes of leukemias based on expression data. Having found such a plane, the SVM can then predict the classification of an unlabeled new sample by mapping it into the feature space and asking on which side of the separating plane the example lies (**Fig. 6**). Then a label is assigned according to its relationship with the decision boundary *(10,19)*. Multi-class SVM classifiers can be built with linear kernels using the library LIBSVM version 2.36 (www.csie.ntu.edu.tw/~cjlin/libsvm/) *(20)*.

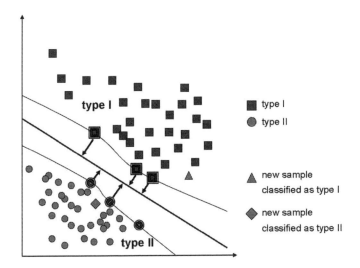

Fig. 6. Classification task. The support vector machine separates a given set of binary labeled training data with a hyperplane that is maximally distant from them (maximal margin). The middle black line is the decision surface defining the borderline between the area of prediction of type I samples (squares) and type II samples (circles). The outer lines precisely meet the constraint. Support vectors marked as critical for the classification task are the points that lie closest to the separating hyperplane.

3.4.6. Functional Gene Annotation: NetAffx Database

The NetAffx database can be used to functionally annotate the probe sets represented on the microarrays. The NetAffx Analysis Center (www.affymetrix.com/analysis/) is an integrated, freely available online resource created by Affymetrix *(21)*. This Web-based application enables researchers to correlate results from experiments with array design and annotation information. It is a dynamic tool and provides access to underlying array content and the design of GeneChip probe arrays, including probe sequences and extensive gene annotations from both Affymetrix and the public domain. It allows the user to search array contents for sequences of interest, review gene and protein characterizations for represented probe sets, and sort transcripts by functional group, metabolic pathway, and disease association. For each cataloged Affymetrix GeneChip microarray, an anchoring databank summarizes all the annotations for the probe sets. The information provided for each probe set falls into two categories: sequence annotations and static information. Sequence annotations refer to the information about the representative sequence for a probe set, including functional annotations for gene title, gene symbol, and cytogenetic bands. The static information for each probe set details the probe sequences, accession numbers, and textual description, and describes what the probes were designed to interrogate. The static probe set data are also depicted graphically.

3.4.7. Software

Software packages from Affymetrix (www.affymetrix.com/support/) are used for principal data acquisition (MAS5), storage (MicroDB), and analysis (DMT). Individual gene expression profiles can also be prepared as Microsoft Excel tables.

The following packages can be applied for identification of differentially expressed genes and classification:

SAM (Stanford University; www-stat.stanford.edu/~tibs/SAM/index.html)
Bioconductor (open source; www.bioconductor.org)
q-value (University of Washington; faculty.washington.edu/~jstorey/qvalue/)
LIBSVM (National Taiwan University; www.scie.ntu.edu.tw/~cjiln/libsvm/).

SAM is available as a Microsoft Excel Add-in. Bioconductor is an open source and open development software project for the analysis and comprehension of genomic data *(22)*. Bioconductor packages provide statistical and graphical methodologies for analyzing genomic data. LIBSVM (Version 2.6) is a software solution for SVM-based classification. The *q*-value software takes a list of *p*-values resultling from the simultaneous testing of many hypotheses and estimates their *q*-values *(13)*. In addition, further third-party software packages can be used for statistical analyses and data visualization:

SPSS (SPSS Inc.; www.spss.com/)
Pathways Analysis (Ingenuity Systems; www. Ingenuity.com)
GeneMaths (Applied Maths, Inc.; www.applied-maths.com)
J-Express (MolMine AS; www. molmine.com/).www.applied-maths.com

4. Notes

1. The whole sample target preparation procedure can be performed in two working days, taking the assay's safe stopping points into account. Day 1 includes isolation of total RNA, synthesis of ds cDNA, cleanup of ds cDNA, and ethanol precipitation overnight. The IVT reaction, cRNA cleanup, quantification, and fragmentation are performed on day 2. After a hybridization cocktail has been prepared, it is either subsequently hybridized to a probe array, or can be stored at −20°C for later use. Throughout all steps, powder-free gloves should be worn. All steps to minimize the introduction of exogenous nucleases should be taken. Water used in the protocols has to be molecular-biology grade. All steps should be performed in nuclease-free 1.5-mL reaction tubes.

Table 8
Template cDNA Used for Each In Vitro
Transcription (IVT) Reaction

μg total RNA	Volume cDNA	Volume H$_2$O
5 μg or less	22 μL	—
6 μg	20 μL	2 μL
7 μg	18 μL	4 μL
8 μg	16 μL	6 μL
9 μg	13 μL	9 μL
10 μg	11 μL	11 μL
Final volume	22 μL	

2. The initial sample homogenization is necessary to reduce the viscosity of the cell lysates. Homogenization shears the high-molecular-weight genomic DNA and other high-molecular-weight cellular components to create a homogeneous lysate. Incomplete homogenization results in inefficient binding of RNA to the silica-gel membrane, and therefore significantly reduces yields.

3. It is important to completely dry the silica-gel membrane before the elution step, because residual ethanol may interfere with downstream enzymatic reactions.

4. Addition of a carrier to nucleic acid precipitations, e.g., 0.5 μL glycogen (20 mg/mL), aids in visualization of the pellet and may increase recovery.

5. Depending on the input total RNA used for cDNA synthesis, the amount of template cDNA used for each IVT reaction can be determined as in **Table 8**.

6. Fragmenting the cRNA target before hybridization to GeneChip probe arrays has been shown to be critical in obtaining optimal assay sensitivity. Affymetrix recommends that the cRNA used in the fragmentation procedure be sufficiently concentrated to maintain a small volume during the procedure. This will minimize the amount of magnesium in the final hybridization cocktail. Thus, the cRNA should reach a minimum concentration of 0.6 μg/μL. Typically, an IVT reaction starting with 5.0 μg of total RNA input for cDNA synthesis yields between 35 and 50 μg biotinylated cRNA. Remaining undiluted and non-fragmented cRNA can be deposited for long-term storage at –80°C.

7. Labeled cRNA targets can be reused. The same hybridization cocktail can be hybridized to a new probe array up to three times. Mostly, the targets are hybridized first to U133A and then to U133B arrays. To prevent leaking of fluids from the cartridge during hybridization and scanning, glue dots should be applied to each of the two septa on the array cartridge.

8. In addition to the conventional probe sets designed to be within the most 3′ end (approx 600 bases of a transcript), additional probe sets in the 5′ region and middle portion (M) of the transcript are also represented for certain housekeeping genes, including GAPD. The signal intensity ratio of the 3′ probe set over the 5′ probe set is often referred to as the 3′/5′ ratio. This ratio gives an indication of

the integrity of the starting RNA, efficiency of first-strand cDNA synthesis, and/ or IVT of cRNA. As recommended by the manufacturer, there is no single threshold cutoff to assess sample quality. Routinely, most users refer to a threshold ratio of less than 3.0 for the most common tissues.

9. As a simple means to relate signal values between arrays, a set of 100 maintenance genes is represented on recent expression microarrays (probe set identifiers from 200000_s_at to 200099_s_at). These normalization controls were originally identified from a data set of HG-U95Av2 hybridizations representing a large number of different tissues and cell lines. The data on these probe sets shared the common characteristic of consistently being called present (P) while exhibiting relatively low signal variation over different sample types *(23)*. Therefore, when scaling data between the HG-U133A and B arrays, an algorithm against these normalization controls, which are represented on both arrays, avoids a skewing of the data and provides an improved alternative tool to global scaling. Specific mask files for these probe sets are available from the manufacturer (www.affymetrix.com). Scaling factors, i.e., the multiplication factor applied to each signal value on an array, will vary across different samples, and there are no set guidelines for any particular sample type. However, if they differ by too much within a set of experiments, this indicates wide variation in the underlying image files, and therefore the analyzed data should be treated with caution.

5. Commentary

The introduction of microarray technology has been a major step towards the comprehensive biological characterization of various diseases, and clearly will allow the identification of yet unknown subentities and even new entities. In particular, it has become clear that distinct cytogenetically defined subtypes in AML carry highly specific gene expression profiles, which can be used to identify these subtypes based on microarray analyses with very high accuracy *(24–27)*. Therefore, it is expected that the routine application of microarrays will significantly improve molecular diagnostics in leukemia and will provide deep insights into the pathogenetic alterations of malignant and nonmalignant hematopoietic cells. In addition, these comprehensive data are anticipated to allow the identification of prognostically relevant markers as well as disease-specific markers that can be applied for programs of monitoring minimal residual disease. Of highest clinical relevance is the capability of microarray approaches to identify pathogenetically essential structures and alterations that can be targeted by future drugs, which hopefully will lead to improved management of these diseases. The accurate diagnosis and subclassification of leukemias is currently based on a comprehensive combination of various methods, including cytomorphology, cytochemistry, multiparameter immunophenotyping, cytogenetics, fluorescence *in situ* hybridization, and quantitative and non-quantitative molecular genetics, which are costly, time-consuming, and require skilled expert-level personnel in centralized reference laboratories. Based on microarray methods, substantial steps forward may be made in the direction of both optimizing the diagnostic capabilities and reducing financial reserves that have to be invested. A significant number of today's diagnostic approaches can be reproduced by gene expression profiling already. However, further large trials are needed to assert the validity of this technology.

References

1. Dugas, M., Schoch, C., Schnittger, S., et al. (2001) A comprehensive leukemia database: integration of cytogenetics, molecular genetics and microarray data with clinical information, cytomorphology and immunophenotyping. *Leukemia* **15,** 1805–1810.
2. Gubler, U. and Hoffman, B. J. (1983) A simple and very efficient method for generating cDNA libraries. *Gene* **25,** 263–269.
3. Hoffmann, E. P. (2004) Expression profiling—best practices for data generation and interpretation in clinical trials. *Nat. Rev. Genet.* **5,** 229–237.
4. Lipshutz, R. J., Fodor, S. P., Gingeras, T. R., and Lockhart, D. J. (1999) High density synthetic oligonucleotide arrays. *Nat. Genet.* **21,** 20–24.
5. Lockhart, D. J., Dong, H., Byrne, M. C., et al. (1996) Expression monitoring by hybridization to high-density oligonucleotide arrays. *Nat. Biotechnol.* **14,** 1675–1680.
6. Mei, R., Hubbell, E., Bekiranov, S., et al. (2003) Probe selection for high-density oligonucleotide arrays. *Proc. Natl. Acad. Sci. USA* **100,** 11,237–11,242.
7. Sambrook, J., Fritsch, E. F., and Maniatis, T. (1989) *Molecular Cloning: A Laboratory Manual* (2nd edition). Cold Spring Harbor Laboratory: Cold Spring Harbor, NY.
8. Slonim, D. K. (2002) From patterns to pathways: gene expression data analysis comes of age. *Nat. Genet.* **32 Suppl.,** 502–508.
9. Golub, T. R., Slonim, D. K., Tamayo, P., et al. (1999) Molecular classification of cancer: class discovery and class prediction by gene expression monitoring. *Science* **286,** 531–537.
10. Yeoh, E. J., Ross, M. E., Shurtleff, S. A., et al. (2002) Classification, subtype discovery, and prediction of outcome in pediatric acute lymphoblastic leukemia by gene expression profiling. *Cancer Cell* **1,** 133–143.
11. Quackenbush, J. (2002) Microarray data normalization and transformation. Nat. Genet. 32 Suppl, 496–501.
12. Tusher, V. G., Tibshirani, R., and Chu, G. (2001) Significance analysis of microarrays applied to the ionizing radiation response. *Proc. Natl. Acad. Sci. USA* **98,** 5116–5121.
13. Storey, J. D. and Tibshirani, R. (2003) Statistical significance for genomewide studies. *Proc. Natl. Acad. Sci. USA* **100,** 9440–9445.
14. Eisen, M. B., Spellman, P. T., Brown, P. O., and Botstein, D. (1998) Cluster analysis and display of genome-wide expression patterns. *Proc. Natl. Acad. Sci. USA* **95,** 14,863–14,868.

15. Jolliffe, I. T. (2002) *Principal Component Analysis.* Springer: New York.
16. Guyon, I., Weston, J., Barnhill, S., and Vapnik, V. (2002) Gene selection for cancer classification using support vector machines. *Machine Learning* **46,** 389–422.
17. Schölkopf, B. and Smola, A. J. (2002) *Learning with Kernels.* MIT Press: Cambridge, MA.
18. Vapnik, V. (1998) *Statistical Learning Theory.* Wiley: New York.
19. Kohlmann, A., Schoch, C., Schnittger, S., et al. (2004) Pediatric acute lymphoblastic leukemia (ALL) gene expression signatures classify an independent cohort of adult ALL patients. *Leukemia* **18,** 63–71.
20. Chang, C. C. and Lin, C. J. (2001) LIBSVM: a library for support vector machines. Software available at www.csie.ntu.edu.tw/~cjlin/libsvm/
21. Liu, G., Loraine, A. E., Shigeta, R., et al. (2003) NetAffx: Affymetrix probesets and annotations. *Nucleic Acids Res.* **31,** 82–86.
22. Dudoit, S., Gentleman, R. C., and Quackenbush, J. (2003) Open source software for the analysis of microarray data. *Biotechniques* **March Suppl.,** 45–51.
23. Warrington, J. A., Nair, A., Mahadevappa, M., and Tsyganskaya, M. (2000) Comparison of human adult and fetal expression and identification of 535 housekeeping/maintenance genes. *Physiol. Genomics* **2,** 143–147.
24. Kohlmann, A., Schoch, C., Schnittger, S., et al. (2003) Molecular characterization of acute leukemias by use of microarray technology. *Genes Chromosomes Cancer* **37,** 396–405.
25. Ross, M. E., Zhou, X., Song, G., Shurtleff, S. A., Girtman, K., Williams, W. K., et al. (2003) Classification of pediatric acute lymphoblastic leukemia by gene expression profiling. *Blood* **102,** 2951–2959.
26. Ross, M. E., Mahfouz, R., Onciu, M., et al. (2004) Gene expression profiling of pediatric acute myelogenous leukemia. *Blood* **104,** 3679–3687.
27. Schoch, C., Kohlmann, A., Schnittger, S., et al. (2002) Acute myeloid leukemias with reciprocal rearrangements can be distinguished by specific gene expression profiles. *Proc. Natl. Acad. Sci. USA* **99,** 10,008–10,013.

15

Classification of AML Using a Monoclonal Antibody Microarray

Richard I. Christopherson, Kerryn Stoner, Nicole Barber, Larissa Belov, Adrian Woolfson, Mike Scott, Linda Bendall, and Stephen P. Mulligan

Summary

A cluster of differentiation (CD) antibody microarray called the DotScan microarray has been developed that enables an extensive immunophenotype to be obtained for a suspension of leukocytes in a single analysis. For a leukemia with a leukemia count of greater than $10 \times 10^9/$ L, the immunophenotype obtained is essentially that of the leukemic clone. The antibody microarray is printed as microscopic (10 nL) dots on a nitrocellulose film on a microscope slide. Cells are captured by the immobilized antibodies and a dot pattern is recorded with an optical array reader giving the immunophenotype of the leukemia. Procedures are being developed that should enable diagnosis of myeloid leukemias by comparison of the dot pattern obtained from an unknown blood sample with a library of consensus patterns for the common leukemias.

Key Words: AML; antibody; array; CD antigen; CD11b; CD13; CD33; CD34; CD117; cell capture; diagnosis; FAB classification; immunophenotype; myeloid leukemia; pattern recognition; prognosis; proteomics; WHO classification.

1. Introduction
1.1. Background

The "cluster of differentiation" (CD) antigens were discovered on leukocytes using monoclonal antibodies that "cluster" for reaction with particular cells. CD numbers have been assigned to these antigens at successive meetings on human leukocyte differentiation antigens (HLDA). At the last meeting, HLD8 in December 2004, 92 new CD antigens were added tot he existing list of 247 (1), bringing the total number to CD339, with more antigens if different variants of the proteins are included (e.g., CD11a, 11b, and 11c). Although the CD antigens have been discovered on leukocytes, they fulfill functions required

From: *Methods in Molecular Medicine, Vol. 125: Myeloid Leukemia: Methods and Protocols*
Edited by: H. Iland, M. Hertzberg, and P. Marlton © Humana Press Inc., Totowa, NJ

by most human cells, such as: cytokine receptors, ion channels, cell–cell inter-actions, adhesion molecules, enzymes, and immunoglobulins.

Using composite immunophenotypic data obtained by flow cytometry pub-lished by a number of laboratories, Nguyen et al. *(2)* were able to distinguish 33 subtypes of leukemia by the expression of 41 different CD antigens. How-ever, such an approach using flow cytometry would be too labor-intensive and expensive for routine diagnoses. We have developed a CD antibody microarray (DotScan) that allows acquisition of extensive immunophenotypes of leuko-cytes from a single analysis *(3)*. The DotScan microarray consists of antibody dots (10 nL) against 82 CD antigens with 14 additional control antigens. Mono-nuclear leukocytes purified on Histopaque are captured by the immobilized antibodies of the microarray giving a dot pattern that represents the immunophenotype of the leukocytes. The DotScan microarray has been suc-cessfully used to immunophenotype myeloid leukemias, lymphoid leukemias, and lymphomas, with more than 1100 samples analyzed from peripheral blood, bone marrow, and lymph nodes. The results obtained from panels of patients have been expressed as frequency plots for expression of CD antigens for the common leukemias: acute myeloid leukemia (AML), chronic myeloid leuke-mia (CML), acute lymphoblastic leukemia (ALL), and chronic lymphocytic leukemia (CLL), as well as a number of B-lymphoproliferative disorders, to determine consensus patterns of CD antigen expression. Data obtained so far strongly suggest that an extensive immunophenotype of a leukemia should be sufficient for diagnosis.

Leukemias are currently classified using four criteria: morphology, limited immunophenotype, cytochemistry, and cytogenetics. AML is a heterogenous leukemia with 8 subtypes using the French–American–British (FAB) classifi-cation (M0-M7) and 16 subtypes using the World Health Organization (WHO) classification *(4)*. Casasnovas et al. *(5)* have reclassified AML from 733 patients into five categories, MA to ME, based upon expression of seven CD antigens within four groups (CD13/CD33/CD117, CD7, CD35/CD36, CD15). Immunophenotyping for these seven CD antigens allowed stratification into clinically relevant subgroups with prognostic factors. Immunophenotyping is useful for assignment of myeloid lineage, but has had a limited application in the subtyping and classification of myeloid leukemias. There are three sub-types of myeloid leukemia with relatively specific immunophenotypes: AML-M0, AML-M6, and AML-M7. Otherwise, there is currently limited correlation between the cellular immunophenotypes of the myeloid leukemias and the FAB *(6)* and WHO classifications *(4)*, and no antigens give consistent prognostic information. Recurrent cytogenetic and molecular abnormalities have increas-ingly been recognized in AML associated with specific clinicopathological entities, and these are incorporated in the WHO classification with morphological differences.

The DotScan microarray also has considerable potential for identifying prognostic factors for leukemia subtypes (e.g., stable or progressive CLL), and whether a leukemia will be susceptible or refractory to a drug, but many more samples are required to define the consensus patterns of CD antigen expression that correlate with these attributes. When myeloid leukemias are analyzed using the DotScan microarray, human AB serum is included to eliminate nonspecific binding of leukocytes to immobilized antibodies via Fc receptors on cells (CD16, CD23, CD32, CD64, and CD89). Data of excellent quality have been obtained for AML samples from panels of patients, but more samples are required to define some of the rarer subtypes of this heterogeneous leukemia.

1.2. Immunophenotyping Techniques

1.2.1. Flow Cytometry

Immunophenotyping of hematological malignancies is typically performed by flow cytometry with gating to identify the leukemic population and then study by fluorescence the antigen profile of these cells *(7,8)*. The subjective placement of electronic gates to establish positive and negative antigen expression results in some variation between laboratories. Less commonly now, immunophenotyping may be performed using a slide-based immunofluorescence or cytochemical technique *(9)* as in cytochemistry. Immunophenotyping of hematological malignancies by flow cytometry typically involves testing for 15–20 antigens to determine cell lineage and leukemic classification.

1.2.2. DotScan Microarray

We have devised a novel microarray of CD antibody dots (10 nL) bound to nitrocellulose on a glass slide, that enables testing for 80–100 antigens in a single, simple assay. The DotScan microarray has been successfully used to immunophenotype lymphoid (B- and T-) and myeloid leukemias. We have analyzed many B-lymphoid leukemias, using mononuclear leukocytes purified on Histopaque, and the results have been definitive, especially for B-cell chronic lymphocytic leukemia (B-CLL), where we have data for 100 patients and a characteristic immunophenotype *(3,10)*. For these leukemias, an extensive immunophenotype (82 CD antigens) should be sufficient for diagnosis. We believe the microarray has considerable potential for identifying prognostic factors in B-CLL, but to date insufficient cases have been analyzed for meaningful correlation, and we are continuing to build the database. In general, there are insufficient data at present to enable discrimination between the rare forms of lymphoid leukemia, but this work is ongoing.

1.2.3. Diagnosis Using an Extensive Immunophenotype

The DotScan microarray is being used to accumulate an extensive patient database of immunophenotypes of myeloid leukemias to establish consensus patterns for the subtypes. It is likely that an extensive immunophenotype will be sufficient to classify subtypes of AML, and that expression patterns may also provide prognostic information not available from the limited immunophenotype currently obtained by flow cytometry. DNA microarrays determine mRNA levels, whereas an extensive immunophenotype determined with the DotScan microarray provides a direct extension of our knowledge of CD antigens and incorporates antibodies currently in diagnostic use. The DotScan microarray identifies cell-surface proteins that correlate directly with cellular function, whereas mRNA levels may not correlate directly with the leukemia. The antigens determined by flow cytometry in a standard immunophenotype for AML represent a narrow range of "lineage specific" markers (**Table 1**). A broader panel of myeloid antigens including adhesion molecules such as CD11(a-c), CD18, CD49(a-f), CD62L, activation markers such as CD71, and a broader panel of myeloid antigens are generally not studied by flow cytometry.

The WHO classification includes five sub-types of AML with cytogenetic abnormalities: *AML/ETO*, inv16, *CBFβ/MYH11*, *PML-RARα*, and MLL; this group will clearly expand with further investigation. These cytogenetic abnormalities may correlate with changes in expression of surface molecules observed as part of an extensive immunophenotype. For example, Munoz et al. *(11)* found differences between AML groups with and without internal tandem duplications (ITD) of the *FLT3* gene. A diagnosis of FAB subtype AML-M5 and expression of monocytic markers CD36 and CD11b were more frequent in *FLT3/ITD*(+) patients, whereas stem cell markers CD34 and CD117 were less common. Myeloid leukemias characterized by specific immunophenotypes are uncommon, but CD13, CD33, and CD117 are expressed in AML-M0 *(12,13)*, glycophorin A (CD235a) in AML-M6, and CD41 and CD61 in AML-M7. Furthermore, the extensive immunophenotype available from the DotScan microarray should result in additional patterns of antigen expression within these subtypes that increase the confidence of classification *(14)*. Other subgroups of AML are likely to have characteristic consensus immunophenotypes. For example, Paietta *(15)* found diagnostic power for acute promyelocytic leukemia (APML) with three antigens—HLA-DR, CD11a, and CD18. Characteristic dot patterns or surface molecule profiles from the DotScan microarray for AMLs may allow classification and diagnosis of a wider range of subtypes. These immunological classifications may not necessarily correspond with previous morphological criteria, and a new classification system may evolve using surface molecule profiles from the DotScan microarray.

Table 1
Monoclonal Antibodies Used in Standard
Immunophenotyping for Acute Leukemias*

Cells or lineage	Surface antigen
Stem	CD34, HLA-DR, CD45
B-	CD19, CD20, CD22, CD79a
T-	CD2, CD3, CD5, CD7
Natural killer	CD16, CD56
Myeloid	CD13, CD33, CD15, CD117, MPO
Erythroid	Glycophorin A
Megakaryoblastic	CD41, CD61

*Modified from **ref. 16**.

2. Materials

1. Glass microscope slides with a film of nitrocellulose (18 × 27 mm, FAST slides) (Schleicher and Schuell, Keene, NH).
2. Antibodies: Coulter and Immunotech (Beckman Coulter, Gladesville, NSW, Australia), Pharmingen (BD Biosciences, North Ryde, NSW, Australia), Biosource International (Monarch Medical, Stafford City, Qld, Australia), Serotec (Australian Laboratory Services, Sydney Markets, NSW, Australia), and Sigma-Aldrich (Castle Hill, NSW, Australia).
3. Bovine serum albumin (BSA): Sigma-Aldrich (Castle Hill, NSW, Australia).
4. Diploma skim milk: Bonlac Foods (Melbourne, Vic., Australia).
5. Histopaque-1077: Sigma-Aldrich (Castle Hill, NSW, Australia).
6. Phosphate-buffered saline (PBS): Sigma-Aldrich (Castle Hill, NSW, Australia).
7. Heat-inactivated human AB serum: Sigma-Aldrich (Castle Hill, NSW, Australia).
8. Formaldehyde: Sigma-Aldrich (Castle Hill, NSW, Australia).

3. Methods

3.1. Construction of CD Antibody Microarrays

1. The procedure is modified from Belov et al. *(3,10)*. A PixSys 3200 Aspirate and Dispense System (Cartesian Technologies, Irvine, CA) is used to construct duplicate microarrays consisting of 96 different 10-nL antibody dots (82 CD antibodies and 14 control antibodies) on FAST nitrocellulose slides.
2. Antibody solutions are reconstituted as recommended, frozen in aliquots at −20°C with 0.1% (w/v) BSA, and used at concentrations ranging from 50 to 1000 µg/mL, as supplied for flow cytometry.
3. After application of the antibody dots (10 nL) in a rectangular array, the nitrocellulose is blocked with 5% (w/v) skim milk in PBS (90 min at room temperature or overnight at 4°C), washed in two changes of water, dried, and stored at 4°C with desiccant.

4. Each batch of slides is tested with cell lines and/or frozen peripheral blood leukocytes or leukemia cells of known immunophenotype to check antibody-binding activities.

3.2. Binding of Leukocytes to the DotScan Microarray

1. The collection of peripheral blood from patients and normal subjects, purification of mononuclear leukocytes on Histopaque-1077, and their immunophenotyping on a CD antibody microarray are described by Belov et al. *(3,10)*.
2. Most lymphoid cell suspensions are tested in PBS containing 1 mM ethylenediamine tetraacetic acid (EDTA), but cells from patients with AML are tested in PBS, without EDTA, containing heat-inactivated human AB serum (2% (v/v), Sigma-Aldrich, St. Louis, MO) to minimize nonspecific Fc receptor binding (*see* **Note 1**).
3. Leukocytes (4–6 × 10^6 cells, *see* **Note 2**) suspended in 300 μL of PBS plus AB serum are incubated at room temperature (20°C) for 60 min.
4. Unbound cells are gently washed off with PBS; then the microarrays are fixed for at least 20 min in PBS containing 3.7% (v/v) formaldehyde, and washed in PBS.
5. Complete instructions on the use of the DotScan microarray are provided with the kits available from Medsaic Pty. Ltd. (Australian Technology Park, Eveleigh, Australia).

3.3. Data Recording and Analysis

Dot patterns of leukocytes captured on the DotScan microarray are recorded using a DotScan array reader and software (*see* **Note 3**). The software quantifies the intensities of each dot from the digital image file and compiles expression profiles as bar charts showing the average intensities above background on an 8-bit grayness scale from 1 to 256 (*see* **Note 4**). **Fig. 1** shows dot patterns obtained for M4 AML from peripheral blood and bone marrow from two different patients. The digital images of the dot patterns obtained with the DotScan array reader (**Fig. 1**) were analyzed using the DotScan software to produce the bar charts shown in **Fig. 2**. The immunophenotype (*see* **Note 5**) of the AML-

Fig. 1. *(opposite page)* Mononuclear leukocytes from patients with acute myeloid leukemia captured on the DotScan microarray: **(A)** antibody location; **(B)** patient 63047, acute myeloid leukemia (AML)-M4 peripheral blood; **(C)** patient 63269, AML-M4 bone marrow. The DotScan microarray contains duplicate antibody microarrays, and the dot intensities are averaged by the software. The numbers in the key provide addresses for the cluster of differentiation (CD) antibodies; mIgG1, mIgG2a, mIgG2b and mIgM are murine isotype control antibodies; TCR α/β, TCR γ/δ, HLA-DR, FMC7, κ, λ, and sIg are antibodies against T-cell receptors α/β and γ/δ, HLA-DR, FMC7, κ-, and λ-immunoglobulin light chains and surface immunoglobulin, respectively. Mabthera (Roche, Hertfordshire, UK) is a humanized monoclonal antibody against CD20. 33 HIM and 34 581 are antibodies 33 HIM 3–4 and 34 581 derived from different hybridoma clones from those for CD33 and CD34 in the main array.

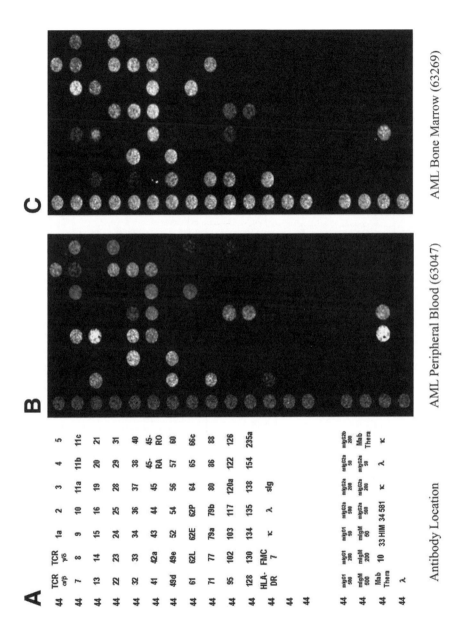

A						
44	TCR αβ	TCR γδ	1a	2	3	4	5
44	7	8	9	10	11a	11b	11c
44	13	14	15	16	19	20	21
44	22	23	24	25	28	29	31
44	32	33	34	36	37	38	40
44	41	42a	43	44	45	45-RA	45-RO
44	49d	49e	52	54	56	57	60
44	61	62L	62E	62P	64	65	66c
44	71	77	79a	79b	80	86	88
44	95	102	103	117	120a	122	126
44	128	130	134	135	138	154	235a
44	HLA-DR	FMC 7	κ	λ	sIg		
44							
44							
44	mIgG1 500	mIgG1 200	mIgG1 50	mIgM 50	mIgG2a 500	mIgG2a 200	mIgG2b 200
44	mIgM 500	mIgM 200	mIgM 50	33 HIM 34 581	mIgG2a 500	mIgG2a 200	Mab Thera
44	Mab Thera	10	κ	λ	κ	λ	κ
44	λ						

Antibody Location

B AML Peripheral Blood (63047)

C AML Bone Marrow (63269)

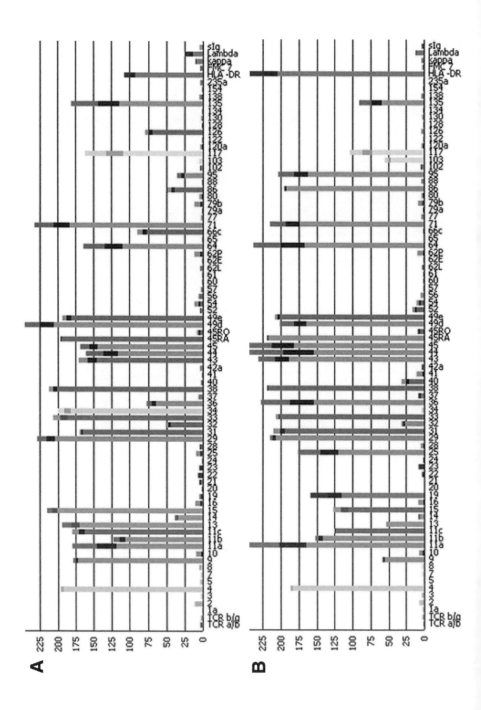

M4 from peripheral blood shows high-level expression of CD antigens in the following descending order of intensities: CD49d, CD29, CD15, CD38, CD71, CD33, CD45RA, CD4, CD34, CD49e, CD13, CD9, CD11c, CD31, CD43, and CD45 (**Fig. 2a**). For the AML-M4 from bone marrow, the following CD antigens are expressed in descending order of intensities: HLA-DR, CD38. CD45RA, CD45, CD29, CD43, CD49e, CD33, CD11a, CD31, CD64, CD44, CD86, CD71, CD36, and CD4 (**Fig. 2b**). This procedure may be used for other disorders affecting myeloid cells, such as CML and myelodysplastic syndromes (MDS; *see* **Notes 5** and **6**). Consensus immunophenotypes can be assigned to each subtype of myeloid leukemia (*see* **Note 7**). Further enhancements of this novel technology are under development (*see* **Notes 8–10**).

4. Notes

1. The dot patterns for myeloid leukemias obtained with the DotScan microarray are optimal when heat-inactivated human AB serum is included to eliminate non-specific binding via Fc receptors. The resulting immunophenotype defines the myeloid lineage and a monoclonal leukemia.
2. Leukocytes must be alive to be captured on the DotScan microarray. Cells that have been frozen at –80°C in dimethylsulfoxide/fetal calf serum may be used if viability is retained.
3. The white dots (**Fig. 1**) represent approx 2000 cells captured on each antibody dot. Cells are captured only by antibodies that are complementary to their surface molecules, and the dot pattern therefore represents the immunophenotype for that population of cells. In **Fig. 1**, dots of high intensity (white) are due to leukemia cells; those of lower intensities are the background of normal peripheral blood leukocytes (PBL).
4. Neutrophil and monocyte precursors in bone marrow provide a significant background for analysis of AML as a result of the expression of CD11a, CD11b, CD11c, CD13, CD15, CD16, CD24, CD33, CD38, CD45RO, CD64, CD66c, CD71, CD88, CD95, and CD128. An additional cell fractionation step, such as selective depletion of granulocyte precursors with Dynabeads coupled to a CD antibody, might reduce the background.
5. Immunophenotyping using the DotScan microarray may be complicated by mul-

Fig. 2. *(opposite page)* Bar charts generated with DotScan software from the digital images of the dot patterns of **Fig. 1**: (**A**) patient 63047; (**B**) patient 63269. Markers routinely used for flow cytometry are shown as pale gray for T-cells, black for B-cells, and dark gray for myeloid cells. All other antibodies are shown in medium gray. Data are shown in "overlay" mode, where intensities for the duplicate dot patterns are superimposed for each antibody. Numbers on the *x*-axis refer to antibodies against the corresponding cluster of differentiation antigens. Values on the *y*-axis are average dot intensities above background on an eight-bit grayness scale from 1 to 256.

tiple subpopulations of myeloid leukemia cells in samples, especially in CML and MDS. In CML, large numbers of leukemic cells are present at multiple stages of myeloid development from blasts through to mature polymorphonuclear neutrophils.

6. For MDS, there are very few circulating leukemic cells; rather, immature cells are displaced from the bone marrow and may contribute to the circulating immunophenotype rather than leukemic cells. Some myeloid leukemia cells do not collect on the Histopaque interface but pass into the denser medium and are not analyzed. If the leukemic cells are in the bone marrow rather than the circulation, there might be a "disease signature" in the circulation from leukocyte precursors displaced from the diseased marrow.

7. We have constructed frequency plots for the subtypes of AML from peripheral blood and bone marrow, but will need more patient samples, particularly from peripheral blood, to establish consensus immunophenotypes for a definitive diagnosis of each subtype of AML.

8. Some of the problems in analyzing AMLs may be resolved by development of alternative methods for isolation of leukocytes, such as use of whole blood lysates, or cell fractionation involving differential centrifugation or selective binding of cells to Dynabeads, lectins, or plastics.

9. Analysis of AMLs with a larger microarray with more CD antibodies would probably identify additional CD antigens that discriminate between myeloid leukemias, granulocytes, and their precursors.

10. When a mixture of cells has been captured on the DotScan microarray, subpopulations of cells can still be distinguished using fluorescent multiplexing. This technique has recently been developed in our laboratory and will be essential for more sophisticated analyses, such as minimal residual disease in leukemias.

Acknowledgment

This research was supported by Medsaic Pty. Ltd. and is subject to intellectual property rights. Information concerning the use of the DotScan microarray may be directed to Medsaic Pty Ltd, Suite 145, National Innovation Centre, Australian Technology Park, Garden Street, Eveleigh, NSW 1430, Australia.

References

1. Mason, D., Andre, P., Bensussan, A., et al. (2002) *Leucocyte Typing VII.* Oxford University Press, Oxford, UK.
2. Nguyen, A. N. D., Milam, J. D., Johnson, K. A., and Banez, E. I. (2000) A relational database for diagnosis of haematopoietic neoplasms using immunophenotyping by flow cytometry. *Am. J. Clin. Pathol.* **113,** 95–106.
3. Belov, L., de la Vega, O., dos Remedios, C. G., Mulligan, S. P., and Christopherson, R. I. (2001) Immunophenotyping of leukemias using a cluster of differentiation antibody microarray. *Cancer Res.* 61, 4483–4489.

4. Jaffe, E. S., Harris, N. L., Stein, H., and Vardiman, J. W. (2001) *Pathology and Genetics of Tumours of Haematopoietic and Lymphoid Tissues. World Health Organisation Classification of Tumours.* IARC Press, Lyon.

5. Casasnovas, R. O., Slimane, F. K., Garand, R., et al. (2003) Immunological classification of acute myeloblastic leukemias: relevance to patient outcome. *Leukemia* **17**, 515–527

6. Bennett, J. M., Catovsky, D., Daniel, M. T., et al. (1976) Proposals for the classification of the acute leukaemias. French-American-British (FAB) co-operative group. *Br. J. Haematol.* **33**, 451–458.

7. Jennings, C. D. and Foon, K. A. (1997) Recent advances in flow cytometry: application to the diagnosis of hematologic malignancy. *Blood* **90**, 2863–2892.

8. Marti, G. E., Stetler-Stevenson, M., and Fleisher, T. (2001) Diagnostic flow cytometry in hematologic malignancies, in *Methods in Molecular Medicine: Hematologic Malignancies: Methods and Techniques,* vol 55 (Faguet, G. B., ed.), Humana Press, Totowa, NJ, pp. 179–215.

9. General Haematology Task Force of BCSH. (1994) Immunophenotyping in the diagnosis of acute leukaemias. *J. Clin. Pathol.* **47**, 777–781.

10. Belov, L., Huang, P., Barber, N., Mulligan, S. P., and Christopherson, R. I. (2003) Identification of repertoires of surface antigens on leukemias using an antibody microarray. *Proteomics* **3**, 2147–2154.

11. Munoz, L., Aventin, A., Villamor, N., et al. (2003) Immunophenotypic findings in acute myeloid leukemia with FLT3 internal tandem duplication. *Haematologica* **88**, 637–645.

12. Bene, M. C., Bernier, M., Casasnovas, R. O., et al. (2001) Acute myeloid leukaemia M0: haematological, immunophenotypic and cytogenetic characteristics and their prognostic significance: an analysis in 241 patients. *Br. J. Haematol.* **113**, 737–745.

13. Catovsky, D. and Matutes, E. (1992) The classification of acute leukaemia. *Leukemia.* **6 Suppl. 2**, 1–6.

14. Suzuki, R., Murata, M., Kami, M., et al. (2003) Prognostic significance of CD7+CD56+ phenotype and chromosome 5 abnormalities for acute myeloid leukemia M0. *Int. J. Hematol.* **77**, 482–489.

15. Paietta, E. (2003) Expression of cell-surface antigens in acute promyelocytic leukaemia. *Best Pract. Res. Clin. Haematol.* **16**, 369–385.

16. Brunning, R. D., Matutes, E., Harris, N. L., et al. (2001) Acute myeloid leukaemia: introduction, in *Pathology and Genetics of Tumours of Haematopoietic and Lymphoid Tissues. World Health Organisation Classification of Tumours* (Jaffe, E. S., Harris, N. L., Stein, H., and Vardiman, J. W., eds), IARC Press, Lyon, pp. 77–81.

16

Methods for the Detection of the *JAK2* V617F Mutation in Human Myeloproliferative Disorders

Peter J. Campbell,* Linda M. Scott,* E. Joanna Baxter,
Anthony J. Bench, Anthony R. Green, and Wendy N. Erber

Summary

A single acquired mutation in the *JAK2* gene has recently been described in human myelo-proliferative disorders, including most patients with polycythemia vera and about half of those with essential thrombocythemia and idiopathic myelofibrosis. Reliable and easily implemented methods for detection of this V617F mutation promise to revolutionize the way these disorders are diagnosed and classified, and may in the future have implications for targeted therapeutics. Two polymerase chain reaction-based methods for detection of the mutation are described here. One method is based on allele-specific amplification of the mutant band, and the other on elimination of a restriction enzyme recognition sequence by the mutation. Both methods are significantly more sensitive than conventional sequencing techniques, and could be readily implemented in a molecular diagnostic laboratory.

Key Words: Myeloproliferative disorder; polycythemia vera; essential thrombocythemia; idiopathic myelofibrosis; *JAK2*; mutation.

1. Introduction

The classic myeloproliferative disorders (MPDs) comprise polycythemia vera (PV), essential thrombocythemia (ET), and idiopathic myelofibrosis (IMF) *(1)*. They are considered clonal stem cell disorders *(2)*, and result in expansion of one or more lineages of bone marrow cells, usually with retention of differentiation capacity. The *sine qua non* of PV is expansion of the red cell mass, with most patients also developing granulocytosis and/or thrombocythemia, whereas ET is generally characterised by an isolated thrombocythemia *(3–5)*. The major clinical manifestations of these disorders are arterial thrombosis, venous thrombosis, and a propensity to hemorrhage, but overall life expectancy

---

* These authors contributed equally to this work.

From: *Methods in Molecular Medicine, Vol. 125: Myeloid Leukemia: Methods and Protocols*
Edited by: H. Iland, M. Hertzberg, and P. Marlton © Humana Press Inc., Totowa, NJ

is not too dissimilar to age- and sex-matched reference populations *(6,7)*. IMF, on the other hand, is dominated by marrow fibrosis, together with signs of extramedullary hematopoiesis, with ensuing bone marrow failure as the condition progresses *(8)*. All three MPDs can transform to acute myeloid leukemia, albeit at low rates, and PV and ET can undergo secondary myelofibrotic transformation. Diagnostic criteria have been controversial *(8–10)*, often relying on excluding other diagnoses that can present with elevated blood counts, and on markers, such as erythropoietin levels and erythropoietin-independent erythroid colony (EEC) growth, tests that are not universally available.

Recently, our understanding of the molecular mechanisms underlying MPDs has been advanced by the description of a mutation in the *JAK2* gene *(11–14)*, a key hematopoietic regulator. When sensitive methods are used for the detection of the V617F mutation, it is found in virtually all cases of PV, and about one-half of cases of ET and IMF *(11)*. The JAK family members (JAK1, JAK2, TYK2, JAK3) act as non-receptor tyrosine kinases, being activated in response to cytokines that utilize cytokine receptor super-family members. Considerable evidence has suggested that ligand binding leads to oligomerization of the receptor chains and their associated JAK proteins, resulting in JAK transphosphorylation and catalytic activation. The JAKs in turn tyrosine-phosphorylate the cytokine receptors, as well as a variety of cellular substrates that are recruited to the activated receptor complexes. The V617F mutation promotes constitutive autophosphorylation of the JAK2 protein, with subsequent activation of downstream effectors *(12,13)*, and leads to erythrocytosis in a murine retrovirus model *(12)*.

Because the V617F mutation is a single mutation that occurs very frequently in MPDs (and not in normal individuals), its reliable detection in a routine laboratory setting will facilitate the diagnostic assessment of patients being evaluated for a possible MPD. Presence of the V617F mutation indicates that the patient has an acquired, clonal hematological disorder and not a reactive or secondary process. Absence of the *JAK2* V617F mutation does not exclude a MPD, because up to 50% of patients with ET and IMF do not have this mutation. The V617F mutation does not help in sub-classifying the type of MPD of a given patient, and thus does not supplant the need for a bone marrow or red cell mass evaluation. The low frequency of the mutation in other disorders, such as acute myeloid leukemia *(15)*, myelodysplasia *(15,16)*, and other cancers *(15)*, also indicates a degree of specificity for PV, ET, and IMF.

MPDs are stem cell disorders in which a proportion of circulating granulocytes are clonally derived. Therefore, they are amenable to mutation analysis on peripheral blood. However, the proportion of clonal granulocytes is variable *(17,18)*. Thus, a molecular test for the V617F mutation must be sufficiently sensitive to detect low levels of clonal granulocytes in a background of normal granulocytes and lymphocytes. Sequencing approaches, which are only capable of detecting a heterozygous mutation when present in greater than 40% of cells, are insufficiently sensitive and may give false-negative results. More sensitive molecular methods are therefore required. We have developed two sensitive methods for detecting the mutation, one based on allele-specific amplification of the mutation in a polymerase chain reaction (PCR), and the other on digestion of the wild-type allele, but not the V617F allele with the restriction enzyme, *Bsa*XI *(11)*. Both methods are capable of sensitively and specifically detecting the mutation, even when present in only 1–10% of cells.

The allele-specific PCR method uses a three-primer system, in which there is a common reverse primer, a mutation-specific forward primer, and a control forward primer (**Fig. 1**). The 3′ end of the mutation-specific primer is the T nucleotide, which is mutated (substituted in place of G) in V617F-positive disease, and the primer also has an intentional mismatch at the third nucleotide from the 3′ end. This increases the specificity of primer binding, helping to ensure that product only amplifies when the mutation is present. The other forward primer amplifies both mutant and wild-type DNA, and acts as a control for the fidelity of the PCR reaction (**Fig. 2**). The advantages of the allele-specific PCR approach are that it is sensitive and not particularly resource-intensive. Potential disadvantages are the fact that it cannot discriminate between heterozygous and homozygous mutation, and the very small chance of false-positive reactions due to mispriming of the mutation-specific primer. One other set of primers has been published that involves a four-primer system *(19)*. That system allows identification of some patients who have homozygous V617F mutation, but the significance of this in a routine diagnostic or clinical setting is yet to be determined.

The restriction enzyme method exploits the observation that the nucleotide change resulting in the V-to-F alteration in *JAK2* perturbs a specific restriction endonuclease recognition sequence. *Bsa*XI recognizes the nonpalindromic sequence, 5′...GGAG(N)$_5$GT...3′, but is unusual in that the enzyme cleaves the DNA twice, on either side of this motif. A 30-bp fragment is produced as a result of endonuclease cleavage, such that the true restriction site is:

```
5′    NNNNNNNGGAGNNNNNGTNNNNNNNNNNNNNN 3′
3′ NNNNNNNNNNCCTCNNNNNCANNNNNNNNNNN 5′
```

with the recognition sequence highlighted in bold. The *Bsa*XI restriction site present within exon 14 of *JAK2* has the sequence:

```
                        *
5′       AAATTATGGAGTATGTGTCTGTGGAGACGA 3′
3′ AAATTTAATACCTCATACACAGACACCTCT 5′
```

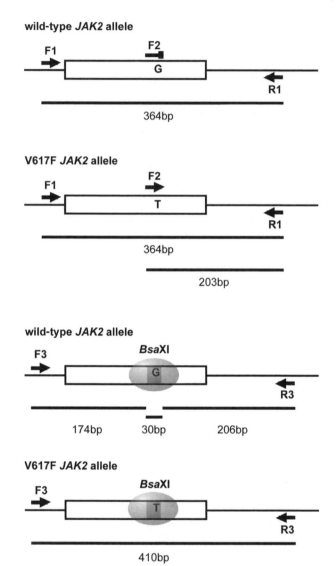

Fig. 1. Allele-specific polymerase chain reaction (PCR) and *Bsa*XI digestion methods for detecting the *JAK2* V617F mutation. (**A**) Allele-specific PCR generates a 364-bp product from wild-type sequence, as a result of amplification from primers F1 and R1. V617F DNA gives a 364-bp product from amplification between F1 and R1 primers, and a 203-bp product as a result of amplification between F2 and R1 primers. (**B**) After amplification with primers F3 and R3, *Bsa*X1 only digests the wild-type sequence (giving 30-, 174-, and 206-bp products), but not the V617F sequence (leaving an undigested 410-bp product). The 174- and 206-bp product co-migrate on a conventional 2% agarose gel.

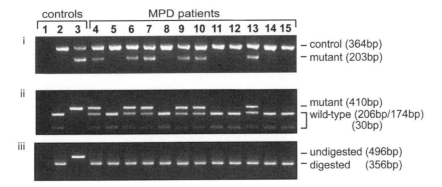

Fig. 2. Controls and patient samples tested with allele-specific polymerase chain reaction (PCR) and *Bsa*XI digestion. Allele-specific PCR (**i**) and *JAK2 Bsa*XI digestion (**ii**) were used to genotype DNA from unfractionated peripheral blood leukocytes from patients with myeloproliferative disorders (MPDs). Lane 1, water; lane 2, granulocyte DNA from V617F-negative control; lane 3, granulocyte DNA from V617F-homozygous control; lanes 4-15, MPD patients. (**iii**) Digestion control using *SCL* genomic fragment containing a *Bsa*XI site. Lane 1, water; lane 2, with enzyme control; lane 3, no enzyme control; lanes 4–15, MPD patients.

The distal G in the recognition motif (that marked by an asterisk) is the nucleotide mutated in V617F-positive MPD patients. As a consequence, *Bsa*XI is unable to cleave within exon 14 of the mutated *JAK2* allele. By amplifying this region of *JAK2*, then digesting the PCR product with *Bsa*XI, a mutant allele (that is, one which does not cut) can be distinguished from an unaffected allele (one which does cut) by gel electrophoresis (**Fig. 2**). A control PCR fragment derived from the *SCL* gene should also be produced from the same DNA sample. This fragment also contains a *Bsa*XI restriction site and acts as a control for complete enzyme digestion.

The advantages of the *Bsa*XI restriction approach are that it is sensitive, and can discriminate between a heterozygous mutation and a homozygous mutation in some applications. Potential disadvantages are that it is more labor-intensive than the allele-specific PCR approach detailed previously and that it may generate false-positives in some cases, as a result of incomplete digestion of a wild-type allele.

In this chapter, we present detailed protocols and notes for both allele-specific PCR and *Bsa*XI restriction approaches.

2. Materials

2.1. Allele-Specific PCR

1. Template DNA, 40 ng/µL, stable at 4°C (*see* **Note 1**).

2. Oligonucleotide primers. For these primers, we make a stock solution at 100 μ*M* and a working solution at 10 μ*M*, diluted in nuclease-free distilled water, and store at –20°C. Sequences (*see* **Note 2**):
   a. Common reverse primer (R1):
      5′-CTGAATAGTCCTACAGTGTTTTCAGTTTCA-3′
   b. Mutation-specific forward primer (F2):
      5′-AGCATTTGGTTTTAAATTATGGAGTATATT-3′
   c. Control forward primer (F1):
      5′-ATCTATAGTCATGCTGAAAGTAGGAGAAAG-3′
3. 10X PCR buffer (Applied Biosystems) supplied with *Taq* polymerase. Store at –20°C.
4. Magnesium chloride (MgCl$_2$), 25 m*M*. Store at –20°C.
5. Deoxynucleoside triphosphates (dNTPs). Stock solution 25 m*M* each dNTP, and working solution 2.5 m*M* each dNTP. Store working solution in small aliquots at –20°C, as repeated freeze-thawing damages the dNTPs.
6. Ultra-pure (deionized) water.
7. AmpliTaq-Gold™ (Applied Biosystems) *Taq* polymerase, 5 U/μL.
8. Thin-walled PCR tubes or PCR plate.
9. MJ Research PTC-200 (or other model or brand) PCR thermal cycler.

2.2. BsaXI Restriction Analysis

1. Template DNA, 40 ng/μL, stable at 4°C.
2. Oligonucleotide primers. Stock solution of each primer is 50 μ*M,* stored at –20°C.
   a. *JAK2*:
      5′-ATCTATAGTCATGCTGAAAGTAGGAGAAAG-3′ (forward; F3)
      5′-ACCTTCTACTTTTAACTTCATTGCTTTCCT-3′ (reverse; R3)
   b. *SCL*:
      5′-TCCTGGGGTCTTCTGTCTTG-3′ (forward)
      5′-CCTGAGAGGCAATGGGAGTA-3′ (reverse)
3. 10X PCR buffer (Applied Biosystems), stored at –20°C.
4. Magnesium chloride (MgCl$_2$), 25 m*M*. Store at –20°C.
5. Deoxynucleoside triphosphates (dNTPs). Stock solution 100 m*M* each dNTP, and working solution 10 m*M* each dNTP, stored at –20°C.
6. Ultra-pure (deionized) water.
7. AmpliTaq-Gold (Applied Biosystems) *Taq* polymerase, 5 U/μL.
8. Thin-walled PCR tubes or PCR plate.
9. *Bsa*XI restriction endonuclease (New England Biolabs, cat. no. R0609, 2 U/μL).
10. MJ Research PTC-200 (or other model or brand) PCR thermal cycler.

3. Methods

3.1. Allele-Specific PCR

1. Aliquot 2 μL template DNA (80 ng/reaction) into PCR tubes or a 96-well plate. Always include a V617F-positive DNA sample, a V617F-negative DNA sample, and water as controls (*see* **Note 3**).

2. Make a master mix for the number of reactions set up with:
   a. Common reverse primer (R1) (10 μ*M*), 5 μL;
   b. Mutation-specific forward primer (F2) (10 μ*M*), 2.5 μL;
   c. Control forward primer (F1) (10 μ*M*), 2.5 μL;
   d. 10X PCR buffer, 5 μL;
   e. Magnesium chloride (25 m*M*), 3 μL;
   f. dNTPs (2.5 m*M* each), 4 μL;
   g. AmpliTaq-Gold polymerase (5 U/μL), 0.5 μL;
   h. Ultra-pure (deionized) water, 25.5 μL;
   i. Template DNA, (2μL).
   Final volume 50 μL. Mix well and aliquot 48 μL into each tube (*see* **Note 4**).
3. Place the tubes or plate into a thermal cycler and PCR amplify using the following program (*see* **Notes 5** and **6**):
   a. 94°C for 11 min (if using AmpliTaq Gold or other hot-start Taq);
   b. 36 cycles of: 94°C for 30 s, 58°C for 30 s, 72°C for 30 s;
   c. 72°C for 6 min;
   d. 4°C thereafter.
4. Run the PCR products for samples and controls on a 1.5% agarose gel with ethidium bromide. The control forward primer and common reverse primer amplifies a 364-bp product from all samples, and the mutation-specific forward primer and common reverse primer amplify a 203-bp product only from V617F-positive DNA (*see* **Note 7** and **Fig. 2i**).

3.2. Bsa*XI Restriction Analysis*

1. Aliquot 2 μL purified template DNA into two individual PCR tubes or wells of a 96-well plate. Alternately, when analyzing individual hematopoietic colonies, aliquot 5 μL crude cell lysate into two individual PCR tubes or wells of a 96-well plate (*see* **Note 8**). Also include V617F-positive and V617F-negative DNA samples as controls (*see* **Note 3**).
2. Make two PCR master mixes: one with primers specific to the *JAK2* gene (F3 and R3), the other with primers specific to the *SCL* gene. The volume of each master mix should be sufficient for the total number of reactions (*n*) to be performed; we generally make enough for 1.1*n* to allow for pipetting inaccuracies. Each reaction consists of:
   a. Forward primer (50 μ*M*), 1.0 μL;
   b. Reverse primer (50 μ*M*), 1.0 μL;
   c. 10X PCR buffer, 5.0 μL;
   d. MgCl$_2$ (25 m*M*), 3.0 μL;
   e. dNTPs (10 m*M* each), 1.0 μL;
   f. *Taq* polymerase (5 U/μL), 0.5 μL;
   g. Water to 50.0 μL final reaction volume.
   Mix well and aliquot 48 μL (45 μL if cell lysate is being used) into each tube or well.
3. Place the tubes or plate in a thermal cycler, and amplify using the following program:

a. 94°C for 11 min;

b. 35 cycles: 94°C for 30 s, 57°C for 30 s, 72°C for 30 s (*see* **Note 9**);

c. 72°C for 6 min;

d. 4°C hold.

4. The PCR products can be used immediately in *Bsa*XI digestion reactions (*see* **Note 10**). A restriction master mix appropriate for the number of reactions to be performed should be made, with each reaction consisting of:

a. 10X digestion buffer (NEB buffer #4), 2.0 μL;

b. *Bsa*XI (2 U/μL), 2.0 μL;

c. Water, 6.0 μL

5. Transfer 10-μL aliquots of the restriction master mix into clean Eppendorf tubes or wells of a 96-well plate, then add 10 μL of each individual PCR reaction. Include a mock-digestion of the V617F-positive control PCR reaction by combining 10 μL PCR product with 8 μL water and 2 μL 10X NEB digestion buffer #4. Briefly spin all digestion reactions in a bench-top centrifuge to concentrate the reagents at the bottom of the tube/well.

6. Digestions are performed at 37°C for 2–4 h (*see* **Note 11**).

7. Analyze all digestion products on a 2% TBE-agarose gel containing ethidium bromide. The pattern of restriction fragments observed for each sample will reflect the JAK2 genotype of each DNA sample (*see* **Notes 12** and **13** and **Fig. 2ii,iii**).

8. Ensure that the *SCL* PCR product is fully digested (*see* **Note 12**).

4. Notes

1. A suitable template for allele-specific PCR includes genomic DNA from purified granulocytes, but we have also successfully used genomic DNA from unfractionated peripheral blood and bone marrow. Note that dilution of the malignant clone with large numbers of wild-type cells (especially lymphocytes) may, in theory, lead to false-negative results. A total of 80 ng of genomic DNA gives strong bands; less than 40 ng may require increased numbers of cycles to detect a band (at the expense of greater chance of false-positive results). Appropriate positive control DNA can be obtained from the HEL cell line, which is V617F-positive, and negative control DNA from the K562 cell line, which is V617F-negative.

2. The mutation-specific primer (F2) contains an intentional mismatch (A instead of G) three nucleotides from the 3' end, which helps reduce mispriming to the wild-type allele.

3. Ideally, PCR amplification reactions should be set up in a designated pre-PCR area to reduce the chance of contamination. Standard precautions, including wearing laboratory gloves and using filter pipet tips and pre-PCR dedicated pipets, should also be observed.

4. The relative concentrations of the three primers do influence the relative strength of the bands. If the mutation-specific band is weak, even in a patient with a high clonal burden of V617F-positive cells, the amount of the mutation-specific for-

ward primer (F2) can be increased relative to the amount of control forward primer (F1). The concentration of $MgCl_2$ may also have to be optimized for an individual laboratory—try a range of concentrations from 0.5 mM to 5.0 mM (= 1.0 µL to 10 µL of 25 mM $MgCl_2$).

5. The choice of annealing temperature is critical to the success of the method. The annealing temperature of 58°C was identified in our laboratory as the highest temperature at which the mutation-specific primer (F2) amplified a product from V617F-positive DNA. Annealing temperatures of 60°C or higher gave no product (failed), whereas annealing temperatures of less than 54°C gave a faint mutant band in normal DNA (false-positive). The calibration of different machines may not be uniform, and thus assessment of a range of annealing temperatures may be required.

6. The number of cycles may have to be increased if the template DNA is limited in quantity or quality.

7. If controls do not give appropriate bands, see **Table 1** for possible explanations and solutions. Often, V617F-positive DNA gives faint bands of higher molecular weight than the control band, but these are not seen with V617F-negative DNA. In our experience, this has not influenced the quality or interpretation of the assay.

8. Suitable templates for *Bsa*XI restriction analysis include genomic DNA from purified granulocytes or unfractionated peripheral blood, although we have also successfully used crude cell lysates prepared from hematopoietic colonies. Genotype analysis of individual colonies by this method avoids the complication of contaminating normal cells present in granulocyte or unfractionated blood samples (*see* **Note 13**). Discrete individual colonies should be removed from the methylcellulose in which they are normally cultured, using a standard pipettor set to a volume of 50 µL. Take care to minimize the amount of methylcellulose aspirated with the colony; this can inhibit subsequent amplification if present in sufficient quantities. The colony can be expelled from the pipet tip by mixing with 100 µL deionized water, previously aliquoted into individual wells of a 96-well plate. DNA of sufficient quality for PCR amplification can be rapidly prepared by incubating this 96-well plate at 100°C for 10 min in a thermal cycler. Samples can either be used immediately, or stored at –20°C. We recommend the use of 5 µL for each PCR reaction.

9. If genotyping hematopoietic colonies, increase the number of PCR cycles from 35 to 45. Because of their small size, PCR products may not be produced from some colonies; in our experience, additional rounds of amplification are unlikely to amplify the *JAK2* exon 14 fragment.

10. In direct comparison experiments, we have found that the use of commercially-available spin columns (to remove salt, and unincorporated nucleotides and oligonucleotide primers) prior to *Bsa*XI restriction is unnecessary.

11. New England Biolabs, the manufacturer of *Bsa*XI, recommends the addition of no more than 2 U of this enzyme with a 16-h incubation period, because of DNA binding. We have observed satisfactory *Bsa*XI restriction with 2 U enzyme after

Table 1
Troubleshooting Allele-Specific Polymerase Chain Reaction (PCR)

Problem	Possible explanations	Suggested solution
No bands	Annealing temperature too high	Try range of annealing temperatures (54–60°C) and choose highest temperature that gives appropriate results.
	Defective reagents or thermal cycler	Retry with fresh reagents and, if possible, on two thermal cyclers.
Control band present but no mutation-specific band with V617F-positive DNA	Annealing temperature too high	Try range of annealing temperatures (54–60°C) and choose highest temperature that gives appropriate results.
	Relative concentration of mutation-specific primer too low	Try increasing amount of mutation-specific primer (up to 5 µL of 10 M primer).
	$MgCl_2$ concentration not optimal	Try range of $MgCl_2$ concentration (1–10 µL of 25 mM solution in a 50-µL reaction).
Mutation-specific band present but no control band with V617F-positive DNA	Homozygous V617F mutation with high clonal burden in granulocytes	No action needed provided V617F-negative control DNA gives control band.
Mutation-specific band present in V617F-negative DNA	Annealing temperature too low	Try range of annealing temperatures (54–60°C) and choose highest temperature that gives appropriate results.
	$MgCl_2$ concentration not optimal	Try range of $MgCl_2$ concentration (1–10 µL of 25 mM solution in a 50-µL reaction).
	Contamination with V617F-positive template or PCR product	Retry with fresh reagents, fresh primers, and clean pipets and plasticware.
Distinct bands of the wrong molecular weight	Amplification of primer dimers	Increase annealing temperature.
Generalized smear of DNA	Too much template DNA	Reduce amount of DNA per reaction.
Bands in the water control	Contamination with V617F-positive template or PCR product	Retry with fresh reagents, fresh primers, and clean pipets and plasticware.

a 1-h incubation at 37°C, although we routinely use 4 U for 4 h to ensure complete digestion.

12. All *SCL* PCR products should digest with *Bsa*XI, generating products of 356 bp, 110 bp, and 30 bp. In contrast, the mock-digestion control sample should remain as a 496-bp fragment. If this 496-bp fragment is ever observed in a PCR sample incubated with *Bsa*XI, incomplete or ineffectual digestion must have occurred, preventing accurate assessment of the *JAK2* locus. We recommend either repeating the restriction analysis with a new supply of *Bsa*XI (in case the current stock has lost its biological activity), or using a commercially available kit to purify the PCR reaction prior to repeating the restriction analysis (*see* **Note 10**).

13. The wild-type (V617F-negative) *JAK2* allele digests with *Bsa*XI to produce products of 206 bp, 174 bp, and 30 bp, whereas the mutant (V617F-positive) *JAK2* allele remains as an undigested 410-bp fragment (**Fig. 2**). As outlined in the Introduction, unfractionated peripheral blood or purified granulocyte samples are likely to consist of a mixture of wild-type cells and cells from the malignant clone, with the ratio varying from patient to patient. This phenomenon prevents discrimination of V617F-heterozygous and V617F-homozygous genotypes. Total peripheral blood or granulocyte samples analyzed by the *Bsa*XI restriction method should therefore be listed as "V617F-positive" if the 410-bp *JAK2* PCR fragment is observed in a reaction in which *Bsa*XI digestion of the *SCL* PCR fragment is complete. However, because cells present within a hematopoietic colony are clonal, the *JAK2* genotype of individual colonies can be determined by the *Bsa*XI restriction pattern. A wild-type colony will have the 206-bp, 174-bp, and 30-bp restriction fragments, a heterozygous V617F colony will have all four restriction fragments (410 bp, 206 bp, 174 bp, 30 bp), and a homozygous V617F will have only the 410-bp restriction fragment.

References

1. Dameshek, W. (1951) Some speculations on the myeloproliferative syndromes. *Blood* **6,** 372–375.
2. Fialkow, P. J., Faguet, G. B., Jacobson, R. J., Vaidya, K., and Murphy, S. (1981) Evidence that essential thrombocythemia is a clonal disorder with origin in a multipotent stem cell. *Blood* **58,** 916–919.
3. Harrison, C. N. and Green, A. R. (2003) Essential thrombocythemia. *Hematol. Oncol. Clin. North. Am.* **17,** 1175–1190.
4. Spivak, J. L., Barosi, G., Tognoni, G., et al. (2003) Chronic myeloproliferative disorders. *Hematology (Am. Soc. Hematol. Educ. Program)* **2003,** 200–224.
5. Tefferi, A., Solberg, L. A., and Silverstein, M. N. (2000) A clinical update in polycythemia vera and essential thrombocythemia. *Am. J. Med.* **109,** 141–149.
6. Marchioli, R., Finazzi, G., Landolfi, R., et al. (2005) Vascular and neoplastic risk in a large cohort of patients with polycythemia vera. *J. Clin. Oncol.* **23,** 2224–2232.
7. Passamonti, F., Rumi, E., Pungolino, E., et al. (2004) Life expectancy and prognostic factors for survival in patients with polycythemia vera and essential thrombocythemia. *Am. J. Med.* **117,** 755–761.

8. Barosi, G., Ambrosetti, A., Finelli, C., et al. (1999) The Italian Consensus Conference on Diagnostic Criteria for Myelofibrosis with Myeloid Metaplasia. *Br. J. Haematol.* **104,** 730–737.
9. Murphy, S., Peterson, P., Iland, H., and Laszlo, J. (1997) Experience of the Polycythemia Vera Study Group with essential thrombocythemia: a final report on diagnostic criteria, survival, and leukemic transition by treatment. *Semin. Hematol.* **34,** 29–39.
10. Pearson, T. C. (2001) Evaluation of diagnostic criteria in polycythemia vera. *Semin. Hematol.* **38,** 21–24.
11. Baxter, E. J., Scott, L. M., Campbell, P. J., et al. (2005) Acquired mutation of the tyrosine kinase JAK2 in human myeloproliferative disorders. *Lancet* **365,** 1054–1061.
12. James, C., Ugo, V., Le Couedic, J. P., et al. (2005) A unique clonal JAK2 mutation leading to constitutive signalling causes polycythaemia vera. *Nature* **434,** 1144–1148.
13. Levine, R. L., Wadleigh, M., Cools, J., et al. (2005) Activating mutation in the tyrosine kinase JAK2 in polycythemia vera, essential thrombocythemia, and myeloid metaplasia with myelofibrosis. *Cancer Cell* **7,** 387–397.
14. Kralovics, R., Passamonti, F., Buser, A. S., et al. (2005) A gain-of-function mutation of JAK2 in myeloproliferative disorders. *N. Engl. J. Med.* **352,** 1779–1790.
15. Scott, L. M., Campbell, P. J., Baxter, E. J., et al. (2005) The V617F JAK2 mutation is uncommon in cancers and in myeloid malignancies other than the myeloproliferative disorders. *Blood,* in press.
16. Steensma, D. P., Dewald, G. W., Lasho, T. L., et al. (2005) The JAK2 V617F activating tyrosine kinase mutation is an infrequent event in both "atypical" myeloproliferative disorders and the myelodysplastic syndrome. *Blood,* in press.
17. el-Kassar, N., Hetet, G., Briere, J., and Grandchamp, B. (1997) Clonality analysis of hematopoiesis in essential thrombocythemia: advantages of studying T lymphocytes and platelets. *Blood* **89,** 128–134.
18. Harrison, C. N., Gale, R. E., Machin, S. J., and Linch, D. C. (1999) A large proportion of patients with a diagnosis of essential thrombocythemia do not have a clonal disorder and may be at lower risk of thrombotic complications. *Blood* **93,** 417–424.
19. Jones, A. V., Kreil, S., Zoi, K., et al. (2005) Widespread occurrence of the JAK2 V617F mutation in chronic myeloproliferative disorders. *Blood,* in press.

17

Overexpression of *PRV-1* Gene in Polycythemia Rubra Vera and Essential Thrombocythemia

Maurizio Martini, Luciana Teofili, and Luigi M. Larocca

Summary

The polycythemia rubra vera 1 gene (*PRV-1*), a member of the urokinase-type plasminogen activator receptor superfamily, is overexpressed in granulocytes isolated from the peripheral blood of patients with polycythemia vera (PV) and essential thrombocythemia (ET). *PRV-1* overexpression is the first reliable molecular marker of these myeloproliferative disorders, and its detection allows us to discriminate PV and ET from secondary erythrocytosis and thrombocytosis. *PRV-1* overexpression can be investigated by several techniques, including Northern analysis, reverse-transcription (RT)-polymerase chain reaction (PCR), and real-time PCR. Among these, RT-PCR is the most rapid, reliable, and feasible method for the detection of *PRV-1* overexpression in highly purified peripheral blood granulocytes.

Key Words: *PRV-1*; polycythemia rubra vera; essential thrombocythemia; reverse transcriptase; PCR.

1. Introduction

Chronic myeloproliferative diseases (CMD) include chronic myelogenous leukemia (CML), polycythemia rubra vera (PV), essential thrombocythemia (ET), and chronic idiophatic myelofibrosis (IM) *(1–5)*. The presence of the Ph chromosome or its molecular equivalent, the BCR-ABL rearrangement, indubitably indicates a diagnosis of CML. In contrast, PV and ET, the most frequent CMD, do not exhibit a typical molecular marker, and their diagnosis may be performed only by excluding all possible causes of secondary erythrocytosis and thrombocytosis *(6,7)*. Recently, Temerinac et al. cloned a novel gene, named *PRV-1*, that is overexpressed in the peripheral blood granulocytes of patients with PV and in some cases of ET *(8)*. The *PRV-1* gene codes for a hematopoietic cell-surface receptor belonging to the superfamily of urokinase-type plasminogen activator receptors *(9)*. In their study, Temerinac et al. car-

From: *Methods in Molecular Medicine, Vol. 125: Myeloid Leukemia: Methods and Protocols*
Edited by: H. Iland, M. Hertzberrg, and P. Marlton © Humana Press Inc., Totowa, NJ

ried out Northern blot analysis on total RNA extracted from granulocytes and *PRV-1* overexpression was detected by using a radio-labeled probe specific for the *PRV-1* gene. Since the *PRV-1* gene cloning, several studies have been published investigating *PRV-1* expression across the various CMD, in an attempt to distinguish them from one another and from secondary erythrocytosis and thrombocytosis *(10–18)*. In most of these studies, the expression of *PRV-1* mRNA was quantified by using a real-time polymerase chain reaction (PCR) analysis *(11–18)*. In contrast, we assessed the expression of *PRV-1* gene through a qualitative approach by using a specific reverse transcriptase PCR *(10)*. Our method requires the crucial isolation of a 95% pure granulocyte population, RNA extraction and DNase treatment, phenol/chlorophorm purification, and then reverse transcription and a specific PCR. PCR products are separated on agarose gels and, after staining with ethidium bromide, the results are visualized under ultraviolet (UV) light. This method represents a rapid and reliable procedure for discriminating patients with PV and ET from patients affected by secondary erythrocytosis and thrombocytosis.

2. Materials

1. Phosphate-buffered saline (PBS): 0.2 g KCl, 8 g NaCl, 0.2 g KH_2PO_4, 1.15 g Na_2HPO_4 (pH 7.4).
2. Hespan: 6% hetastarch in 0.9% NaCl (DuPont Pharma, Willington DE).
3. Ficoll-Hypaque (Pharmacia Biotech, Uppsala, Sweden).
4. TRIZOL reagent, stored at 4°C (Invitrogen, Carlsbad, CA).
5. Chloroform.
6. Isopropyl alcohol.
7. 75% ethanol (in diethylpyrocarbonate [DEPC]-treated water).
8. RNase-free water (treated with 0.01% DEPC).
9. Deoxyribonuclease I, amplification grade (Invitrogen).
10. 10X DNase I reaction buffer: 200 mM Tris-HCl (pH 8.4), 20 mM $MgCl_2$, 500 mM KCl.
11. 25 mM ethylenediamine tetraacetic acid (EDTA), pH. 8.0.
12. Phenol/chloroform/isoamyl alcohol (25:24:1).
13. Ammonium acetate (7.5 M).
14. Ethanol (100%).
15. Oligo(dT)$_{12-18}$ (0.5 µg/µL).
16. 10X reverse-transcription (RT) buffer: 200 mM Tris-HCl (pH 8.4), 500 mM KCl.
17. 25 mM $MgCl_2$.
18. 0.1 M dithiothreitol (DTT).
19. 10 mM dNTP mix (10 mM each dATP, dCTP, dGTP, dTTP).
20. SuperScript II RT (50 U/µL) (Invitrogen).
21. RNaseOUT Recombinant Ribonuclease Inhibitor (40 U/µL).
22. *Escherichia coli* RNase H (2 U/µL).
23. Taq DNA Polymerase in Storage Buffer A (5 U/µL) (Promega, Madison WI).

24. 10X reaction buffer A without $MgCl_2$: 50 mM Tris-HCl (pH 8.0), 100 mM NaCl, 0.1 mM EDTA, 1 mM DTT, 50% glycerol, and 1% Triton X-100. (Promega).
25. Oligonucleotide primers (10 pM) (Invitrogen).
26. Agarose and electrophoresis equipment.
27. 10X TBE buffer: 890 mM Tris, 890 mM boric acid, 0.01 M EDTA (pH 8.3).
28. Ethidium bromide (10 mg/mL).

3. Methods

The following methods outline (1) the purification of peripheral blood granulo-cytes, (2) RNA extraction and DNase treatment, (3) reverse transcription and test-ing to verify the presence of cDNA, and (4) *PRV-1* amplification and detection.

3.1. Purification of Peripheral Blood Granulocytes

Purification of peripheral blood granulocytes is described under **Subhead-ings 3.1.1.** and **3.1.2.** This includes (a) the collection and storage of peripheral blood and (b) the purification of granulocytes.

3.1.1. Collection and Storage of Peripheral Blood

Fifteen milliliters of peripheral blood are collected in sodium citrate and stored at 4°C, until they can be diluted with an equal amount of Ca^{2+}- and Mg^{2+}-free PBS.

3.1.2. Purification of Peripheral Blood Granulocytes

1. In order to remove red cells, mix 1 mL of Hespan with 7 mL of cell suspension and then sediment for 90 min at room temperature.
2. Harvest the upper layer containing all the nucleated cells, transfer it into a new tube, and centrifuge at 1200g for 10 min at 4°C.
3. Wash the pellet twice with 10 mL of PBS and resuspend the pellet in 9 mL of PBS. Then carefully layer the cell suspension over 5 mL Ficoll-Hypaque density gradient, and centrifuge at 1800g for 20 min.
4. Recover all the cells at the bottom of the vial. This population should consist of over 95% granulocytes (*see* **Note 1**). Wash these cells twice in 10 mL of PBS with centrifugation at 1200g for 10 min.
5. Resuspend the pellet of highly purified granulocytes in 1 mL of Trizol reagent. Samples suspended in Trizol can be stored prior to *PRV-1* analysis for several months at –80°C, or for 2 mo at –20°C.

3.2. RNA Extraction of Highly Purified Granulocytes and DNase Treatment

RNA extraction and DNase treatment is delineated under **Subheadings 3.2.1.–3.2.3.** This includes (a) the extraction of granulocyte total RNA, and its measurement by spectrophotometry, (b) DNase treatment, (c) phenol/chloro-form purification, and a second spectrophotometric measurement of RNA.

3.2.1. Extraction of Granulocyte Total RNA

1. Incubate the samples (stored in Trizol) for 5 min at room temperature.
2. Add 0.2 mL of chloroform, shake vigorously for 3 min, and centrifuge at 11,000g for 15 min at 4°C.
3. After centrifugation, the sample forms three phases: a red-colored lower phase, a white interphase, and a colorless upper phase that contains total RNA. Transfer approx 75–80% of the upper phase into a new tube and add 0.5 mL of isopropyl alcohol.
4. Store the sample for 2 h at –20°C to facilitate RNA precipitation, then centrifuge at 11,000g for 10 min at 4°C.
5. Discard the supernatant
6. Wash the RNA pellet with 1 mL of 75% ethanol (in DEPC-treated water), mix by vortexing, and then centrifuge at 11,000g for 15 min at 4°C.
7. Remove the 75% ethanol and dry the RNA pellet at RT.
8. Resuspend the pellet in 30 μL of RNase-free water.
9. To quantify and to control for the quality of total RNA, each sample is subjected to spectrophotometric analysis.

3.2.2. DNase Treatment

1. Add 1 μg of RNA to 1 μL of amplification-grade DNase I (Invitrogen), 1 μL of 10X DNase I reaction buffer, and RNase-free water up to a final volume of 10 μL.
2. Incubate the mixture for 15 min at room temperature, then stop the reaction by adding 1 μL of 25 mM of EDTA (pH 8) and by heating the sample for 10 min at 65°C.

3.2.3. Phenol/Chloroform Purification and RNA Spectrophotometric Measurement

1. After DNase treatment, dilute total RNA (10 μL) with 90 μL of RNase-free water and add 100 μL of phenol/chloroform/isoamyl alcohol (25:24:1).
2. Vortex vigorously to obtain a lactescent mixture.
3. Centrifuge at 11,000g at 4°C for 10 min. After centrifugation, the mixture forms two phases. Carefully transfer the upper phase, which contains the RNA, into a new tube with 0.5 vol of ammonium acetate 7.5 M and 2 vol of 100% ethanol.
4. Incubate the sample for 2 h at –20°C, then centrifuge at 11,000g at 4°C for 10 min. The RNA forms a transparent pellet at the bottom of the tube.
5. Discard the supernatant, wash the pellet with 500 μL of 75% ethanol (in DEPC-treated water), and centrifuge at 11,000g for 5 min at 4°C.
6. Remove the supernatant, dry the RNA at room temperature, then resuspend the RNA in 8 μL of RNase-free water. To quantify and to control for the quality of total RNA, each sample is subjected to spectrophotometric analysis.

3.3. Reverse Transcription and Testing to Verify the Presence of cDNA

3.3.1. Reverse Transcriptase Reaction

1. Mix the total RNA that has been subjected to DNase treatment (8 μL for each sample) with 1 μL of dNTPs and 1 μL of Oligo(dT)$_{12–18}$.
2. Incubate the tube at 65°C for 5 min, then place the sample on ice for 2 min.
3. Add 9 μL of reaction mixture composed by 2 μL of 10X reverse transcriptase buffer, 4 μL of 25 mM MgCl$_2$, 2 μL of 0.1 M DTT, and 1 μL RNaseOUT to each RNA/primer mixture, mix gently, and incubate at 42°C for 2 min.
4. Then, add 1 μL (50 U) of SuperScript II RT to each tube except for the no RT control, mix, and incubate at 42°C for 50 min.
5. Stop the reaction by heating at 70°C for 15 min.
6. Add 1 μL of RNase H into each tube and incubate for 20 min at 37°C.
7. Store at –20°C.

3.3.2. Test to Verify the Presence of cDNA

Reverse transcribed RNA (cDNA) is amplified with primers for the house-keeping gene β-actin to control for the presence of cDNA in each sample (*see* **Note 2**).

1. Amplify 3 μL of cDNA in a reaction mix containing specific primers for the β-actin gene (1 μmol/L of each primer), 1 unit of Taq DNA polymerase, 200 μmol/L of dNTPs, 2.5 μL of 10X Reaction Buffer A, 1.5 mM MgCl$_2$, and water to a final volume of 25 μL. The β-actin-specific oligonucleotide primers (forward 5′-TAC ATG GGT GGG GTG TTG AA-3′; reverse 5′-AAG AGA GGC ATC CTC ACC CT-3′) will amplify a 234-bp fragment.
2. The PCR conditions are as follows: one cycle of 3 min at 95°C, followed by 36 cycles at 95°C for 40 s, 55°C for 40 s, 72°C for 40 s, and a final cycle of 3 min at 72°C.
3. Separate the PCR products on a 2% agarose gel in 1X TBE buffer.
4. After staining with ethidium bromide, visualize the PCR products under UV light (**Fig. 1**).

3.4. PRV-1 *Amplification and Detection*

1. Amplify 3 μL of cDNA in a reaction mix containing specific primers for *PRV-1* (1 μmol/L of each primer), 1 U of Taq DNA polymerase, 200 μmol/L of dNTPs, 3 μL of 10X Reaction Buffer A, 1.5 mM MgCl$_2$, and water to a final volume of 30 μL. The *PRV-1*-specific primers (sense 5′-CAG TTT GGG ACA GTT CAG C-3′; antisense 5′-AAA GCG GGA GGG AGT TAA C-3′) will amplify a 286-bp fragment.
2. The PCR conditions are as follows: one cycle of 5 min at 95°C, followed by 31 cycles

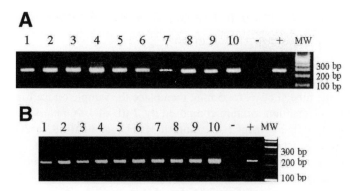

Fig. 1. *PRV-1* overexpression in essential thrombocythemia (ET) and polycythemia rubra vera (PV). (**A**) *PRV-1* mRNA in patients with ET (lanes 1–5) and PV (lanes 6–10). Negative control (water) and positive control (previously tested and sequenced cDNA) are indicated with – and +, respectively. (**B**) β-actin expression indicates cDNA integrity in the same samples. MW indicates molecular-weight marker.

at 95°C for 40 s, 54°C for 40 s, 72°C for 40 s, and a final cycle of 3 min at 72°C.
3. Separate the mixture on a 2% agarose gel in 1X TBE buffer.
4. After staining with ethidium bromide, visualize the PCR products under UV light (**Fig. 1**) (*see* **Notes 3–6**).

4. Notes

1. Purification of peripheral blood granulocytes is a crucial step in this method. In fact, several studies show that *PRV-1* is absent in normal mature peripheral blood granulocytes, whereas it is expressed in promyelocytes and monocytes. Peripheral blood mononuclear cells contain 2–6% of monocytes, and it is therefore essential to use our protocol, which assures a 95% or greater granulocyte purification, in order to avoid false-positive cases. The purity of the granulocyte population should be assessed by microscope examination of Wright-Giemsa-stained slides.
2. Amplification of the β-actin gene (or other housekeeping genes) constitutes an important step in this method. In fact, using this test it is possible verify the presence of cDNA after the reverse transcriptase step, and then eliminate samples without cDNA. In this control amplification, we use both an internal negative control (water) and a positive control (previously tested cDNA).
3. Sometimes after PCR for *PRV-1* amplification, we have detected a nonspecific band on the gel. This band (approx 450 bp long) is due to DNA contamination in the sample resulting from the failure of DNase treatment (**Fig. 2**). In this case, it is necessary to repeat the DNase treatment. Moreover, the first time this assay is employed, it is advisable to sequence the PCR product to guarantee that the sequence of the amplified product matches the sequence of *PRV-1* cDNA, reported in GenBank (accession number AF146747). We always utilize negative (water) and positive (previously tested and sequenced cDNA) controls in this

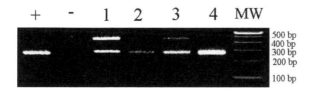

Fig. 2. Nonspecific band generated by the *PRV-1* amplification procedure. *PRV-1* mRNA in patients with PV (lanes 1–4). Lanes 1 and 3 show a nonspecific band (approx 450 bp in length). Negative control (water) and positive control (previously tested and sequenced cDNA) are indicated with – and +, respectively. MW indicates molecular-weight marker.

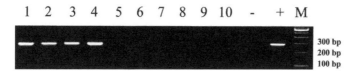

Fig. 3. *PRV-1* overexpression in several types of leukocytosis. *PRV-1* mRNA in patients with acute postsurgical secondary leukocytosis (lanes 1–4), inflammatory/infectious secondary locytosis (lanes 5–6), chronic myeloid leukemia (lane 7), infectious mononucleosis (lane 8), and myelodysplastic syndrome (lanes 9–10). Negative control (water) and positive control (previously tested and sequenced cDNA) are indicated with – and +, respectively. MW indicates molecular-weight marker.

    assay.

4. In our original paper, all cases that were negative for *PRV-1* expression by UV detection were further analyzed and validated by hybridization with a specific radiolabeled PRV-1 probe in order to exclude false-negative results *(10)*. Because samples were never found to be negative at UV examination but positive with radioactive hybridization, we have discontinued this procedure. In conclusion, UV detection represents an easy, sensitive, and reproducible method to detect *PRV-1* overexpression in highly purified peripheral blood granulocytes.

5. We have also used an alternative, and more specific, pair of oligoprimers to detect *PRV-1* overexpression. These primers (forward 5′-CCA CAG ACG GGT CAT GAG CG-3′; reverse 5′-GGG CTG TGG GGC CCA AAG-3′), were used under the following conditions: 95°C for 40 s, 55°C for 40 s and 72°C for 45 s; this produced a 395-bp fragment. The PCR buffer and the oligoprimer, dNTP, and MgCl$_2$ concentrations for this amplification were the same as described in the standard method (*see* **Subheading 3.4.**). The results of *PRV-1* overexpression obtained with these alternative primers were the same as those obtained with the original primers; however, the alternative primers produced a weaker PCR product.

6. We have found *PRV-1* overexpression in several patients affected by secondary leukocytosis *(10)*. The clinical history and laboratory data generally permit discrimination of these false-positive cases from PV and ET (**Fig. 3**).

References

1. Dameshek, W. (1951) Some speculations on the myeloproliferative syndromes. *Blood* **6**, 372–375.
2. Adamson, J. W., Fialkow, P. J., Murphy, S., Prchal, J. F., and Steinmann, B. A. (1976) Polycythemia vera: stem-cell and probable clonal origin of the disease. *N. Engl. J. Med.* **295**, 913–916.
3. Jacobson, R. J., Salo, A., and Fialkow, P. J. (1978) Agnogenic myeloid metaplasia: a clonal proliferation of hematopoietic stem cells with secondary myelofibrosis. *Blood* **51**, 189–194.
4. Fialkow, P. J., Jacobson, J. R., Singer, J. W., Sacher, R. A., McGuffin, R. W., and Neefe, J. R. (1980) Philadelphia chromosome (Ph1)-negative chronic myelogenous leukemia (CML): a clonal disease with origin in a multipotent stem cell. *Blood* 56, 70–73.
5. Fialkow, P. J., Faguet, G. B., Jacobson, R. J., Vaidya, K., and Murphy, S. (1981) Evidence that essential thrombocythemia is a clonal disorder with origin in a multipotent stem cell. *Blood* **58**, 916–919.
6. Berlin, N. I. (1975) Diagnosis and classification of the polycythemias. *Semin. Hematol.* **12**, 339–351.
7. Murphy, S., Iland, H., Rosenthal, D., and Laszlo, J. (1986) Essential thrombocythemia: An interim report from the Polycythemia Vera Study Group. *Semin. Hematol.* **23**, 177–182.
8. Temerinac, S., Klippel, S., Strunck, E., et al. (2000) Cloning of PRV-1, a novel member of the uPAR receptor superfamily, which is overexpressed in polycythemia rubra vera. *Blood* **95**, 2569–2576.
9. Klippel, S., Strunck, E., Busse, C.E., Behringer, D. and Pahl, H.L. (2002) Biochemical characterization of PRV-1, a novel hematopoietic cell surface receptor, which is overexpressed in polycythemia rubra vera. *Blood* **100**, 2441- 2448.
10. Teofili, L., Martini, M., Luongo, M., et al. (2002) Overexpression of the Polycythemia Rubra Vera-1 Gene in Essential Thrombocythemia. *J. Clin. Oncol.* **20**, 4249–4254.
11. Johansson, P., Andreasson, B., Safai-Kutti, S., et al. (2003) The presence of a significant association between elevated PRV-1 mRNA expression and low plasma erythropoietin concentration in essential thrombocythaemia. *Eur. J. Haematol.* **70**, 358–362.
12. Liu, E., Jelinek, J., Pastore, Y. D., Guan, Y., Prchal, J. F., and Prchal, J. T. (2003) Discrimination of polycythemias and thrombocytoses by novel, simple, accurate clonality assays and comparison with PRV-1 expression and BFU-E response to erythropoietin. *Blood* **101**, 3294–3301.
13. Kralovics, R., Buser, A. S., Teo, S. S., et al. (2003) Comparison of molecular markers in a cohort of patients with chronic myeloproliferative disorders. *Blood* **102**, 1869–1871.
14. Klippel, S., Strunck, E., Temerinac, S., et al. (2003) Quantification of PRV-1 mRNA distinguishes polycythemia vera from secondary erythrocytosis. *Blood* **102**, 3569–3574.

15. Florensa, L., Besses, C., Zamora, L., et al. (2004) Endogenous erythroid and mega-karyocytic circulating progenitors, HUMARA clonality assay, and PRV-1 expression are useful tools for diagnosis of polycythemia vera and essential thrombocythemia. *Blood* **103,** 2427–2428.
16. Cilloni, D., Carturan, S., Gottardi, E., et al. (2004) Usefulness of the quantitative assessment of PRV-1 gene expression for the diagnosis of polycythemia vera and essential thrombocythemia patients. *Blood* **103,** 2428.
17. Tefferi, A., Lasho, T. L., Wolanskyj, A. P., and Mesa, R. A. (2004) Neutrophil PRV-1 expression across the chronic myeloproliferative disorders and in secondary or spurious polycythemia. *Blood* **103,** 3547–3548.
18. Griesshammer, M., Klippel, S., Strunck, E., et al. (2004) PRV-1 mRNA expression discriminates two types of essential thrombocythemia. *Ann. Hematol.* **83,** 364–370.

18

Chimerism Analysis Following Nonmyeloablative Stem Cell Transplantation

Thomas Lion and Franz Watzinger

Summary

Molecular monitoring of hematopoietic chimerism has become a routine diagnostic approach in patients after allogeneic stem cell transplantation. Chimerism testing permits the documentation and surveillance of engraftment and facilitates early detection of impending graft rejection. In patients transplanted for treatment of malignant hematological disorders, monitoring of chimerism can provide an early indication of incipient disease relapse. The investigation of chimerism has therefore become an indispensable tool for the management of patients during the posttransplant period. Growing use of nonmyeloablative conditioning, which is associated with prolonged duration of mixed hematopoietic chimerism, has further increased the clinical importance of chimerism analysis. At present, the most commonly used technical approaches to the investigation of chimerism include microsatellite analysis by polymerase chain reaction and, in the gender-mismatched transplant setting, fluorescence *in situ* hybridization analysis of sex chromosomes. The investigation of chimerism within specific leukocyte subsets isolated from peripheral blood or bone marrow samples by flow-sorting or magnetic bead-based techniques provides more specific information on processes underlying the dynamics of donor/recipient chimerism. Moreover, cell subset-specific analysis permits the assessment of impending complications at a significantly higher sensitivity, thus providing a basis for earlier treatment decisions.

Key Words: Chimerism; microsatellites; FISH; leukocyte subsets; flow-sorting; graft rejection; relapse.

1. Introduction

Investigation of donor- and recipient-derived hematopoiesis (chimerism) by molecular techniques facilitates the monitoring of engraftment kinetics in patients after allogeneic stem cell transplantation. The analysis of chimerism during the immediate posttransplant period permits early assessment of successful engraftment or graft failure (*1,2*). Patients receiving reduced intensity (nonmyeloablative) conditioning regimens have an increased risk of graft

From: *Methods in Molecular Medicine, Vol. 125: Myeloid Leukemia: Methods and Protocols*
Edited by: H. Iland, M. Hertzberg, and P. Marlton © Humana Press Inc., Totowa, NJ

rejection, particularly if they are transplanted with T-cell-depleted grafts *(3)*. The monitoring of residual recipient T-cells in peripheral blood (PB) can provide timely indication of impending allograft rejection and, in patients with leukemia, impending disease recurrence by revealing an increasing proportion of recipient-derived cells *(4,5)*. Polymerase chain reaction (PCR)-based chimerism assays analyzing highly polymorphic microsatellite (short tandem repeat) markers permit the detection of residual autologous cells at a sensitivity of approx 1–5% *(6–11)*. When investigating chimerism in total leukocyte preparations from PB, this level of sensitivity may not be sufficient to allow early assessment of impending complications. It is possible to overcome this problem by investigating chimerism in specific leukocyte subsets of interest, isolated by flow-sorting or by immunomagnetic bead separation. Because residual recipient-derived cells can be detected within the individual leukocyte fractions with similar sensitivity, it is possible to identify and monitor minor autologous populations that escape detection in total PB leukocyte samples. The overall sensitivity of chimerism assays achievable by investigating specifically enriched leukocyte subsets is in the range of 0.1–0.01% *(4)*, i.e., one to two logs higher than analysis of total leukocyte preparations.

1.1. Prediction of Graft Rejection by the Monitoring of Chimerism Within Lymphocyte Subsets

Patients who receive reduced intensity conditioning reveal persisting leukocytes of recipient genotype more commonly than patients after myeloablative conditioning. The higher incidence of mixed or recipient chimerism may be attributable both to cells of myeloid and lymphoid lineages *(3)*. In patients who receive T-cell-depleted grafts, there is a strong correlation with the presence of mixed or recipient chimerism within T-cells (CD3+) and NK-cells (CD56+). Detection of mixed chimerism within lymphocyte populations is associated with an increased risk of late rejection *(3,4)*. In most instances, serial analysis reveals an increasing recipient-specific allelic pattern prior to overt graft rejection *(3–5)*. The correlation between the observation of mixed or recipient chimerism and graft rejection was shown to be higher for natural killer (NK) cells than for T-helper (CD3+/CD4+) or T-suppressor (CD3+/CD8+) cells *(3)*. Patients displaying recipient chimerism in CD56+ cells between days +14 and +35 appear to have an extremely high risk of graft rejection. By contrast, virtually all patients who experience late graft rejection show pure donor genotype within the myeloid (CD14+ and CD15+) cells during the same period *(3)*. Hence, the observation of recipient chimerism within the CD56+ cell subset is highly predictive for the occurrence of late graft rejection. These findings underscore the importance of cell subset analysis in post-transplant chimerism testing.

1.2. Detection of Imminent Relapse by Serial Analysis of Leukemia Lineage-Specific Chimerism

Investigation of entire leukocyte fractions from PB has been shown to reveal reappearance of autologous cells (mixed chimerism) before the diagnosis of relapse *(5)*, thus providing a basis for timely initiation of treatment, which usually includes the reduction or withdrawal of immunosuppressive therapy or the administration of donor lymphocyte infusions (DLI). In some instances, however, analysis of chimerism within total leukocytes may not show any changes indicative of impending relapse *(1,4)*. By contrast, serial investigation of specific leukocyte subsets derived from PB or bone marrow (BM) reveals informative changes in most patients who later experience hematological relapse. These patients reveal either persistence or reappearance of autologous allelic patterns within cell populations expected to harbor leukemic cells, if present. Occasionally, however, the only observation made before hematological relapse is lineage-specific chimerism kinetics suggestive of graft rejection *(4)*. This observation may be attributable to the loss of the graft-vs-leukemia effect associated with rejection of the allograft.

1.3. Technical Aspects

Despite the recent introduction of single-nucleotide polymorphism (SNP) analysis by real-time PCR for the investigation of chimerism *(12,13)*, short tandem repeats (STRs) have remained the most commonly used source of polymorphic markers in the human genome for quantitative assessment of donor/recipient hematopoiesis after allogeneic stem cell transplantation. The exploitation of SNP markers for chimerism testing is a promising approach, which can provide a sensitivity superior to STR analysis by PCR, but currently available techniques lack the precision required for monitoring of chimerism kinetics in the range between 1% and 100% donor/recipient cells. Within this range, STR-PCR and, in the sex-mismatched transplant setting, fluorescence *in situ* hybridization (FISH) analysis of the X and Y chromosomes *(14)*, are presently the techniques providing the greatest accuracy in quantitative investigation of chimerism. As outlined previously, the overall sensitivity and the clinical utility of diagnostic information can be greatly increased by performing the analysis of chimerism in specific leukocyte fractions isolated from peripheral blood or bone marrow. In this chapter, particular emphasis has therefore been put on the technical requirements of lineage-specific investigation of chimerism.

2. Materials

2.1. Isolation of Cell Subsets by Flow-Sorting

1. White blood cell counter.
2. Refrigerated centrifuge: Megafuge 1.0 (Heraeus).

3. Flow-sorter: FACS-Aria (Beckton Dickinson).
4. 50-mL polypropylene conical tubes (Beckton Dickinson).
5. 15-mL polypropylene conical tubes (Beckton Dickinson).
6. Fluorescence-activated cell sorting (FACS) tubes: 5-mL polystyrene tubes (Becton Dickinson).
7. Filters: 40 μm mesh (Nybolt).
8. Red blood cell (RBC) lysis buffer: 8.3g NH_4Cl, 1g $KHCO_3$ per liter; pH is adjusted to 7.4 with buffer (citrate-HCl pH = 4.00 or citrate-NaOH pH = 6.00 [Merck]).
9. Phosphate-buffered saline (PBS): 7.597 g NaCl, 1.245 g $Na_2HPO_4 \cdot 2H_2O$, 0.414 g $NaH_2PO_4 \cdot H_2O$ per liter.
10. MOPC-21 (lyophilized reagent, Sigma M7894).
11. Fetal calf serum (FCS) (Sebak).
12. Penicillin/streptomycin (PS) (Gibco).
13. Na-azide (Merck).
14. MOPC-21 solution: 5 mg lyophilized reagent/5 mL PBS containing 2% FCS/PS 1:100 vol/10% Na-azide.
15. Monoclonal antibodies (MAB):
   a. Syto 41: stains all nucleated cells (Eubio).
   b. 8 fluorescein isothiocyanate (FITC): stains CD8, suppressor T-cell marker (Dako).
   c. 56PE: stains CD56, NK-cell marker (Becton Dickinson).
   d. 3ECD: stains CD3, T-cell marker (Instrument Laboratory).
   e. 45PerCP: stains CD45, pan-leukocyte marker (Becton Dickinson)
   f. 4PE-Cy7: stains CD4, helper T-cell marker (Becton Dickinson).
   g. 71APC: stains CD71, normocyte marker (transferrin receptor, Becton Dickinson).
   h. 14APC-Cy7: stains CD14, monocyte marker (Becton Dickinson).
   i. 15FITC: stains CD15, granulocyte marker (Dako).
   j. 33 PE: stains CD33, myeloid cell marker (Becton Dickinson).
   k. 19ECD: stains CD19, B-lymphocyte marker (Instrument Laboratory).
   l. 34 PE-Cy7: stains CD34, stem cell marker (Becton Dickinson).
16. RPMI 1640 medium without L-glutamine (Gibco).

2.2. Purification of DNA

2.2.1. Purification of DNA From Peripheral Blood or Bone Marrow

1. Spectrophotometer.
2. Benchtop centrifuge.
3. Qiagen DNA Blood Mini Kit (Qiagen, Hilden, Germany).

2.2.2. Purification of DNA From Nails

1. Washing solution: 0.5% sodium dodecyl sulfate (SDS) and 0.5 M NaOH.
2. Distilled water (dH$_2$O) (DNAse free).

3. Extraction buffer: 1X TBE, 1.4% SDS, 0.15 M NaCl, 28 mM dithiothreitol (DTT), and 68 µg/mL proteinase K.
4. Phenol.
5. Chloroform/isoamylalcohol 25:1.
6. 3M Na-acetate, pH 5.2.
7. Ethanol (absolute).
8. Ethanol 70%.

2.2.3. Purification of DNA From Cell Subsets Isolated by Flow-Sorting

2.2.3.1. VARIANT A: QIAGEN COLUMN EXTRACTION

1. Benchtop centrifuge.
2. Thermoblock (Eppendorf).
3. Qiagen DNA Blood Mini Kit (Qiagen, Hilden, Germany)—includes protease, AL buffer, washing buffers AW1 and AW2, and elution buffer AE.
4. Ethanol (absolute).

2.2.3.2. VARIANT B: PROTEINASE K LYSIS

1. Eppendorf centrifuge.
2. Waterbath or heating block.
3. 1 M Tris-HCl buffer—molecular-biology grade, premade (Sigma).
4. 10 mM Tris-HCl (pH 8.0), made from the above buffer; dilute the Tris with dH_2O only.
5. Proteinase K, molecular-biology grade (nuclease-free) (Boehringer); dilute to 100 µg/mL in 10 mM Tris-HCl (pH 8.0).

2.3. STR-PCR and Capillary Electrophoresis With Fluorescence-Assisted Detection (see Note 1)

1. PCR cycler (PE2400, PE9600; Applied Biosystems, Foster City, CA).
2. Benchtop centrifuge.
3. Capillary electrophoresis instrument equipped for analysis of fluorescence signals (ABI310/ABI 3100, Avant Genetic Analyzer, Applied Biosystems).
4. Genomic DNA.
5. 10X buffer (including: Tris-HCl, KCl, $(NH_4)_2SO_4$, 15 mM $MgCl_2$, pH 8.7) (Qiagen).
6. 25 mM $MgCl_2$ (Qiagen).
7. dNTPs (Invitrogen, Carlsbad, CA).
8. STR-locus-specific primers (forward or reverse primer labeled with a fluorescence dye (FAM, HEX, or NED; Applied Biosystems) (*see* **Table 1**).
9. HotStar Taq Polymerase (Qiagen).
10. Deionized formamide (Applied Biosystems).
11. GeneScan-500 ROX Size Standard (Applied Biosystems).
12. 10X GA Buffer (including EDTA) (Applied Biosystems).
13. 310 Genetic Analyzer Performance Optimized Polymer 4 (POP-4) or 3100 POP-4 Performance Optimized Polymer (Applied Biosystems).

Table 1
Selected Microsatellite Loci

	Locus	Marker	CHLC accession	Chrom. location	Type	Het	Alleles	PCR products lenghth (in bp)	Primer sequences 5'-3'
1	D3S3045	GATA84B12	32627	3	TetNR	0,82	7	176–208	Forw.: ACCAAATGAGACAGTGGCAT Rev.: ATGAGGACGGTTGACATCTG
2	D4S2366	GATA22G05	31823	4	TetNR	0,79	7	120–144	Forw.: TCCTGACATTCCTAGGGTGA Rev.:AAAACAAATATGGCTCTATCTATCG
3	D12S1064	GATA63D12	40934	12	TetNR	0,82	8	173–201	Forw.: ACTACTCCAAGGTTCCAGCC Rev.: AATATTGACTTTCTCTTGCTACCC
4	D16S539	GATA11C06	715	16	TetNR	0,76	12	148–172	Forw.: GATCCCAAGCTCTTCCTCTT Rev.: ACGTTTGTGTGTGCATCTGT
5	D17S1290	GATA49C09	40873	17	TetNR	0,84	9	170–210	Forw.: GCCAACAGAGCAAGACTGTC Rev.: CGAAACAGTTAAATGGCCAA

The most informative set of short tandem repeat (STR) loci from the authors' laboratory, which has provided an adequate marker in the majority of all donor/recipient constellations tested. A series of successful marker sets from different European laboratories has been recently published (*6–11*). Abbreviations: Chrom = chromosomal; TetNR = tetranucleotide repeat marker; Het = heterozygosity. For the selection of appropriate markers for initial genotyping and subsequent analysis of chimerism (*see also* **Notes 21–24, 28**).

14. 310 Genetic Analyzer Capillaries 47 cm × 50 μm or 3100-Avant Capillary Array 36 cm (Applied Biosystems).

2.4. FISH Analysis of X and Y Chromosomes for Chimerism Analysis in the Sex-Mismatched Transplant Setting

1. Eppendorf centrifuge.
2. Coated slides with 12 chambers (Roth Lactan).
3. Cover slips for individual chambers (*see* **Note 2**).
4. Glass jars for incubation of slides.
5. Heating plate.
6. Humid chamber (*see* **Note 3**).
7. Incubator (37°C).
8. Water bath (72°C).
9. Glass cover slips: 24 × 60 mm.
10. Fluorescence microscope equipped with appropriate filters for Spectrum Green, Spectrum Orange, and DAPI.
11. Ethanol 70%, 85%, 96%.
12. 1X Phosphate-buffered saline (PBS).
13. Pepsin (Sigma).
14. Pepsin solution: 50 μg/mL in 0.01 N HCl; freshly prepared, prewarmed at 37°C.
15. Formaldehyde fixative: 1% formaldehyde, 1X PBS, 50 mM $MgCl_2$ (store at 4°C in darkness).
16. Deionized water.
17. X and Y chromosome-specific DNA probe solution: CEP X spectrum orange/Y spectrum green DNA Probe Kit (# 7J2050, VYSIS).
18. Rubber cement (Marabu).
19. 0.25X sodium saline citrate (SSC).
20. Tween-20 (Pharmacia).
21. Washing solution : 0.4X SSC, 0.2% Tween-20.
22. Vectashield mounting medium with DAPI (H-1200, Vector).
23. Immersion oil for fluorescence microscopy.

3. Methods
3.1. Isolation of Cell Subsets by Flow-Sorting

1. Starting material is peripheral blood (PB), usually anticoagulated with EDTA, or bone marrow (BM), usually anticoagulated with heparin.
2. Determine the white blood cell count (WBC) using any available equipment and determine the PB/BM volume required for the following steps (*see* **Note 4**).
3. Transfer the appropriate volume (containing 4×10^6 cells) to a 50-mL tube and add 10 vol of RBC lysis buffer.
4. Incubate in a refrigerator at 4°C until lysis is complete (5–10 min).
5. Centrifuge for 10 min at 400g in a refrigerated centrifuge at 4°C.
6. Remove the supernatant and resuspend the pellet in 10 mL PBS.

7. Centrifuge for 10 min at 400g in a refrigerated centrifuge at 4°C.
8. Remove the supernatant and resuspend the pellet of nucleated cells (NC) in 1–2 mL PBS.
9. Determine the number of NC/µL using any available equipment.
10. Transfer 10^6 NC for each monoclonal antibody (MAB) labeling reaction in a volume not exceeding 500 µL to a 15-mL tube for subsequent staining.
11. Add 60 µL MOPC-21 solution per 10^6 cells, then vortex briefly.
12. Incubate the tubes in a refrigerator at 4°C for 20 min (*see* **Note 5**), then add the respective monoclonal antibody (MAB) cocktails in a volume of 60 µL:
    a. Cocktail 1 (for flow-sorting of CD4, CD8, NK-cells, and nucleated red cells): Syto41/8FITC/56PE/3ECD/45PerCP/4PE-Cy7/71APC/14APC-Cy7.
    b. Cocktail 2 (for flow-sorting of granulocytes, monocytes, B–lymphocytes, and CD34 cells): Syto41/15FITC/33PE/19ECD/45PerCP/34PE-Cy7/71APC/14APC-Cy7.
13. Vortex briefly, then incubate in a refrigerator at 4°C for 30 min.
14. Remove excess MAB by adding approx 5 mL of RPMI culture medium containing 2% FCS and PS 1:100 vol, then vortex briefly.
15. Centrifuge for 10 min at 400g in a refrigerated centrifuge at 4°C.
16. Remove supernatant and resuspend the pellet in 200 µL RPMI/2%FCS/PS.
17. Filter the cell suspension through 40-µm mesh into a FACS tube.
18. Isolate 4000 cells per population, whenever possible.
19. Collect individual cell populations in Eppendorf tubes (*see* **Note 6**).

3.2. Purification of DNA

*3.2.1. DNA Extraction From Peripheral Blood or Bone Marrow (see **Note 7**)*

1. Use Qiagen DNA Blood Mini Kit according to the manufacturer's recommendations.
2. Quantify DNA yield by spectrophotometry.
3. Use 10 ng of DNA as template in individual PCR reactions.

*3.2.2. DNA Extraction From Nails (see **Note 8**)*

1. Collect nail clippings from 1 to 10 fingers (or toes).
2. Place the nail sample in a 1.5-mL Eppendorf tube.
3. Add washing solution, then vortex briefly.
4. Pulse spin (Eppendorf centrifuge, maximum speed).
5. Aspirate washing solution.
6. Add approx 1 mL dH$_2$O.
7. Vortex briefly.
8. Pulse spin.
9. Aspirate dH$_2$O.
10. Repeat **steps 6–9** once.
11. Add extraction buffer, and incubate the sample at 56°C overnight (or over the weekend, if convenient).

12. Upon complete (or partial) digestion of the nails, extract the DNA using standard phenol/chloroform extraction and ethanol precipitation.

3.2.3. DNA Extraction From Flow-Sorted Cell Subsets (see **Note 9**)

3.2.3.1. VARIANT A: QIAGEN COLUMN EXTRACTION

1. Resuspend with 200 µL PBS, then add 200 µL AL buffer.
2. Vortex for 15 s.
3. Add 20 µL protease, then vortex the solution briefly.
5. Incubate at 70°C for 10 min.
6. Add 210 µL ethanol (absolute), then vortex briefly.
7. Apply the solution to the spin column.
8. Centrifuge and wash the sample according to the standard Qiagen protocol.
9. Collect DNA with 100 µL of elution buffer (*see* **Note 10**).

3.2.3.2. VARIANT B: PROTEINASE K LYSIS

1. Collect flow-sorted cells in 50 µL Tris-buffer.
2. Add 10 µL of 100 µg/mL proteinase K (PK).
3. Incubate for a minimum of 1 h at 56°C.
4. Vortex and spin down liquid briefly.
5. Incubate for 10 min at 95°C to inactivate the PK.
6. Vortex and spin down in Eppendorf centrifuge at full speed for 30 s to separate the DNA supernatant from the cellular debris.
7. Use 10–30 µL of the supernatant as template for the PCR reaction (avoid aspiration of the cellular debris in the pellet to prevent inhibition of the PCR reaction).

3.3. STR-PCR and Capillary Electrophoresis With Fluorescence-Assisted Detection for Chimerism Analysis (see Note 11 and Fig. 1)

1. Set up the PCR reactions in a total volume of 50 µL as follows:
   dH$_2$O: 5.5 µµL
   10X buffer: 5.0 µµL
   MgCl$_2$ (25 m*M*): 1.0 µL
   dNTPs (from 2.5 m*M* stocks): 4.0 µL
   Primers (from 2.5 pmol/µL stocks): 4.0 µL
   Qiagen Taq Polymerase (from 5 units/µL stock): 0.5 µL
   DNA (*see* **Note 12**): 30.0 µL
   Total volume: 50.0 µL
2. Perform PCR amplification under the following cycling conditions:
   Initial denaturation at 95°C: 15 min
   32 cycles including denaturation at 94°C: 60 s
   annealing at 54°C: 45 s
   extension at 72°C: 90 s
   Final extension step at 72°C: 7 min
   Eliminate split peaks by adding an additional extension step at 60°C: 45 min
   (*see* **Note 13**).

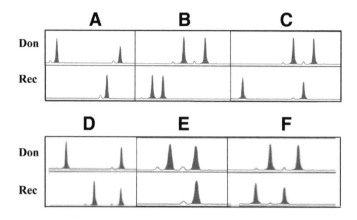

Fig. 1. Examples of allelic constellations in the donor and the recipient. The examples displayed represent a number of possible signal combinations as revealed by initial genotyping of donor- and recipient-derived DNA by a series of six different microsatellite markers prior to allogeneic stem cell transplantation. **A–D** represent constellations rendering the respective markers eligible for the follow-up of chimerism in this patient. In the constellations shown, the recipient and donor are either homozygous or heterozygous, but the recipient alleles are located outside the area of donor allele stuttering (*see* **Note 17**). In **C**, one of the recipient alleles is located in the stutter region of a donor allele, but the second recipient allele is not. In **D**, donor and recipient share one allele, but each has one unique allele not affected by stutter peak formation. **E–F** represent examples of constellations not eligible for follow-up: in **E**, the homozygous recipient has no signal distinguishable from donor alleles; in **F**, both recipient peaks are in the stutter region of donor peaks. Abbreviations: Don = Donor; Rec = Recipient.

3. Prepare PCR products for loading onto the capillary electrophoresis apparatus by setting up a mixture of 13.7 μL HiDi Formamide (deoinized), 0.3 μL ROX, and 1.0 μL PCR product.
4. Denature the PCR products by incubating the tubes at 95°C for 2 min.
5. Let the samples cool down to room temperature prior to capillary electrophoresis.
6. Load samples to ABI 310/3100-Avant Genetic Analyzer (*see* **Note 14**).
7. Adjust the electrophoresis time ("run time") according to the length of the analyzed PCR products (*see* **Note 15**).
8. Apply the GeneScan software (supplied with ABI310/3100 apparatus) to analyze the PCR products.
9. Use the height (or area) of individual peaks to calculate donor/recipient chimerism by employing the formulas indicated in **Fig, 2** (*see* **Note 16**).

Commonly encountered problems and recommended measures are outlined in **Notes 17–20**.

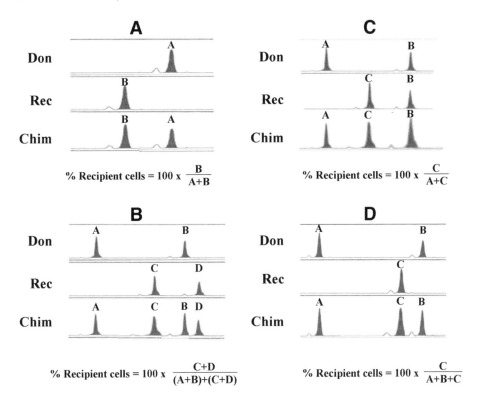

Fig. 2. Calculation of chimerism in percent recipient T-cells. **A–D** show paradigms for the calculation of chimerism. In the formulas indicated, the letters A–D represent either peak heights or areas (*see* **Note 16**). Alleles shared between donor and recipient (**C**, allele B) are disregarded in the calculation. Abbreviations: Don = Donor; Rec = Recipient; Chim = Chimeric situation.

Microsatellites for initial genotyping and selection of markers for the follow-up of chimerism are described in **Table 1** and **Notes 21–24**.

3.4. FISH Analysis of X and Y Chromosomes for Chimerism Analysis in the Sex-Mismatched Transplant Setting (see *Fig. 3*)

3.4.1. Application of Cells to the Slide(s)

1. Centrifuge cell suspension (e.g., flow-sorted cell populations) in Eppendorf tubes for 10 min at approx 4000g.
2. Remove supernatant, leaving about 5 µL liquid in the tube.
3. Resuspend cells and apply the suspension to an appropriately labeled chamber on the slide.
4. Air-dry the slide(s) at room temperature (RT) for at least 2 h.

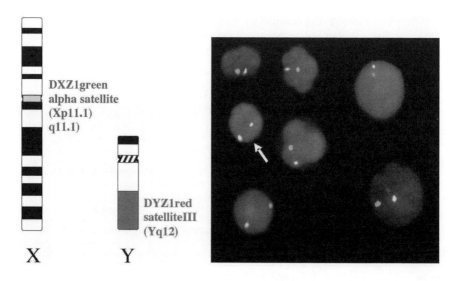

Fig. 3. Detection of male and female cells by fluorescence *in situ* hybridization. In the sex-mismatched transplantation setting, cells of donor and recipient origin can be detected by fluorescence *in situ* hybridization (FISH) based on the use of probes specific for the X and Y chromosomes. The probes are labeled with different dyes, e.g., green for the X chromosome and red for the Y chromosome, as shown in this example. In interphase nuclei, female cells (arrow) display two green signals (XX), while the remaining six male cells show one green and one red signal (XY). This technique permits accurate quantification of donor and recipient derived hematopoietic cells.

3.4.2. Pretreatment of Cells

1. Perform fixation of the air-dried slide(s) by passing through an ethanol series (70%, 85%, 96%), each step for 3 min, then air-dry slide(s) at RT.
2. Permeabilize the cells by incubating the slide(s) in pepsin solution for 20 min at 37°C.
3. Transfer the slide(s) to 1X PBS for 5 min at room temperature.
4. Incubate the slide(s) in the formaldehyde fixative for 10 min at room temperature (in darkness).
5. Transfer the slide(s) to 1X PBS for 5 min at room temperature.
6. Briefly rinse the slide(s) with deionized water.
7. Dehydrate the cells by incubating in an ethanol series (70%, 85%, 96%), each step for 3 min, then air-dry the slide(s) at room temperature.

3.4.3. Hybridization

1. Apply 0.6 µL of the DNA probe solution to each chamber.
2. Cover each chamber with a fitting cover slip (avoid bubble formation).
3. Seal each slip with rubber cement.

4. Allow the cement to dry completely at room temperature in darkness (*see* **Note 25**).
5. For denaturation of target DNA and probes, place the slide(s) on a heating plate at 73°C for 5 min.
6. For hybridization, transfer the slide(s) to a humid chamber within an incubator at 37°C for 4–48 h (*see* **Note 26**).

3.4.4. Stringency Washes and Counterstaining of Cells

1. Carefully remove the rubber cement and cover slip(s) from the slide(s). Avoid scratching.
2. Incubate the slide(s) in 0.25X SSC at 72°C for 2 min.
3. Incubate the slide(s) in washing solution at room temperature for approx 5 min (allows cooling of slide(s) to room temperature).
4. Rinse slide(s) with deionized water.
5. Counterstain cells by adding 15 µL Vectashield mounting medium per slide (across all chambers).
6. Apply a glass cover slip to the slide.
7. Store in darkness at 4°C until analysis (*see* **Note 27**).

3.4.5. Analysis by Fluorescence Microscopy

Whenever possible, evaluate at least 500 nuclei to calculate the percentage of male/female cells in the sample with adequate precision (*see* **Fig. 3** and **Note 28**).

4. Notes

1. The main advantages of automated fluorescence-based detection of microsatellite markers over the use of conventional polyacrylamide gel electrophoresis (PAGE) include greater precision and easier performance of quantitative analysis, reduced manual handling of PCR products, and higher sensitivity.
2. Use, e.g., overhead transparency cut to appropriate size.
3. Use, e.g., a metal box with lid containing wet filter paper.
4. We use a total of 4×10^6 nucleated cells (NC) per patient sample for cell sorting. The total blood volume required is therefore based on the WBC count.
5. The incubation at 4°C minimizes nonspecific staining by blocking nonspecific antigen-binding regions.
6. If the subsequent DNA extraction is performed by proteinase K lysis, the cells should be collected in a small amount of buffer, e.g., 50 µL Tris, as indicated, in order to avoid the need for a DNA-concentrating step.
7. Capillary electrophoresis-based product analysis seems to be sensitive to variations in DNA template quality. Therefore, it is necessary to use isolation protocols yielding high-quality DNA in order to obtain reproducible results and satisfactory sensitivity. DNA isolation kits (e.g., from Qiagen) have proven to be adequate for this application.
8. Initial genotyping for the detection of informative STR loci is usually performed using peripheral blood (PB) from the recipient and PB or bone marrow (BM)

from the donor. In some instances, no cell material is available from the allograft recipient before transplantation. To identify an appropriate genetic marker for the monitoring of chimerism, assessment of the patient's genotype is necessary, but PB can no longer be used due to the presence of donor cells. We have tested cell material from different sources to identify patient-specific genetic finger-prints. Epithelial cells derived from the oral mucosa or from the skin may contain donor leukocytes. In fact, buccal swabs were demonstrated to contain granulo-cytes of donor origin already during the first days after SCT, before they were detected in PB (*15*, and our own unpublished observations). The same applies to cells isolated from urinary sediment. Hair provides a reliable source of endog-enous DNA, but may not be available in patients after several courses of chemo-therapy. Nail clippings were found to be an ideal source of patient DNA in this setting. They are readily available in all patients, and sufficient quantities of good-quality DNA adequate for PCR genotyping can be obtained from approx 5 mg nail material. Usually, clippings of fingernails from both hands yield 20–50 mg of material, providing 10–25 µg of DNA by using the procedure indicated.

9. The amount of cells within individual fractions isolated by flow-sorting ranges mostly between 2000 and 10,000, but may occasionally be as low as a few hun-dred. A technique permitting efficient DNA extraction from small cell numbers is therefore required. We try to obtain 4000 cells per cell fraction in order to have sufficient amounts of DNA for PCR analysis. The use of a modified protocol for the Qiagen DNA Blood Mini Kit provides very pure DNA, but the yields are relatively low, albeit sufficient for subsequent PCR. The DNA extraction based on cell lysis and proteinase K treatment is simpler, faster, and cheaper. The DNA yields are virtually quantitative, as determined by real-time PCR analysis of con-trol genes, but the quality (purity) of DNA may not be adequate in all instances (i.e., may not work equally well with all primer combinations).

10. The volume of elution buffer should be kept low in order to provide DNA con-centrations adequate for subsequent PCR analysis. The eluate can be re-applied to the spin column in attempts to increase the DNA yield. Alternatively, if the yields do not provide sufficient amounts of DNA for PCR analysis, addition of a carrier to the cell lysate prior to application to the spin column may be warranted.

11. The employment of capillary electrophoresis instruments requires less hands-on time than conventional gel electrophoresis due to the automated loading of samples, electrophoresis, and measurement of fluorescence signals. However, the capacity of devices with a single capillary and an average electrophoresis time of 20–30 min per sample may be a limiting factor for sample throughput. The efficiency can be improved by loading PCR products of different chimerism assays onto the capillary and analyzing all fragments in the same run. This can be done when primers for amplification of various microsatellite loci are labeled with different dyes, thus permitting easy identification of the products after elec-trophoresis (*16*). These considerations are certainly of relevance at major diag-nostic centers, where high sample throughput is required. Alternatively, instruments with multiple capillaries can be used. Currently, the overall cost of

capillary electrophoresis with fluorescence-based detection of PCR products is considerably higher than conventional analysis using polyacrylamide gel electrophoresis.

12. The amount of template DNA in the PCR reactions can play a role in the achievable sensitivity of the assay. Most investigators use 50–100 ng of template (corresponding to approx $7.5–15 \times 10^3$ diploid human cells), a quantity readily available when analyzing chimerism within the entire white blood cell population. In such instances, it is feasible to reproducibly detect residual recipient cell populations in the range of 1% (i.e., approx 100 cells). This level of sensitivity may not be readily achievable, however, when specific white blood cell fractions isolated by flow-sorting or by magnetic bead separation are investigated. In these instances, only small cell numbers are available for DNA isolation, yielding no more than 1–30 ng of DNA (corresponding to approx 150–4500 cells). Although 1% sensitivity (equivalent to detecting about 45 cells or less) can be reached even in this experimental setting, it is more common to achieve sensitivities of approx 3–5%. Despite the slightly decreased sensitivity of assays using low cell numbers as starting material, the overall sensitivity in detecting minor autologous cell fractions within specifically enriched leukocyte populations is generally one to two logs higher than chimerism analysis in whole white blood cell preparations.

13. Split peaks (*see* **Fig. 4C**): Several DNA polymerases can catalyze the addition of a single nucleotide (usually adenosine) to the 3′-ends of double-stranded PCR amplicons. This nontemplate addition leads to the generation of PCR products that are one base pair longer than the actual target sequence. In order to avoid the occurrence of split peaks that are one base apart due to inefficient nucleotide addition, a terminal cycling step at 60°C for 45 min is included in the PCR profile. This step provides the polymerase with extra time to complete nucleotide addition to all double-stranded PCR products, thus usually preventing formation of split peaks.

14. The injection parameters need to be adjusted according to the yield of the PCR reaction and generally range between 5 and 15 s injection time and 1–6 kV. Usually, samples are run using different parameters in order to achieve optimal sensitivity. The peak height of the dominant alleles should be approx 5000 rfu to permit detection of subdominant alleles at a sensitivity of approx 1%, because the lower limit of detection (i.e., signal above noise) is approx 50 rfu. Quantitative analysis is possible only if the detected peaks are not off-scale (indicated by the apparatus). In some instances, very high peaks (saturated signals) are not recognized and indicated by the software as being off-scale, and appear as double peaks (tip of the peak is bent down) (*see* **Fig. 4E**).

15. A run time of 20 min is sufficient for PCR products up to approx 400 bp in size, 30 min are adequate for products up to approx 600 bp.

16. Quantification of the degree of mixed chimerism is often carried out relative to a patient-specific standard curve established from serial dilutions of pre-transplant recipient in donor DNA. For each patient, standard curves are produced for one or more informative microsatellite markers. For quantitative analysis of donor

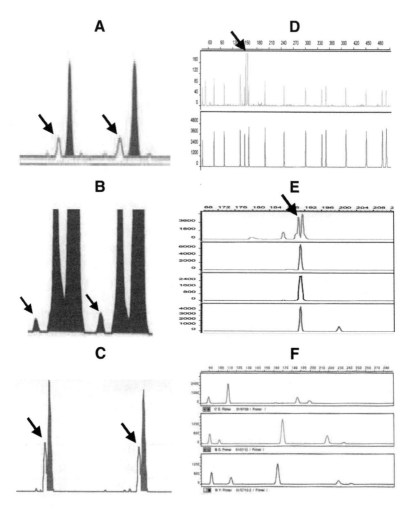

Fig. 4. Nonspecific peaks occurring in polymerase chain reaction-based microsatellite analysis by capillary electrophoresis with fluorescence detection. (**A**) Stutter peaks (arrows) (*see* **Note 17**). (**B**) Second stutter peaks. The main peaks are extremely high and display very high stutter peaks migrating one repeat unit in front of the main peaks. In such instances, second stutter peaks may occur (arrows), which migrate two repeat units in front of the main peaks (*see* **Note 17**). (**C**) Split peaks (arrows) (*see* **Note 13**). (**D**) Bleeding-through peaks of the ROX standard (red; bottom row), which are visible also in the channel used for analysis of the patient sample (green; upper row). The arrow points at the specific peak; all other peaks are bleed-through signals from the ROX standard (*see* **Note 18**). (**E**) Saturated peak with bleed-through signals. The peak (arrow) is not recognized as being off-scale, but appears as a split peak (*see* **Note 14**). Moreover, the strong signal leads to bleeding-through in all other color channels (bottom three rows) (*see* **Note 18**). (**F**) Dye-associated spurious

and recipient alleles, both peak height and peak area can in principle be used. The formula used for calculating the degree of (most commonly recipient) chimerism is based on the quotient between recipient and donor allele peak heights or areas. The mode of quantitative analysis may differ between individual centers *(17)*. Some investigators select only one unique allele from each recipient and donor for the calculation. Like many others, we include all unique recipient and donor alleles in the calculation, while shared alleles are excluded *(18)*. The formulas used are indicated in **Fig. 2**.

17. The so-called stutter peaks resulting from polymerase slippage during the amplification of microsatellite loci typically migrate at a distance of one repeat unit in front of the parent allele and may interfere with specific allelic peaks (*see* **Fig. 4A**). This problem must be accounted for by judicious marker selection. As a general rule, informative donor and recipient alleles must be separated by at least two repeat units to prevent interference with stutter peaks. Occasionally, a second stutter allele, located at a distance of two repeat units from the main peak, may be present (*see* **Fig. 4B**). If the second stutter is of relevant height—i.e., more than 1% of the main peak—another marker should be selected for chimerism analysis. The problem of second stutter peaks can be circumvented by selecting a marker that provides donor and recipient peaks separated by more than two repeat units. In general, tetra- and pentanucleotide repeat markers (i.e., microsatellite loci displaying a repeat motif of four and five nucleotides in length, respectively) yield less prominent stutter peaks and are therefore preferred over di- and trinucleiotide repeat markers (i.e., microsatellite loci displaying a repeat motif of two and three nucleotides in length, respectively).

18. In certain instances, so-called bleed-through signals *(19)* may be observed, which may affect the interpretation of results. When using very high injection parameters, the ROX standard (red) may result in signals visible in analyses of PCR products labeled by HEX (green) (*see* **Fig. 4D**). The same phenomenon may occur in multiplex PCR reactions combining primers labeled by different dyes or in the presence of extremely high signals (*see* **Note 14**), where false (bleed-through) signals may be observed in different color windows (*see* **Fig. 4E**).

19. The occurrence of dye-associated nonspecific peaks *(20)* is a problem peculiar to the fluorescence-based technology discussed (*see* **Fig. 4F**). Apparently, the fluorescent dyes FAM, HEX, and NED may give rise to formation of multiple template-independent peaks at positions characteristic for each dye. The peaks can be relatively high and migrate in a range similar to that of many microsatellite markers. The signals may therefore interfere with specific microsatellite peaks

---

Fig. 4. *(continued)* peaks (*see* **Note 19**) may occasionally be observed. Upper row: FAM-related peaks (positions at 89 bp, 110 bp, 162 bp [barely visible in this picture], 186 bp, and 199 bp); middle row: HEX-related peaks (positions at 90 bp, 100 bp, 169 bp, 218 bp, and 236 bp); bottom row: NED-related peaks (positions at 91 bp, 113 bp, 163 bp, 230 bp, and 242 bp).

and thus compromise the analysis of chimerism. There is currently no clear explanation for this phenomenon. If this problem is observed, a feasible approach to its elimination is having primers for each microsatellite locus labeled with different fluorescent dyes and selecting a primer/dye combination that does not show any interference between the specific alleles of the marker used and the dye-associated peak positions.

20. In addition to the occurrence of nonspecific peaks, as outlined in **Notes 13** and **17–19**, other problems may lead to the appearance of extra signals. Conversely, the problem of faint or absent peaks may also occur. Some of the common causes and possible measures are listed in **Table 2**.

21. Only a limited number of highly polymorphic microsatellite loci need to be tested to provide an informative marker in virtually all donor/recipient constellations. In matched sibling and haploidentical transplants, more markers are generally required in order to differentiate between donor and recipient cells as compared to the unrelated setting. The screening panels used at most centers include 6–15 microsatellite markers. Genotyping with a panel of 3–7 markers is often sufficient to reveal allelic differences between recipient- and donor-derived cells suitable for the analysis of chimerism.

22. The criteria for the selection of informative markers are not uniformly defined *(21)*. Ideally, at least one unique donor and recipient allele should be present to render a marker eligible for chimerism testing. For the monitoring of residual recipient hematopoiesis only, the presence of a unique recipient allele distinguishable from the donor allele(s) could be regarded as the minimum requirement.

23. As a result of preferential amplification of short fragments during PCR cycling, minor recipient cell populations may be detected with greater sensitivity if the informative recipient alleles are shorter in length than any donor allele. Although microsatellite markers usually show relatively small differences in length between alleles, amplification efficiencies may nevertheless differ significantly and therefore have an impact on the sensitivity of the assays.

24. Investigation of a posttransplant DNA sample with multiple microsatellite markers may improve the reproducibility and accuracy of quantitative chimerism analysis. The accuracy of quantitative chimerism assays can be increased by testing each sample with more than one marker and calculating mean values *(18)*. Some investigators therefore perform clinical testing of chimerism with commercial multiplex kits facilitating co-amplification of several microsatellite markers in a single PCR reaction *(16)*. However, the advantages indicated above are counterbalanced by significantly higher cost of consumables and lower sensitivity resulting from the high number of different fragments co-amplified. Most diagnostic centers therefore rely on the use of singleplex PCR reactions for chimerism analysis. Multiplex PCR assays are sometimes used for initial recipient/donor genotyping to select one or more informative markers for the monitoring of chimerism. If posttransplant DNA samples are tested by more than one microsatellite marker, amplification is usually performed in separate PCR reactions.

Table 2
Commonly Encountered Problems in Chimerism Calculation and Recommended Measures

Possible cause	Recommended measure
Extra signals:	
Contamination with extraneous DNA	Use appropriate precautions and controls (aerosol-resistant pipette tips)
DNA input too high	Decrease amount of template DNA or reduce the number of Polymerase chain reaction (PCR) cycles
Sample not completely denatured	Heat sample to 93°C for 3 min before capillary electrophoresis
Faint or no signals:	
Impure DNA: Presence of inhibitors	Test different extraction methods combined with filtration of DNA through a spin column
Insufficient template DNA	Increase amount of DNA template
Primer concentration too low	Increase primer concentration
Incorrect PCR program	Check the PCR program
Wrong MgCl$_2$ concentration	Test different concentrations of MgCl$_2$

25. Rubber cement must be completely dry to avoid leakage of probe solution. The incubation is performed in darkness to avoid fading of fluorescence.

26. Hybridization for 4 h is sufficient, but may be carried out overnight or even over the weekend (for convenience) without any negative effect.

27. Under the storage conditions indicated, the fluorescence remains stable for years, thus permitting analysis of the slides at any later time point.

28. The reported average sensitivity in detecting minor (in most instances recipient-derived) cell populations using different microsatellite markers ranges from 1 to 5%. The sensitivity may to a large extent depend on the size (i.e., amplicon length) of the informative recipient allele(s), the allelic constellation, and the number of alleles co-amplified. In practice, however, some markers from the panels used at individual centers tend to provide higher sensitivity than others and are therefore used preferentially.

Acknowledgments

Supported by the Österreichische Kinderkrebshilfe. The authors wish to acknowledge the contribution of the following colleagues from the CCRI, Vienna, Austria: Dieter Printz and Gerhard Fritsch (flow-sorting), Margit König (FISH analysis), Helga Daxberger and Sandra Preuner (STR-PCR and capillary electrophoresis).

References

1. Dubovsky, J., Daxberger, H., Fritsch, G., et al. (1999) Kinetics of chimerism during the early post-transplant period in pediatric patients with malignant and nonmalignant hematologic disorders: implications for timely detection of engraftment, graft failure and rejection. *Leukemia* **13**, 2060–2069.
2. Pérez-Simón, J. A., Caballero, D., Lopez-Pérez, R., et al. (2002) Chimerism and minimal residual disease monitoring after reduced intensity conditioning (RIC) allogeneic transplantation. *Leukemia* **16(8)**, 1423–1431.
3. Matthes-Martin, S., Lion, T., Haas, O. A., et al. (2003) Lineage-specific chimerism after stem cell transplantation in children following reduced intensity conditioning: potential predictive value of NK-cell chimerism for late graft rejection. *Leukemia* **17(10)**, 1934–1942.
4. Lion, T., Daxberger, H., Dubovsky, J., et al. (2001) Analysis of chimerism within specific leukocyte subsets for detection of residual or recurrent leukemia in pediatric patients after allogeneic stem cell transplantation. *Leukemia* **15**, 307–310.
5. Bader, P., Kreyenberg, H., Hoelle, W., et al. (2004) Increasing mixed chimerism is an important prognostic factor for unfavorable outcome in children with acute lymphoblastic leukemia after allogeneic stem-cell transplantation: Possible role for pre-emptive immunotherapy? *J. Clin. Oncol.* **22(9)**, 1696–1705.
6. Chalandon, Y., Vischer, S., Helg, C., Chapuis, B., and Roosnek, E. (2003) Quantitative analysis of chimerism after allogeneic stem cell transplantation by PCR amplification of microsatellite markers and capillary electrophoresis with fluorescence detection: the Geneva experience. *Leukemia* **17**, 228–231.
7. Schraml, E., Daxberger, H., Watzinger, F., and Lion, T. (2003) Quantitative analysis of chimerism after allogeneic stem cell transplantation by PCR amplification of microsatellite markers and capillary electrophoresis with fluorescence detection: the Vienna experience. *Leukemia* **17**, 224–227.
8. Kreyenberg, H., Holle, W., Mohrle, S., Niethammer, D., and Bader, P. (2003) Quantitative analysis of chimerism after allogeneic stem cell transplantation by PCR amplification of microsatellite markers and capillary electrophoresis with fluorescence detection: the Tuebingen experience. *Leukemia* **17**, 237–240.
9. Acquaviva, C., Duval, M., Mirebeau, D., Bertin, R., and Cave, H. (2003) Quantitative analysis of chimerism after allogeneic stem cell transplantation by PCR amplification of microsatellite markers and capillary electrophoresis with fluorescence detection: the Paris-Robert Debre experience. *Leukemia* **17**, 241–246.
10. Hancock, J. P., Goulden, N. J., Oakhill, A., and Steward, C. G. (2003) Quantitative analysis of chimerism after allogeneic bone marrow transplantation using immunomagnetic selection and fluorescent microsatellite PCR. *Leukemia* **17**, 247–251.
11. Koehl, U., Beck, O., Esser, R., et al. (2003) Quantitative analysis of chimerism after allogeneic stem cell transplantation by PCR amplification of microsatellite markers and capillary electrophoresis with fluorescence detection: the Frankfurt experience. *Leukemia* **17(1)**, 232–236.

12. Maas, F., Schaap, N., Kolen, S., et al. (2003) Quantification of donor and recipient hemopoietic cells by real-time PCR of single nucleotide polymorphisms. *Leukemia* **17(3)**, 621–629.

13. Fredriksson, M., Barbany, G., Liljedahl, U., Hermanson, M., Kataja, M., and Syvänen, A. C. (2004) Assessing hematopoietic chimerism after allogeneic stem cell transplantation by multiplexed SNP genotyping using microarrays and quantitative analysis of SNP alleles. *Leukemia* **18**, 255–266.

14. Najfeld, V., Burnett, W., Vlachos, A., Scigliano, E., Isola, L., and Fruchtman, S. (1997) Interphase FISH analysis of sex-mismatched BMT utilizing dual color XY probes. *Bone Marrow Transplant* **19(8)**, 829–834.

15. Thiede, C., Prange-Krex, G., Freiberg-Richter, J., Bornhauser, M., and Ehninger, G. (2000) Buccal swabs but not mouthwash samples can be used to obtain pretransplant DNA fingerprints from recipients of allogeneic bone marrow transplants. *Bone Marrow Transplant* **25(5)**, 575–577.

16. Thiede, C., Bornhäuser, U., Brendel, C., et al. (2001) Sequential monitoring of chimerism and detection of minimal residual disease after allogeneic blood stem transplantation (BSCT) using multiplex PCR amplification of short tandem repeat-markers. *Leukemia* **15**, 293–302.

17. Lion, T. (2003) Summary: reports on quantitative analysis of chimerism after allogeneic stem cell transplantation by PCR amplification of microsatellite markers and capillary electrophoresis with fluorescence detection. *Leukemia* **17(1)**, 252–254.

18. Thiede, C. and Lion, T. (2001) Quantitative analysis of chimerism after allogeneic stem cell transplantation using multiplex PCR amplification of short tandem repeat markers and fluorescence detection. *Leukemia* **15**, 303–306.

19. Moretti, T. R., Baumstark, A. L., Defenbaugh, D. A., Keys, K. M., Smerick, J. B., and Budowle, B. (2001) Validation of short tandem repeats (STRs) for forensic usage: performance testing of fluorescent multiplex STR systems and analysis of authentic and simulated forensic samples. *J. Forensic Sci.* **46(3)**, 647–660.

20. Schraml, E. and Lion, T. (2003) Interference of dye-associated fluorescence signals with quantitative analysis of chimerism by capillary electrophoresis. *Leukemia* **17(1)**, 221–223.

21. Thiede, C., Borhäuser, M., and Ehninger, G. (2004) Evaluation of STR informativity for chimerism testing-comparative analysis of 27 STR systems in 203 matched related donor recipient pairs. *Leukemia* **18**, 248–254.

Index